THERAPEUTIC STRATEGIES IN HYPERTENSION

THERAPEUTIC STRATEGIES IN HYPERTENSION

Edited by

George L. Bakris

CLINICAL PUBLISHING

OXFORD

Clinical Publishing
an imprint of Atlas Medical Publishing Ltd

Oxford Centre for Innovation
Mill Street, Oxford OX2 0JX, UK

Tel: +44 1865 811116
Fax: +44 1865 251550
E-mail: info@clinicalpublishing.co.uk
Web: www.clinicalpublishing.co.uk

Distributed by:

Marston Book Services Ltd
PO Box 269
Abingdon
Oxon OX14 4YN, UK

Tel: +44 1235 465500
Fax: +44 1235 465555
E-mail: trade.orders@marston.co.uk

First published 2006

A catalogue record for this book is available from the British Library

ISBN 1 904392 41 5

Project manager: Gavin Smith
Typeset by Mizpah Publishing Services Private Limited, Chennai, India
Printed by Biddles Limited, Kings Lynn, Norfolk, UK

Contents

Contributors

Surender K. Arora, MD, Assistant Instructor, Division of Endocrinology, Diabetes and Hypertension, SUNY-Downstate and Kings County Hospital, Brooklyn, New York, USA

George L. Bakris, MD, Professor and Vice-Chairman, Department of Preventive Medicine, Director, Hypertension/Clinical Research Center, Rush University Medical Center, Chicago, Ilinois, USA

Andrew E. Briglia, DO, Assistant Professor of Medicine, Division of Nephrology, Department of Medicine, University of Maryland School of Medicine, Baltimore, Maryland, USA

Brent M. Egan, MD, Department of Medicine, Medical University of South Carolina, Charleston, South Carolina, USA

William J. Elliott, MD, PhD, Professor of Preventive Medicine, Internal Medicine and Pharmacology, Department of Preventive Medicine, Rush Medical College of RUSH University Medical Center, Chicago, Ilinois, USA

John M. Flack, MD, MPH, Professor and Interim Chairman of Internal Medicine, Division of Clinical Epidemiology and Translational Research and Endocrinology, Metabolism and Hypertension, Department of Internal Medicine, Wayne State University School of Medicine and the Detroit Medical Center, Detroit, Michigan, USA

Philip B. Gorelick, MD, MPH, John S. Garvin Professor and Head, Director, Centre for Stroke Research, Department of Neurology and Rehabilitative Medicine, The University of Illinois at Chicago, Chicago, Illinois, USA

Willa A. Hsueh, MD, Professor of Medicine, Chief, Endocrine Division, Department of Medicine, UCLA Medical Center, Los Angeles, California, USA

Nitin Khosla, MD, Rush University Medical Center, Department of Preventive Medicine, Hypertension/Clinical Research Center, Chicago, Ilinois, USA

Gérard M. London, MD, Chief, Department of Nephrology, Manhes Hospital Fleury-Mérogis, France

Samy I. McFarlane, MD, MPH, Associate Professor, Chief, Division of Endocrinology, Diabetes and Hypertension, SUNY-Downstate and Kings County Hospital, Brooklyn, New York, USA

Samar A. Nasser, PA-C, MPH, Physician Assistant, Division of Clinical Epidemiology and Translational Research, Department of Internal Medicine, Wayne State University and the Detroit Medical Center, Detroit, Michigan, USA

Shannon M. O'Connor, BS, Research Assistant, Division of Clinical Epidemiology and Translational Research, Department of Internal Medicine, Wayne State University and the Detroit Medical Center, Detroit, Michigan, USA

Laura L. Pedelty, PhD, MD, Assistant Professor of Neurology, Department of Neurology and Rehabilitative Medicine, The University of Illinois at Chicago, Chicago, Illinois, USA

Mahboob Rahman, MD, MS, Associate Professor of Medicine, Division of Nephrology and Hypertension, Case Western Reserve University, University Hospitals of Cleveland, Cleveland VA Medical Center, Cleveland, Ohio, USA

Rekha Ramamurthy, MD, Fellow, Endocrinology Section, Department of Medicine, Feinberg School of Medicine, Northwestern University, Chicago, Ilinois, USA

Arash Rashidi, MD, Fellow, Division of Nephrology and Hypertension, Case Western Reserve University, University Hospitals of Cleveland, Cleveland VA Medical Center, Cleveland, Ohio, USA

Luis M. Ruilope, MD, Associate Professor of Medicine, Head, Hypertension Unit, 12 de Octubre Hospital , Madrid, Spain

Michel E. Safar, PhD, PU-PH Consultant, Diagnosis Center, Hôtel-Dieu Hospital, Paris, France

Moro O. Salifu, MD, MPH, FACP, Associate Professor, Program Director, Division of Nephrology, SUNY-Downstate Medical Center, Brooklyn, New York, USA

Pantelis Sarafidis, MD, Rush University Medical Center, Department of Preventive Medicine, Hypertension/Clinical Research Center, Chicago, Ilinois, USA

Neil J. Stone, MD, FAHA, FACC, Professor of Clinical Medicine (Cardiology), Feinberg School of Medicine, Northwestern University, Consultant Cardiologist, Lipidologist Medical Director, Vascular Center of Bluhm Cardiovascular Institute, Northwestern Memorial Hospital, Chicago, Ilinois, USA

Matthew R. Weir, MD, Professor of Medicine, Director, Division of Nephrology, Department of Medicine, University of Maryland School of Medicine, Baltimore, Maryland, USA

1

Is there an ideal strategy for achieving blood pressure goals?

L. M. Ruilope, G. L. Bakris

INTRODUCTION

It is well recognized that blood pressure (BP) control remains well short of the goals recommended by guidelines [1, 2]. In clinical practice a percentage of control above 30% (for a goal lower than 140/90 mmHg) is rarely seen [3]. For a similar BP goal control values above 40% have been described in hospital-based hypertension units [4] and the percentage has been as high as 60% in some clinical trials like the Antihypertensive and Lipid Lowering Treatment to Prevent Heart Attack (ALLHAT) [5] study. However, in the last two instances, if a goal lower than 130/80 mmHg had been considered according to guidelines, e.g. when associated clinical conditions (ACC), diabetes and chronic kidney disease are present, adequate BP control seen is less than 20% in hypertension units [4] and the same is probably applicable for most clinical trials. All these facts have led to the conclusion that attaining an adequate BP goal is difficult in particular for systolic BP. They have also forced the consideration that what guidelines consider as adequate BP control could represent an elusive target in daily clinical practice [6]. The aim of this chapter is briefly to review the feasibility of new strategies directed towards attaining better BP control in daily clinical practice.

WHEN TO INITIATE PHARMACOLOGICAL INTERVENTION: THE CONCEPT OF THRESHOLD BLOOD PRESSURE REVISITED

Both the level of BP and its consequences rise continuously if arterial hypertension is not adequately treated. Progression from pre-hypertension into established hypertension is a well-known fact [7]. Later on, and if hypertension is not controlled, it progresses to more advanced stages and causes the well-known increase in cardiovascular (CV) and renal damage [8]. Defining the most effective threshold BP at which to start pharmacological intervention could impede the evolution of arterial hypertension, thus avoiding the progression of CV disease. A direct pharmacological intervention, accompanied by lifestyle changes, is contemplated if BP levels are above the limit defining stage 2 in arterial hypertension (>160/100 mmHg). In the remaining cases, threshold BP is defined by the persistence of BP values above 140/90 mmHg after a period of adequately performed lifestyle changes. On the other hand, both JNC7 and ESH–ESC Guidelines [1, 2] recognize the existence of compelling indications that suggest starting treatment even when BP levels are in the range of pre-hypertension. This is the case when target organ damage (TOD) or ACC are present. However, in daily clinical practice the threshold BP at which pharmacological therapy is

Luis M. Ruilope, MD, Associate Professor of Medicine, Head, Hypertension Unit, 12 de Octubre Hospital, Madrid, Spain

George L. Bakris, MD, Professor and Vice-Chairman, Department of Preventive Medicine, Director, Hypertension/Clinical Research Center, Rush University Medical Center, Chicago, Ilinois, USA

started differs and intervention frequently takes place when BP levels are clearly above the levels recommended by guidelines. Moreover, once pharmacological therapy is started, clinical inertia [9] greatly contributes to the lack of good BP control due to the acceptance by doctors of elevated BP levels as adequate for the patient.

THE CONCEPT OF ARTERIAL HYPERTENSION PREVENTION THROUGH PHARMACOLOGICAL INTERVENTION

The possibility of preventing the development of arterial hypertension by producing lifestyle changes, in particular reducing obesity, has been demonstrated [10]. Pharmacological intervention directed at preventing the development of arterial hypertension (BP > 140/90 mmHg) has recently been suggested [11]. The Trial of Preventing Hypertension (TROPHY) study tested the hypothesis that pharmacological treatment of pre-hypertension prevents or postpones stage 1 hypertension. The study contemplated a follow-up of 4 years; during the first two, candesartan, an angiotensin receptor blocker (ARB), was compared to placebo and in the last two, all patients received placebo. Active therapy decreased the risk of developing stage 1 hypertension by 66.3% ($P < 0.001$) during the first two years. At the end of the study, the risk was still reduced by 15.6% ($P < 0.007$) in those patients who had received the active medication.

The transition from pre-hypertension into established hypertension reflects, in part, ongoing changes such as arteriolar hypertrophy [12] and endothelial dysfunction [13]. In this sense, pre-hypertension is characterized by the existence of elevations in plasma norepinephrine and plasma renin concentrations [14, 15] that could promote growth and endothelial dysfunction. Regression of arteriolar hypertrophy has been shown to occur when treatment with an angiotensin-converting enzyme inhibitor (ACE-I) or an ARB are given [16, 17]. This does not occur in the presence of a β-blocker. These data stress that earlier intervention with drugs in daily clinical practice could facilitate the attainment of much better BP control, facilitated by regression of the vascular changes accompanying the increase in BP since the initial stages of the process.

Conversely, it has been demonstrated that BP within the range of pre-hypertension is associated with an elevated risk of CV disease [18, 19] beyond that which is attributable to accompanying conditions such as diabetes, TOD or established CV disease and partly attributable to the association of pre-hypertension with other CV risk factors [20, 21]. Early pharmacological intervention in arterial hypertension must then be contemplated in order to diminish the early development of CV disease.

HOW TO INITIATE PHARMACOLOGICAL THERAPY: WHICH MONOTHERAPY AND WHEN TO USE COMBINATION THERAPY

An apparent discrepancy in the choice of the first step drug exists between JNC7 [1] and the ESH–ESC [2] Guidelines. JNC7 defends the use of diuretics in most people as first step therapy to get a significant diminution of the great risk that accompanies elevated BP and to do it at the lowest cost. On the contrary, the ESH–ESC Guidelines defend the need for individual therapy in each patient admitting that any drug available can be considered as suitable for first step therapy. The demonstration that arterial hypertension is the number one risk factor for mortality in developed as well as developing countries [22] fits well with the concept of JNC7. However, the fact that nowadays pre-hypertension correlates particularly well with insulin resistance [23] forces the consideration that the benefit of simply lowering BP at medium-term may not be enough to correct the risks associated with elevated BP. In fact, targeting pre-diabetes in hypertensive patients has recently been described [24] and it represents a situation frequently seen in clinical practice, in which the choice of the antihypertensive drug is relevant to promoting, preventing or retarding the development of diabetes.

It is also true that the discussion about which monotherapy is most effective seems inadequate if we consider the elevated percentage of patients requiring combination therapy to obtain adequate BP control. Only 22–24% of people in clinical trials actually achieve BP goals with monotherapy. In fact, unwanted metabolic effects of some antihypertensive drugs are attenuated when used in combination with members of other classes of antihypertensive agents, in particular with drugs that suppress the renin–angiotensin system (RAS) [25]. The possibility of using a combination, either free or fixed, from the beginning of pharmacological therapy in hypertensive patients is contemplated in both guidelines [1, 2]. Implementing this possibility will probably contribute to improvements in BP control due to the better ability of a combination therapy to lower BP.

IS THERE A DIFFERENT RESPONSE TO THERAPY DEPENDING ON AGE? BRITISH GUIDELINES REVISITED

Recently, a new version of the British Society of Hypertension Guidelines [26] has been published. The recommended choice of the first antihypertensive drug is based on the fact that hypertensives can be broadly classified as 'high-renin' and 'low-renin'. Drugs can be divided according to their effects on the RAS into those with capacity to inhibit ACE-I/ARB (A) or β-blockers (B) and those without effects on the system, calcium antagonists (C) and diuretics (D). As can be seen in Figure 1.1, patients younger than 55 with the highest RAS activity should receive a drug from group A or B as the first drug, while those older than 55 should receive one from group C or D. The need for combination should be covered by adding a drug of the other group (C or D for A or B and *vice versa*).

If three drugs are required, A + C + D should be the ideal combination. This algorithm of treatment is based on previous experience of the authors indicating that BP control is more successful following the recommendations of the British Guidelines [27].

For comparison, an algorithm put forward for those with kidney disease and/or diabetes that integrates both the JNC7 and ESC–ESH Guidelines is noted in Figure 1.2. In contrast to the British Guidelines, which focus on the general hypertensive patient, this algorithm

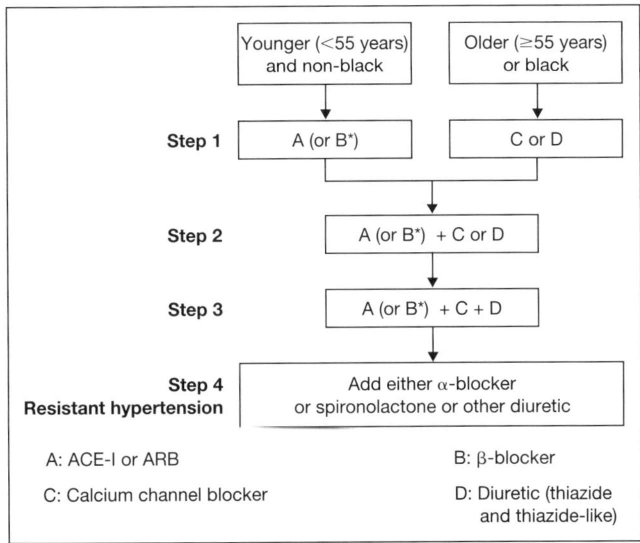

Figure 1.1 Recommendations for combining BP lowering drugs (AB/CD rule) (with permission from [26]). *Combination therapy involving B and D may induce more new onset diabetes compared with other combination therapies.

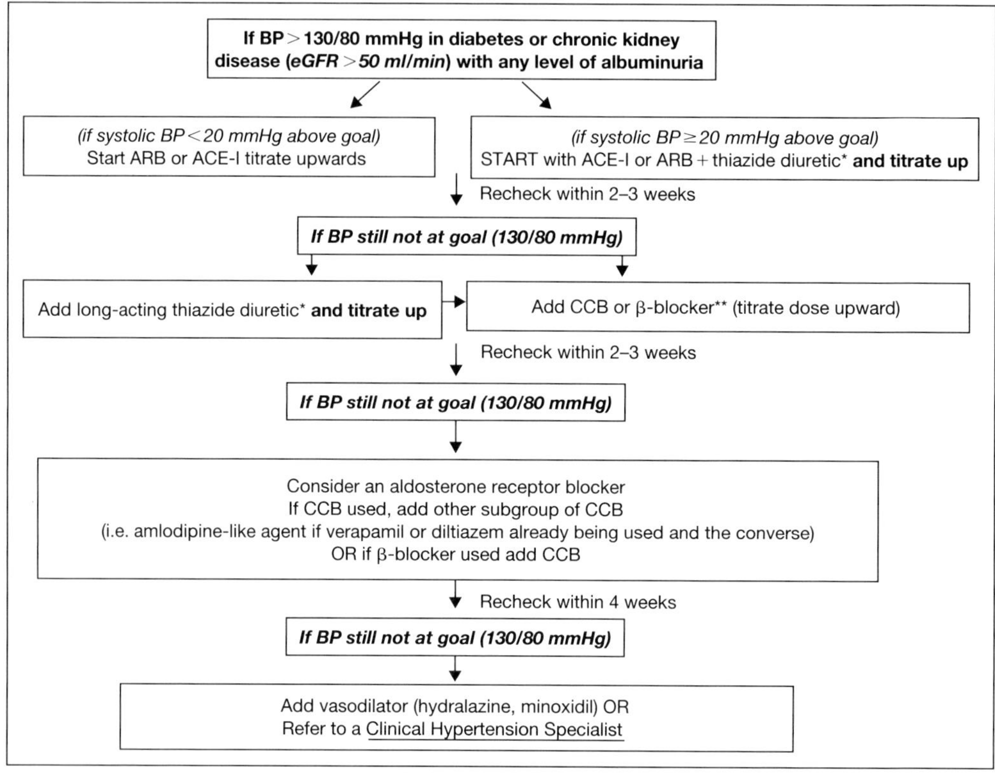

Figure 1.2 Exercise caution over the use of high doses of diuretics. If a β-blocker is prescribed then it should be combined with a DHP CCB. *If estimated GFR is <50 ml/min, then a loop diuretic should be used, either furosemide (2–3 times daily) or torosemide (1–2 times daily). If estimated GFR is ≥ 50 ml/min, then a thiazide-like diuretic could be used.[28] **Carvedilol has been shown to be beneficial in renal impairment and outcome studies. Other β-blockers are not excluded, however, there are no renal outcome data to support the use of atenolol in such patients and only limited data to support metoprolol (AASK trial, Toprol XL). Additionally, other α-/β-blockers such as labetolol, may be useful but have not been studied in this population. eGFR = estimated glomerular filtration rate (most currently accepted method for Stages 2–4- modified MDRD formula (GFR calculator can be found: www.kidney.org; www.nephron.com and multiple other websites); BP = blood pressure; ARB = angiotensin II receptor blocker; ACE-I = angiotensin-converting enzyme inhibitor; CCB = calcium channel blocker; DHP CCB = dihydropyridine calcium channel blocker; RAAS = renin–angiotensin–aldosterone system.

focuses on the most prevalent concomitant diseases in older hypertensive patients with a focus on achieving the BP goal [28].

PREDICTORS OF A POOR RESPONSE TO ANTIHYPERTENSIVE THERAPY: THE GREATER THE CV DAMAGE, THE POORER THE RESPONSE TO DRUG TREATMENT

Several factors have been identified as potential impediments to the attainment of adequate BP control. Several of them are related to an inadequate lifestyle in particular diet containing an excessive amount of salt, an excessive number of calories facilitating an increase in body weight, excessive alcohol intake, or a low intake of fruit and vegetables (Table 1.1.) Other factors are related to inadequate doses of antihypertensive drugs and inadequate combinations, or to accompanying therapies interfering with antihypertensive therapy. However, the degree of CV and renal involvement as a consequence of the increase in BP is

Table 1.1 Lifestyle modifications and effects on BP

Modification	*Approximate SBP reduction (range)*
Weight reduction	5–20 mmHg/10 kg weight loss
Adopt DASH eating plan	8–14 mmHg
Dietary sodium reduction	2–8 mmHg
Physical activity	4–9 mmHg
Moderation of alcohol consumption	2–4 mmHg

With permission from [1].

Table 1.2 Patient characteristics associated with lower adherence

Demographics
- African-American race

Social/environmental
- Lack of insurance or access
- Active substance use
- Homelessness
- Poor social support
- Doubt efficacy of medication
- Confidentiality concerns

Lack of knowledge
- Benefits of BP and other treatment regimen
- Need for EPO and Vitamin D therapy
- Resistance

Psychological factors beliefs
- Poor self-efficacy
- Two aspects of the Health Belief Model:
  (1) having *greater perceived* benefits from therapy
  (2) having *fewer perceived* barriers to treatment

an important predictor of the need for multiple antihypertensive therapies. The presence of ACC or advanced TOD preclude a more difficult control of BP and the need of more medication to do it [29]. An aggressive attitude is required in the treatment of these patients because the adequate level of control is lower than 130/80 mmHg.

POOR LONG-TERM ADHERENCE AS THE MAIN CAUSE OF POOR BLOOD PRESSURE CONTROL

Long-term adherence to medication regimens is a critical part in considering pharmacotherapy strategy so as to ensure maximum reduction in morbidity and mortality for renal and CV related conditions [30, 31]. It is clear that acceptance of the patient, family, physician and healthcare system all play a role in ensuring optimal adherence to a given medical regimen. Lower socio-economic groups and African-Americans have the lowest adherence rates regardless of educational level [32, 33]. Older people, as well, are not as adherent to medications. This is primarily related to issues of side-effects and cost [34]. A number of approaches have been proposed to improve medication adherence but the one approach that appears to be optimal is a systems (team) approach, where a system is put into place that incorporates the healthcare system, pharmacist, physician, ancillary healthcare

Table 1.3 Non-patient-related factors associated with medication adherence

Provider-related barriers to adherence
Mistrust of provider
Provider's interpersonal skills
Provider's experience/expertise
Medication-related barriers to adherence
Fit with lifestyle
Complexity/pill burden
Dose frequency
Side-effects
Duration

Table 1.4 Guidelines to improve maintenance of antihypertensive therapy

Be aware of the problem and be alert for signs of inadequate intake of medications
Articulate the goal of therapy with few or no side-effects
Educate the patient
Maintain contact with the patient
Keep care inexpensive and simple
Prescribe according to pharmacological principles
Be willing to stop and substitute unsuccessful therapy
Anticipate and address side-effects
Continue to add effective and tolerated drugs
Provide feedback and validation of success
Summarized with permission from [35].

professional and the patient with their family. Table 1.2 lists the common barriers to patient adherence to antihypertensive medications. Table 1.3 lists non-patient related factors associated with changes in medication adherence. It is clear that a physician needs to think about modifying all these factors when considering optimizing the treatment of a given patient.

Many patients do not take their prescribed medications. In most surveys, one-quarter to one-half of patients have abandoned their antihypertensive drugs one year after starting therapy [35]. It is also true that many physicians do not prescribe all the required medications required to control BP in their patients [9]. The reasons for a low compliance and for such a poor long-term adherence are diverse but in particular poor tolerability has been claimed as one of the most important. Table 1.4 summarizes guidelines directed towards improving maintenance of antihypertensive therapy according to Kaplan [36].

IF AN EARLIER INTERVENTION IS REQUIRED, WHO SHOULD RECEIVE THE MESSAGE? THE RELEVANCE TO PRIMARY CARE MEDICINE AND PUBLIC HEALTH AUTHORITY

CV and renal disease have been described as a continuum [37] starting with the detection of CV and renal risk factors, followed by the detection of TOD and finally by ACC and eventually death. It is clear that lifestyle interventions can clearly delay development of hypertension as well as reduce CV risk. It is inadequate for only physicians and healthcare professionals to discuss such issues; public health authorities also need to intervene and set up an economic system that reinforces health behaviour. As a paradigm, this has occurred in Finland with a dramatic reduction in CV events in the last decade.

REFERENCES

1. Chobanian AV, Bakris GL, Black HR *et al.* The Seventh Report of the Joint National Committee on Prevention, Detection, Evaluation, and Treatment of High Blood Pressure. The JNC 7 Report. *JAMA* 2003; 289:2560–2571.
2. Guidelines Committee. 2003 European Society of Hypertension–European Society of Cardiology guidelines for the management of arterial hypertension. *J Hypertens* 2003; 21:1011–1053.
3. Borghi C, Dormi A, D'Addato S, Gaddi A, Ambrosioni E. Brisighella Heart Study Working Party. Trends in blood pressure control and antihypertensive treatment in clinical practice. *J Hypertens* 2004; 22:1707–1716.
4. Banegas JR, Segura J, Ruilope LM *et al.*, on behalf of the CLUE Study Group Investigators. Blood pressure control and physician management of hypertension in hospital hypertension units in Spain. *Hypertension* 2004; 43:1338–1344.
5. The ALLHAT Officers and Coordinators for the ALLHAT Collaborative Research Group. Major outcomes in high-risk hypertensive patients randomized to angiotensin-converting enzyme inhibitor or calcium channel blocker vs diuretic. *JAMA* 2002; 288:2981–2997.
6. O'Rorke JE, Richardson WS. Evidence based management of hypertension: what to do when blood pressure is difficult to control. *BMJ* 2001; 322:1229–1232.
7. Vasan RS, Larson MG, Leip EP *et al.* Assessment of frequency of progression to hypertension in non-hypertensive participants in the Framingham Heart Study: a cohort study. *Lancet* 2001; 358:1682–1686.
8. Perera GA. Hypertensive vascular disease. *J Chronic Dis* 1955; 1:33–42.
9. Phillips LS, Branch WT, Cook CB *et al.* Clinical inertia. *Ann Intern Med* 2001; 135:825–834.
10. He J, Whelton PK, Appel LJ *et al.* Long-term effects of weight loss and dietary sodium reduction on incidence of hypertension. *Hypertension* 2000; 35:544–549.
11. Julius S, Nesbitt SD, Egan BM *et al.* Feasibility of treating prehypertension with an angiotensin-receptor blocker. *N Engl J Med* 2006; 354:1685–1697.
12. Folkow B. Physiological aspects of primary hypertension. *Physiol Rev* 1982; 62:347–504.
13. Panza JA, Casino PR, Kilcoyne CM, Quyyumi AA. Role of endothelium-derived nitric oxide in the abnormal endothelium dependent vascular relaxation of patients with essential hypertension. *Circulation* 1993; 87:1468–1474.
14. Esler M, Julius S, Zweifler A *et al.* Mild high-renin essential hypertension: neurogenic human hypertension? *N Engl J Med* 1977; 296:405–411.
15. Julius S, Krause L, Schork NJ *et al.* Hyperkinetic borderline hypertension in Tecumseh, Michigan. *J Hypertens* 1991; 9:77–84.
16. Schiffrin EL, Deng LY, Larochelle P. Progressive improvement in the structure of resistance arteries of hypertensive patients after 2 years of treatment with an angiotensin I-converting enzyme inhibitor: comparison with effects of a betablocker. *Am J Hypertens* 1995; 8:229–236.
17. Schiffrin EL, Deng LY. Comparison of effects of angiotensin I-converting enzyme inhibition and β-blockade for 2 years on function of small arteries from hypertensive patients. *Hypertension* 1995; 25:699–703.
18. Vasan RS, Larson MG, Leip BP *et al.* Impact of high-normal blood pressure on the risk of cardiovascular disease. *N Engl J Med* 2001; 345:1291–1297.
19. Kshirsagar AV, Carpenter M, Bang H *et al.* Blood pressure usually considered as normal is associated with an elevated risk of cardiovascular disease. *Am J Med* 2006; 119:133–141.
20. Julius S, Jamerson K, Mejia A, Krause L, Schork N, Jones K. The association of borderline hypertension with target organ changes and higher coronary risk: Tecumseh Blood Pressure study. *JAMA* 1990; 264:354–358.
21. Nesbitt SD, Julius S, Leonard D, Egan BM, Grozinski M. Is low-risk hypertension fact or fiction? Cardiovascular risk profile in the TROPHY study. *Am J Hypertens* 2005; 18:980–985.
22. Ezzati M, Lopez AD, Rodgers A, Hoorn SV, Murray CJL, and the Comparative Risk Assessment Collaborating Group. Selected major risk factors and global and regional burden of disease. *Lancet* 2002; 360:1346–1360.
23. Cordero A, Laclaustra M, Leon M *et al.* Prehypertension is associated with insulin resistance state and not with an initial renal function impairment. A Metabolic Syndrome in Active Subjects in Spain (MESYAS) Registry substudy. *Am J Hypertens* 2006; 19:189–196.
24. Segura J, Campo C, Ruilope LM, Rodicio JL. Do we need to target 'prediabetic' hypertensive patients? *J Hypertens* 2005; 23:2119–2125.
25. Mancia G, Grassi G, Zanchetti A. New-onset diabetes and antihypertensive drugs. *J Hypertens* 2006; 24:3–10.

26. Williams B, Poulter NR, Brown MJ *et al*. The BHS guidelines working party, for the British Hypertension Society. British Hypertension Society guidelines for hypertension management 2004 (BHS-IV): summary. *BMJ* 2004; 328:634–640.
27. Brown MJ, Cruickshank JK, Dominiczak A *et al*. Better blood pressure control: how to combine drugs. *J Hum Hypertens* 2003; 17:81–86.
28. Kjeldsen SE, Bakris GL, Giles TD *et al*. Consensus statement: the kidney and cardiovascular risk factors – implications for management. *J Hypertens*ion, submitted.
29. Pepine CJ, Kowey PR, Kupfer S *et al*. INVEST Investigators. Predictors of adverse outcome among patients with hypertension and coronary artery disease. *J Am Coll Cardiol* 2006; 47:547–551.
30. Balkrishnan R. The importance of medication adherence in improving chronic-disease related outcomes: what we know and what we need to further know. *Med Care* 2005; 43:517–520.
31. Ekman I, Andersson G, Boman K *et al*. Adherence and perception of medication in patients with chronic heart failure during a five-year randomised trial. *Patient Educ Couns* 2006; 61:348–353.
32. Dennehy EB, Suppes T, Rush AJ *et al*. Does provider adherence to a treatment guideline change clinical outcomes for patients with bipolar disorder? Results from the Texas Medication Algorithm Project. *Psychol Med* 2005; 35:1695–1706.
33. Ibrahim SA. Hypertension and medication adherence among African Americans: a potential factor in cardiovascular disparities. *J Natl Med Assoc* 2003; 95:28–29.
34. Elliott WJ. Optimizing medication adherence in older persons with hypertension. *Int Urol Nephrol* 2003; 35:557–562.
35. McInnes GT. Integrated approaches to management of hypertension. *Am Heart J* 1999; 138:S252–S255.
36. Kaplan N. In: Kaplan N (ed.). *Clinical Hypertension*. Lippincott Williams & Wilkins, Philadelphia, 2002.
37. Dzau V, Braunwald E. Resolved and unresolved issues in the prevention and treatment of coronary artery disease: a workshop consensus statement. *Am Heart J* 1991; 121:1244–1263.

2

Should metabolic syndrome patients with 'stage 2' pre-hypertension receive antihypertensive therapy?

B. M. Egan

INTRODUCTION

Metabolic syndrome (MS) affects ~3/8 of adults with high normal blood pressure (BP), i.e. 130–139/85–89 mmHg, which is the upper distribution of pre-hypertension 'Stage 2' pre-hypertension (PHT2). PHT2, as compared to normal BP (<120/80 mmHg), approximately doubles cardiovascular disease (CVD) risk independently of progression to hypertension and comorbid risk factors. MS raises CVD ~40% independently of age, total or low density lipoprotein (LDL)-cholesterol and cigarettes, although including BP and high density lipoprotein (HDL) minimizes independent impact. Nevertheless, MS patients with PHT2 are at significant CVD risk, which raises the question 'Should their BP be treated pharmacologically'?

PHT2 patients with diabetes or nephropathy should receive antihypertensive treatment according to the Seventh Report of the Joint National Committee of Prevention, Detection, Evaluation and Treatment of High Blood Pressure (JNC7). Framingham 10-year coronary heart disease risk calculations suggest non-diabetic PHT2 patients, irrespective of other risk factors, do not benefit from pharmacological reduction of BP unless values <120/80 mmHg are obtained, whereas modelling of NHANES I data suggest benefit from a 12 mmHg reduction. Clinical trials are needed to resolve this question. MS–PHT2 patients who are obese, African-American, microalbuminuric or have impaired fasting glucose or glucose tolerance are at greater risk and are likely beneficiaries of antihypertensive therapy. Renin–angiotensin system blockade, which can lower BP and reduce risk for diabetes and progressive nephropathy, is especially attractive. For 'lower risk' MS–PHT2 patients, lifestyle measures, while generally less effective than pharmacotherapy, can reduce multiple risk factors and CVD. Patients with MS–PHT2 can rapidly progress to hypertension, diabetes, and nephropathy. Regular follow-up is required to reinforce lifestyle change, detect progression to hypertension, diabetes, or nephropathy and provide antihypertensive therapy when progression occurs.

CLINICAL EPIDEMIOLOGY OF PRE-HYPERTENSION

Pre-hypertension represented a new BP category in JNC 7 defined as a BP of 120–139/80–89 mmHg (Table 2.1). In this discussion, we will focus mainly on the upper end of pre-hypertension or readings in the 130–139/85–89 mmHg range. BP readings in this range will

Brent M. Egan, MD, Department of Medicine, Medical University of South Carolina, Charleston, South Carolina, USA

Table 2.1 Classification of hypertension and approximate percentage and numbers of adults in the USA in each BP category [1–6]

BP category	*BP range, mmHg*	*~% adults*[1]	*~N adults*[1]	*~N with MS*
Normal (optimal)	<120/<80	~40	~87 000 000	~13 000 000
Pre-hypertension				
Stage 1 (normal)	120–129/80–84	~18	~39 000 000	~10 000 000
Stage 2 (high normal)	130–139/85–89	~12	~26 000 000	~10 000 000
Stage 1 hypertension	140–159/90–99	~21	~45 000 000	~39 000 000[2]
Stage 2 hypertension	≥160/≥100	~9	~20 000 000	

Terms in parenthesis ( ) indicate JNC6 designation. BP = Blood pressure; *N* = number; ~ = approximation; MS = metabolic syndrome; 1 = lower half and 2 = upper half pre-hypertensive BPs.
[1]Percents and numbers are estimates from the references cited and are rough approximations provided for illustrative purposes to highlight the magnitude of the public health problem presented by BP and MS with a focus on high normal BP. Estimates based on ~217 000 000 adults (US Census Press Release July, 2003).
[2]Includes both Stage 1 and Stage 2 hypertension.

be referred to as PHT2 rather than high normal BP, since these individuals are at increased risk for both progression to established hypertension and CVD independently of progression to hypertension. In other words, 'high normal BP' is not 'normal' but is predictive of future hypertension and carries many of the risks associated with hypertension. While excess cardiovascular risk is also associated with BP values in the lower or 'Stage 1' pre-hypertensive range, i.e. 120–129/80–84 mmHg, the magnitude of the excess risk is approximately half that of the upper pre-hypertensive range.

Pre-hypertension affects ~31% of US adults based on extrapolations from NHANES 1999–2000 [1]. The age-adjusted prevalence of pre-hypertension is higher in men at 39% than in women at 23% [2]. The number of pre-hypertensive individuals is estimated at 45–69.7 million [1–5]. Since the percentage of adults with pre-hypertension and hypertension is approximately equal, one could roughly estimate that 130 000 000 Americans are either pre-hypertensive or hypertensive, i.e. 65 000 000 with each condition [1, 6]. Approximately three of eight individuals with pre-hypertension, or roughly 12% of adults, have high normal BP as defined in JNC6 as readings from 130–139/85–89 mmHg [3]. The prevalence of high normal BP or PHT2 among 347 978 men screened for the Multiple Risk Factor Intervention Trial (MRFIT) was even higher at ~22% [7]. The greater prevalence of PHT2 in MRFIT than the general population is probably explained mainly by the higher prevalence in men than women and in the age group screened, i.e. 35–57 years of age than in younger or older subjects [3, 4].

PRE-HYPERTENSION AND PROGRESSION TO HYPERTENSION

Patients with borderline hypertension, high normal BP, and pre-hypertension are at increased risk for the development of hypertension [8–12]. In fact, Robinson and Brucer [8] used the term 'pre-hypertensive' in 1939 for systolic BPs of 120–139 mmHg based on evidence that most future hypertensive patients originated from this group and that these individuals had higher mortality rates [8]. In 1945, Levy and colleagues [9] observed that borderline hypertension approximately doubled the risk of future hypertension. A relative resting tachycardia also doubled the risk of future hypertension. Individuals with both borderline hypertension and resting tachycardia were at 4-fold greater risk of future hypertension than were normotensive individuals with normal resting heart rates.

More recently, Julius and colleagues reported that more than 10% of patients with high normal BP (PHT2) progress to established hypertension annually [10]. Leitschuh and co-authors documented that pre-hypertensive men and women in the Framingham Heart Study were twice as likely to develop hypertension as their counterparts with normal BP, which reinforces the earlier findings of Robinson and Brucer [8] and Leitschuh and co-workers [11]. The risk of hypertension among those with 'high normal' BPs rose to three times that of the normotensive group when an age-adjusted proportional hazards model was used. Weingarden also documented a 3-fold greater risk of developing hypertension among participants in the longitudinal British Health and Lifestyle Survey with 'high normal' as compared to normal BP values at the initial examination [12].

PRE-HYPERTENSION-2 AND CARDIOVASCULAR DISEASE RISK

Patients with PHT2 are more likely to progress to hypertension, which is a well-established risk factor for cardiovascular and renal diseases [8, 13, 14]. Moreover, patients with PHT2 are more likely than normotensive individuals to be overweight, hyperinsulinaemic, dyslipidaemic and insulin resistant [2, 15, 16]. The dyslipidaemia in patients with 'high normal' BP is similar to that associated with the MS and is characterized by hypertriglyceridaemia, reduced concentrations of the cardioprotective HDL cholesterol and increased numbers of small LDL cholesterol particles [16, 17]. 'High normal' BP is also associated with increased levels of fibrinogen, plasminogen activator inhibitor-1, multiple adipokines and inflammatory cytokines including C-reactive protein as well as endothelial dysfunction, left ventricular hypertrophy, diastolic dysfunction, and decreased coronary flow reserve [15, 18–25].

In view of the array of cardiovascular risk factors associated with PHT2, it is not surprising that these patients are at greater risk for cardiovascular and renal diseases than individuals with normal or 'optimal' BP [7, 8, 26–28]. In fact, roughly 90% or more of patients with PHT2 have at least one other major risk factor for CVD [2, 27, 29]. For example, in NHANES 1999–2000, patients with pre-hypertension were 1.83 (1.30–2.58) times more likely to have at least one additional 'above-optimal' risk factor than normotensive individuals [2]. The presence of multiple concomitant risk factors raises a clinically important question: 'Is "high normal" BP or PHT2 independently associated with increased risk for cardiovascular morbidity and mortality?'

CARDIOVASCULAR DISEASE RISK IN PATIENTS WITH 'STAGE 2 PRE-HYPERTENSION'

The risk of CVD associated with PHT2 has been assessed in at least five cohort studies in the USA. These five studies included participants that were demographically and geographically dissimilar [7, 26–28, 30]. Moreover, there were significant variations in the methods for defining and ascertaining CVD and the number of covariates used to discern the independent relationship between PHT2 and CVD risk. Despite important methodologic differences between the five cohort studies, four of them provided evidence for a significant, positive and independent contribution of PHT2 to CVD risk (Table 2.2) [7, 26–28]. The fifth, the Strong Heart Study, documented an independent relationship of the entire pre-hypertensive range to a higher incidence of CVD compared to normotensives. In the other four studies, the independent risk associated with BP readings in the lower end or Stage 1 pre-hypertensive range was approximately half that of PHT2.

Framingham [26]

In the Framingham Heart Study, 'high normal' BP, in contrast to optimal BP (<120/80 mmHg), was associated with a significantly greater risk for CVD based on results of cardiovascular risk factor-adjusted Cox proportional hazards regression model. The hazard ratio for CVD

Table 2.2 Cardiovascular risk associated with Stage 2 hypertension and estimates of number needed to treat to prevent a major cardiovascular event in 10 years

Study	*Hazard ratio*[1] *PHT2 vs NT*	*Absolute difference %/year*[2] *PHT2 vs NT*	*NNT (10 years)*	
			50%[4]	*100%*[4]
ARIC [28]	2.33, 1.85–2.92	~0.42%	48	24
Framingham [26]	Men 1.6, 1.1–2.2	~0.54% (0.43%)[3]	47	23
	Women 2.5, 1.6–4.1	~0.51% (0.25%)[3]	80	40
NHANES I [27]	1.42, 1.09–1.84	~0.53%	38	19
NHEFS 1 [64]			46 (26)[5]	23 (13)[5]
Strong Heart[6] [30]	1.80, 1.28–2.54	~0.61%	33	17
MRFIT [7]	CHD 1.66 (fatal) CVA 2.14 (fatal)	~0.09%[7]	222	111

NNT = Number needed to treat.
[1]Hazard ratio from cardiovascular risk factor-adjusted Cox proportional hazards regression model.
[2]Estimated absolute difference in cardiovascular event rates, unadjusted unless otherwise specified.
[3]Age-adjusted absolute difference in cardiovascular events.
[4]NNT assuming 50% or 100% efficacy of antihypertensive therapy in reducing excess CVD risk.
[5]Numbers in parenthesis represent adjustment for regression dilution bias from error in systolic BP measurement of 0.53 [65].
[6]All pre-hypertensives with BPs 120–139/80–89 mmHg included [30].
[7]Risk-adjusted absolute difference in mortality rates for fatal CHD and fatal stroke combined.

associated with 'high normal' BP was significant for both men (1.6; 95% confidence interval [CI] 1.1−2.2) and women (2.5; 1.6−4.1).

In this report, subjects with hypertension or CVD at the baseline examination were excluded leaving 6859 subjects for analysis [26]. CVD was defined by the total of fatal cardiovascular events and non-fatal myocardial infarction, stroke, and congestive (chronic) heart failure. The hazard ratios in men and women were adjusted for multiple confounders including age, body mass index (BMI), smoking status, and diabetes. Moreover, BP category and other risk factors were included as time-dependent covariates in the model, so that the independent risk for CVD associated with 'high normal' BP could be more precisely determined. In the Framingham cohort, 'high normal' BP, in comparison to optimal BP, was independently associated with approximately 2-fold greater risk of CVD.

NHANES I [27]

In the NHANES I conducted in 1971−1975, a subset of 14 407 participants were selected for the National Health Examination and Follow-up Study (NHEFS I). This group was evaluated at four subsequent time periods over 18 years with the last evaluation in 1992. The status of 90% of 11 195 survivors was ascertained at the 1992 evaluation. The report on cardiovascular risk associated with pre-hypertension from this dataset included 8986 participants (4616 with hypertension, 2708 with pre-hypertension, 1662 with normal BP).

Cardiovascular events in this study were defined as a composite of myocardial infarction, stroke, and congestive heart failure. At each follow-up evaluation, participants were asked whether a doctor told them they had a heart attack, stroke, or heart failure. Positive answers were counted as a new event for the relevant time period. In addition, in-patient hospital records, nursing home records, and death certificates were reviewed for these diagnoses.

The cardiovascular risk associated with pre-hypertension was ascertained before and after controlling for age and several categorical variables including gender, race, diabetes mellitus, obesity (BMI ≥30 kg/m^2), total cholesterol >200 mg/dl at the baseline examination, smoking status (current or ever), physical activity (self-report of no or little leisure time physical activity), and previous CVD (self-report).

PHT2, in NHANES I participants, was associated with approximately 2-fold greater risk for CVD in unadjusted analyses (hazard ratio 2.13; 95% CI 1.64–2.76). After adjustment for age and the categorical covariates noted, the Cox proportional hazard ratio was attenuated but remained significant (1.42; 95% CI 1.09–1.84). In this report, the lower end of pre-hypertension (Stage 1) was associated with a significantly higher rate of CVD before but not after adjustment for comorbid risk factors.

ARIC Study [28]

In the Atherosclerosis Risk in Communities (ARIC) Study, the Cox proportional hazard ratio for incident CVD with high normal BP was 2.33 (95% CI 1.85–2.92) with normal BP as the reference. ARIC Study participants were excluded from this analysis if they had hypertension, were taking antihypertensive medications, or had prevalent coronary heart disease or stroke at the initial examination. A total of 8960 individuals from the baseline examination were included in this report. Incident CVD was defined as incident coronary heart disease or incident stroke based on a systematic review of participant hospitalizations only.

In order to estimate more precisely the CVD risk associated with PHT2, analyses were adjusted for demographic variables including age, gender and ethnicity. The mean follow-up of participants in the ARIC Study was nearly 12 years, during which time several key risk factors are likely to change including the transition of a significant proportion of individuals with PHT2 to established hypertension. To isolate more precisely the specific effect of PHT2 on cardiovascular risk, several risk factors were analysed as time-dependent covariates, including systolic and diastolic BP, HDL cholesterol, LDL cholesterol, smoking status, BMI, physical activity, and use of cholesterol-lowering medications.

After adjusting for demographic factors and time-dependent covariates, PHT2 was associated with a greater than 2-fold (2.33; 95% CI 1.85–2.92) increased risk for CVD in ARIC Study paricipants. The lower end of pre-hypertension in this report was also independently associated with significantly higher CVD risk (1.69; 95% CI 1.37–2.09).

Strong Heart Study [30]

Among 2629 American-Indians in the Strong Heart Study who were free from hypertension and CVD, the 12-year incidence of combined fatal and non-fatal CVD was assessed. Adjustment was made for multiple confounders (age, gender, BMI, waist circumference, LDL and HDL cholesterol, triglyceride, physical activity, smoking, and alcohol use) in a Cox proportional hazards model. Using this model, the hazard ratio for CVD among non-diabetic pre-hypertensives was 1.8 (1.23–2.54) and for diabetic pre-hypertensives was 3.70 (2.66–5.15) compared to non-diabetic normotensives.

MRFIT [7]

Among 77 248 men with 'high normal' BP in the Multiple Risk Factor Intervention Trial, there were 2140 deaths from coronary heart disease. The hazard ratio for coronary heart disease mortality was 1.61 greater in men with PHT2 than with normal (optimal) BP. The hazard ratio for coronary heart disease was 1.66 (1.56–1.77) for systolic BP 130–139 mmHg and 1.48 (1.39–1.57) for diastolic BP 85–89 mmHg. The proportional hazards regression model was stratified by clinic and adjusted for several variables including age, race, income, cholesterol, self-reported cigarette smoking, and use of medications for diabetes. In MRFIT, the lower end of pre-hypertension, i.e. 120–129/80–84 mmHg, was associated with approximately half the excess coronary heart disease risk seen with PHT2.

Among the same group of men with PHT2 in MRFIT, the hazard ratio for stroke in men with PHT2 was 2.14 compared to men with normal (optimal) BP. As was observed with coronary heart disease, the hazard ratio for stroke associated with systolic BP 130−139 mmHg tended to be higher than for diastolic BP 85−89 mmHg (2.33; 95% CI 1.87−2.92 vs 1.76; 95% CI 1.45−2.15).

SYNOPSIS OF COHORT STUDIES ON CARDIOVASCULAR DISEASE RISK ASSOCIATED WITH STAGE 2 PRE-HYPERTENSION

Four separate cohort studies have documented that PHT2, and a fifth the entire range of pre-hypertension, is significantly, positively, and independently associated with CVD with hazard ratios that range from ~1.4 to 2.3 times greater than for demographically comparable individuals with normal (optimal) BP [7, 26–28, 30].

From a clinical perspective, absolute event rates for CVD in patients with PHT2 are important in estimating the benefit of treatment, which is captured in the number needed to treat. While the number needed to treat will be addressed in greater detail later, the absolute risks associated with PHT2 will be summarized now.

In the Framingham Study, the 'crude' cumulative 10-year incidence of a first cardiovascular event was greater in women with PHT2 (6.4%; 95% CI 4.8−8.0%) than with normal BP and (1.3%; 95% CI 0.8−1.8%). This translates to an absolute difference of 5.1% or ~0.51% annually. Men with PHT2 also had a higher cumulative 10-year incidence of first cardiovascular event (10.3%; 95% CI 8.3−12.1%) than men with normal BP (4.9%; 95% CI 3.5−6.2%) for an absolute difference of 5.4% or ~0.54% annually.

In ARIC, the cumulative incidence of CVD in patients with PHT2 was 12% over 12 years vs 7% with normal BP for a difference of ~0.42% annually. In the NHANES I cohort follow-up, the respective numbers were ~17% vs ~8% over 17 years for a difference of ~0.53% annually. In the Strong Heart Study, the absolute CVD event rates/1000 person-years or events/100 persons over 10 years were 7.3 for non-diabetic normotensives, 13.4 for non-diabetic pre-hypertensives, 19.3 for diabetic normotensives, and 26.5 for diabetic pre-hypertensives. The absolute difference per 100 persons over 10 years between non-diabetic normotensives and non-diabetic pre-hypertensives was 6.1% or 0.61% annually. Thus, in the four cohort studies cited, patients with PHT2 [26–28] and pre-hypertension [30] experience ~0.5% per year higher rates of cardiovascular events than individuals with normal BP. In contrast to these four studies that included fatal and non-fatal stroke and heart disease and/or heart failure [26–28, 30], in MRFIT the cumulative incidence of fatal coronary heart disease and stroke over 15 years was 2.84% among men with PHT2 compared to 1.5% in men with normal BP – an absolute difference of 1.34% or just under 0.1% annually.

CLINICAL EPIDEMIOLOGY OF METABOLIC SYNDROME

Metabolic syndrome (MS) was first defined provisionally by the World Health Organization (WHO) in 1998 and finalized at the 'Geneva Convention' in 1999 [31, 32]. MS was also defined in 2001 by the National Cholesterol Education Program (NCEP) III panel [33]. The WHO and NCEP criteria for defining the MS have some similarities yet several differences (Table 2.3).

METABOLIC SYNDROME DEFINITION AND PREVALENCE

When both definitions are applied to the same individuals in various cohorts, there are substantial similarities in classification but also important differences, particularly for

Table 2.3 World Health Organization (WHO) and National Cholesterol Education Program (NCEP) definitions of MS

WHO MS definition
• Insulin resistance (type 2 diabetes, IFG, IGT)
• Any two of the following:
–BP >140/90 mmHg or antihypertensive medication
–Plasma triglycerides >150 mg/dl
–HDL <35 mg/dl for men; <40 mg/dl for women
–BMI >30 and/or waist-to-hip (W/H) circumference ratio >0.9 for men or >0.85 for women
–Urinary albumin >20 mg/min; urine albumin/creatinine >30 mg/g
NCEP III MS definition
• Waist circumference >40" for men or >34.5" for women
• Serum triglycerides ≥150 mg/dl
• HDL cholesterol <40 mg/dl for men; <50 mg/dl for women
• BP ≥130/85 mmHg (PHT2 or greater)
• Fasting glucose >110 mg/dl

African-American men [34–36]. Insulin resistance and MS are often used interchangeably. In this regard, the WHO definition of MS is more strongly related to insulin resistance than the NCEP definition [36].

As noted, the concordance between MS defined by either National Cholesterol Education Program (NCEP) III or World Health Organization criteria is relatively high. Among 8608 participants in the NHANES 1988–1994 survey, the age-adjusted prevalence of the MS was 23.9% with NCEP III and 25.1% with WHO criteria [34]. Moreover, 86.2% of all individuals were categorized as either having or not having the MS by both definitions. Among the various race and gender subgroups, the incidence of MS was generally similar for both definitions. The greatest disparity in prevalence of MS between the two definitions was observed for African-American men in whom 16.5% met NCEP III and 24.9% met WHO criteria. By WHO criteria, African-American men had the highest prevalence of microalbuminuria (≥20 mg albumin/gram creatinine) at nearly 19%, which is not included in the NCEP III definition.

Based on the results of NHANES III the prevalence of the MS rises from roughly 5% of lean to 25% of overweight and 50–60% of obese adults [37]. While the merits of the MS as a medically important designation have been debated, the fact that the prevalence of the MS in adults is very strongly related to BMI implicates overweight, obesity, and adipocyte biology as common themes underlying cardiovascular risk factor clustering [38]. Thus, lifestyle and pharmacological strategies for preventing or attenuating age-related weight gain and for facilitating sustained weight loss emerge as logical interventions for preventing and managing MS-related risk and disease [39].

DIFFERENTIAL RELATIONSHIP OF PRE-HYPERTENSION AND HYPERTENSION WITH OVERWEIGHT, OBESITY AND THE METABOLIC SYNDROME

The prevalence of hypertension increases from 15.3% in lean people with a BMI <25 kg/m^2 to 27.8% in overweight individuals with BMI 25.0–29.9 and 42.5% among obese subjects with BMI ≥30. While overweight and obesity also increase risk for pre-hypertension, the prevalence of pre-hypertension is relatively constant at 31.7%, 30.6%, and 32.9% of adults in each of the three BMI categories, respectively [1].

In NHANES III and NHANES 1999–2000, the prevalence of MS increased from approximately 15% in normotensive people to 30% in pre-hypertensive individuals and 60% in hypertensive patients [40]. The differential relationship of pre-hypertension and hypertension to obesity is important when considering the association of each with the MS. In other words, the greater prevalence of MS in hypertensive than pre-hypertensive patients is likely explained in part by proportionately fewer lean and more obese hypertensive than pre-hypertensive patients. Obviously, patients in the lower half of the pre-hypertensive range do not meet the BP criterion for MS defined by NCEP III, which also contributes to a lower prevalence of MS in pre-hypertensives than hypertensives.

Additional evidence supports the notion that weight is very strongly related to MS in a subset of 151 patients with high normal BP participating in the Trial of Preventing Hypertension (TROPHY) Study with high normal BP; ~3/8 had the MS [41]. In this cohort, the prevalence of MS rose from ~5% of lean to ~38% of overweight and ~55% of obese subjects. These data suggest that the proportion of lean and obese subjects with high normal BP and MS is strongly linked to overweight and obesity in a manner similar but not identical to that for the general population [37].

METABOLIC SYNDROME AND RISK OF CARDIOVASCULAR DISEASE

The independent relationship of MS to coronary heart disease and cardiovascular mortality is a topic of debate. In 1209 Finnish men, the NCEP and WHO definitions of MS were associated with a 2.27 and 2.83 relative risk, respectively for CVD mortality after adjustment for age, LDL cholesterol, smoking, alcohol intake, socio-economic status, family history of coronary heart disease, white blood cell count and serum fibrinogen concentration [42].

Similarly, in a composite analysis of 6158 women and 5356 from 11 European cohort studies with a median follow-up period of 8.8 years, MS by WHO criteria was associated with a relative risk for cardiovascular mortality of 2.26 in men and 2.78 in women after adjustment for age, blood cholesterol, and smoking [43]. However, among 12 089 participants in the ARIC Study, the components of MS, defined by NECP III criteria that best predicted CVD risk were BP and HDL cholesterol [44]. In this cohort, most of the CVD risk associated with the MS was accounted for by the Framingham risk score. In a prospective study of 5128 men in Britain followed for 20 years, the Framingham risk score was a better predictor of coronary heart disease than MS defined by NCEP III criteria [45]. In this report, MS was a better predictor of diabetes than the Framingham risk score.

When viewing the various reports in the aggregate, it appears that MS, as defined by NCEP III criteria, adds little, if anything, to the prediction of coronary heart disease or CVD when BP and HDL cholesterol are included in the model together with other usual predictors, e.g. age, gender, LDL cholesterol and cigarette smoking. Of note, NCEP III does not include microalbuminuria in definition of MS. In another report that defined MS using WHO criteria, microalbuminuria was the MS criterion most strongly related to relative risk for cardiovascular death (2.80; 95% CI 1.62–2.64) [46]. Microalbuminuria has been identified as a significant independent predictor of CVD in other studies, which argues for its inclusion in predictive models [47]. This may be especially important for ethnic groups such as African-Americans that have a higher prevalence of microalbuminuria [34], which may lead to significant underestimation of MS risk when this risk factor is excluded. Microalbuminuria is, in fact, strongly related to the number of NCEP III MS risk factors [48].

METABOLIC SYNDROME, MICROALBUMINURIA AND CHRONIC KIDNEY DISEASE

In NHANES III, more than 6000 participants were included in both the chronic kidney disease (CKD) and microalbuminuria analyses [48]. The prevalence of microalbuminuria, defined as an albumin/creatinine ratio of 30–300 mg albumin/gram creatinine, increased linearly as a function of MS risk factors from 0 to 5, rising from 3.0% with no risk factors, to 9.8% with three risk factors and 20.1% with all five risk factors. Microalbuminuria, in turn, is related to multiple traditional and novel risk factors, with many of these linked to the metabolic/insulin resistance syndrome [49]. MS patients were 2.6 (95% CI 1.7–4.0) times more likely to have CKD, defined by estimated glomerular filtration rates <60 ml/min, than those without the syndrome [48]. When compared to individuals with 0–1 MS risk factors, patients with three, four, and five risk factors were 3.3, 4.2, and 5.8 times more likely to have CKD and comparable risk ratios for manifesting microalbuminuria.

PATHOPHYSIOLOGY OF OBESITY, METABOLIC SYNDROME, MICROALBUMINURIA AND CHRONIC KIDNEY DISEASE

Evidence strongly supports an association between obesity, MS, microalbuminuria and CKD [48–50]. Furthermore, extant scientific observations provide insight into pathophysiological mechanisms linking obesity and MS with microalbuminuria and CKD. However, the evidence is not uniformly consistent and the relative contributions of various mechanisms remain largely undefined.

RENAL AND GLOMERULAR HAEMODYNAMICS

Overweight, obesity, and MS are strongly related [50]. Several, but not all, studies identified increased renal blood and plasma flow, increased glomerular filtration rates, and particularly an increased filtration fraction in overweight and obese compared to normal weight subjects and in animal models of obesity [51–54]. Of interest, central or abdominal obesity, which is characteristic of patients with insulin resistance and MS, appears more closely associated with renal abnormalities than total or peripheral adiposity [55, 56].

The increased filtration fraction in obese subjects suggests dilation of the afferent arteriole and/or constriction of the efferent arteriole resulting in a relatively greater glomerular capillary hydrostatic pressure. Several factors present in obese subjects, and especially insulin-resistant subjects, e.g. hyperglycaemia, hyperinsulinaemia, and hyperglucagonaemia, are associated with afferent arteriolar dilation, whereas increased activity of the renin–angiotensin system [14, 57] contributes to relative efferent arteriolar constriction. Collectively, these changes facilitate glomerular hyperfiltration and increase urine albumin excretion.

CARDIOVASCULAR AND RENAL DISEASE RISKS RELATED TO METABOLIC SYNDROME

To the extent that the risk factors used to define MS are included in other predictive models, it is not surprising that the MS designation would not materially improve the prediction of CVD. Before dismissing the MS as a non-entity, it may be worthwhile to note that the MS clearly identifies individuals that are at increased risk for CVD and, if not already diabetic, for future diabetes. Patients with PHT2 and MS are at 2–4-fold greater risk for CVD than demographically matched individuals with normal BP who do not have the MS.

Patients with PHT2 and the MS are also at significantly greater risk for progression to hypertension and diabetes, which further amplifies risk for cardiovascular and renal diseases. The MS is strongly related to obesity, sedentary lifestyles, and dietary variables. The MS designation should, therefore, serve to focus attention on lifestyle and pharmacologic therapies that prevent or treat obesity as primary strategies for the prevention and treatment of the MS.

CLINICAL EPIDEMIOLOGY OF 'STAGE 2' PRE-HYPERTENSION AND METABOLIC SYNDROME

In the preceding sections, we have reviewed studies addressing the prevalence of PHT2, MS and their co-occurrence. While the prevalence of pre-hypertension is associated with overweight and obesity, the link is not as strong as for excess weight and hypertension [1, 2]. Since MS is very powerfully related to overweight and especially obesity, one would predict a closer relationship of hypertension than pre-hypertension to MS. In fact, analysis of the two most recent NHANES confirms this expectation, with MS prevalence increasing from ~15% of normotensive indivdiuals to 30% of pre-hypertensive and 60% of hypertensive patients [40].

In this review, we also examined the relationship of PHT2 and MS to CVD, and to a lesser extent, to renal disease. Four cohort studies in the USA have identified a significant, positive, and independent association between PHT2 and CVD risk, which ranges from ~1.4 to 2.3-fold increase compared to normal (optimal) BP [7, 26–28]. MS is also associated with a 2–3 fold increased risk for cardiovascular and renal diseases [42, 43, 48]. The cardiovascular risk associated with MS is attenuated and may disappear completely when controlling for most of the variables in the syndrome including BP, HDL cholesterol, and glucose as well as age, gender, total and LDL cholesterol, and cigarette smoking [44, 45]. Nevertheless, statistical adjustments cannot minimize the fact that MS patients with PHT2 represent a group at high relative and absolute risk for cardiovascular and renal disease.

The data suggest that PHT2 contributes in a positive, clinically significant, and statistically independent manner to excess CVD; hence the question: Should these patients receive antihypertensive pharmacotherapy? In the next section, we will address this fundamentally relevant clinical issue.

SHOULD METABOLIC SYNDROME PATIENTS WITH 'STAGE 2' PRE-HYPERTENSION RECEIVE ANTIHYPERTENSIVE THERAPY?

To date, not one randomized, controlled, clinical trial has addressed this important clinical question. The clinical relevance of the question regarding antihypertensive therapy in MS patients with PHT2 is manifold. First, the individual MS patient with PHT2 is at significant absolute risk for CVD, particularly over periods of 10 years of more. Although the typical clinical trial is completed in 4–5 years, the lifespan of many participants in these trials extends 5–20 years or more beyond the period of investigation. Results from the Framingham, ARIC, NHANES I, Strong Heart (all pre-hypertensives) and MRFIT cohorts clearly document that absolute risk continues to diverge between subjects with normal and PHT2 range BP readings as the duration of follow-up lengthens [7, 26–28, 30].

To evaluate the potential benefits of antihypertensive pharmacotherapy in MS patients with PHT2, we will re-examine data from four of these studies including Framingham, ARIC, NHANES I follow-up NHEFS I, and Strong Heart (Table 2.2). The cumulative 10-year incidence of a first cardiovascular event in the Framingham cohort was greater in women and men with PHT2 with absolute age-adjusted difference in incidence of 2.5% for women and 4.3% for men [26]. If we assume that antihypertensive therapy produced optimal BPs among those with PHT2 and that treatment eliminated 50% of the excess risk, then the number needed to treat over 10 years to prevent one incident event would be ~80 (100/[2.5/2]) for women and ~47 (100/[4.3/2]) for men. Obviously, if antihypertensive therapy were to eliminate 100% of the excess risk, then the number needed to treat would decline to ~40 (100/2.5) for women and ~23 (100/4.3) for men. Similar projections have been made for number need to treat using the ARIC, NHANES 1 and Strong Heart Study data (Table 2.2).

This conceptual approach to assessing benefit of antihypertensive therapy probably underestimates the positive effect of lowering BP in patients with MS and PHT2, since more than 1/2 would progress to hypertension during this time without treatment, which approximately doubles risk again [8, 10]. Patients who progress to hypertension would be at even greater risk during the transition and during any period of loss to follow-up or delay in starting antihypertensive therapy. In this regard, a consistent observation in several antihypertensive trials is that treatment is highly successful in preventing progression to higher pressure levels [58, 59]. Moreover, in a meta-analysis that included twelve trials, five placebo-controlled and one with a calcium channel blocker comparator, angiotensin-converting enzyme inhibitors and angiotensin receptor blockers were associated with a 25% reduction of incident type 2 diabetes mellitus [60]. Overall, the protection against progression to diabetes mellitus afforded by angiotensin receptor blockers and converting enzyme inhibitors was roughly comparable in the placebo-controlled and active comparator trials.

Since diabetes approximately doubles CVD risk, reduction of incident diabetes and the attendant risk would be another benefit of specific classes of antihypertensive agents [61]. Some evidence suggests that diuretic-induced diabetes does not further increase cardiovascular risk in prospective, randomized, controlled trials of hypertensive patients [62]. However, from a practical point, it has not been argued that patients who develop diabetes on diuretic therapy do not need to be monitored or treated for their hyperglycaemia. Consequently, the time, inconvenience, stress and cost burdens to patients who develop diabetes on diuretic therapy are substantial even if one accepts the argument that cardiovascular risk is not increased. Moreover, the risk of drug-induced diabetes mellitus may well be significant but only manifest over periods of time longer than the typical randomized, controlled trial [63].

Projections from NHEFS I on the number of JNC6 risk group B and C patients with PHT2 are more 'optimistic' than my 'crude', i.e. non-biostatistician, projections from the Framingham, ARIC, and Strong Heart Study data [26]. The estimated benefit for patients with 'high normal' BP, or PHT2, and at least one additional major cardiovascular risk factor, i.e. JNC6 risk group B, is relevant to our discussion, since this group is arguably at comparable or even less risk than non-diabetic patients with the MS [64]. In other words, JNC6 risk group B with PHT2 should provide a relatively conservative estimate of the benefits of antihypertensive therapy for MS patients with the same BP level.

Ogden and colleagues estimated benefit of treatment assuming a 12 mmHg reduction BP over 10 years in NHEFS I [65]. They projected that the number needed to treat of risk group B patients with PHT2 to prevent one cardiovascular event was 13. These estimates assumed that the intervention was 100% effective in eliminating the risk associated with a 12 mmHg BP elevation and included a correction of 0.53 for regression dilution bias due to imprecision in measuring systolic BP. Without correction for regression dilution bias, the estimated number needed to treat for risk group B was 23.

The efficiency of antihypertensive therapy in reducing excess risk is a vitally important question. The Framingham 10-year coronary heart disease risk calculation recommended by NCEP/Adult Treatment Panel (ATP) III assumes that treated individuals have a higher risk than untreated persons at the same BP for all values 120/80 mmHg or higher [66]. For example, in men with systolic BP 130–139 mmHg, one risk point accrues if BP is untreated and two risk points are added if BP is treated. Similarly, with systolic BP 120–129 mmHg, untreated men receive zero risk points and treated men receive one risk point. Thus, a treatment-induced reduction in systolic BPs from the 130 s to 120 s mmHg range does not confer any projected coronary heart disease benefit in men. Using this model, systolic BP must be lowered to <120 mmHg (optimal) in men with PHT2 to reduce risk one point.

Based on the NCEP III/Framingham risk calculator, antihypertensive therapy can have a significant adverse effect on total risk factor points for coronary heart disease in women [66]. Lowering systolic BP from the 130 s to the 120 s is not neutral as in men but actually increases the risk score by one point in women. Nevertheless, as was seen with men, lowering BP to <120 mmHg in women reduces total points by one in women with high normal BP.

The Framingham 10-year risk coronary heart disease risk score assumes that antihypertensive therapy does not fully reverse the effect of elevated BP and/or that there is a risk of antihypertensive medications unless values are reduced to <120 mmHg [66]. As a practical matter, for many patients, especially those in the upper end of the 130–139 mmHg systolic range, it is likely that two agents would be required in many, if not most, patients in order to reduce systolic BP to <120 mmHg. In contrast, a 12 mmHg reduction in systolic BP with a single agent is feasible [65], particularly if the clinician and patient are willing to titrate to higher doses and to switch between an angiotensin-converting enzyme inhibitor or angiotensin receptor blocker to a calcium channel blocker, e.g. if the desired BP response is not achieved [67, 68]. Unfortunately, at this time, data are simply unavailable to resolve definitively the discrepancies in projected benefit of antihypertensive treatment for patients with MS and PHT2.

RECOMMENDATION FOR BLOOD PRESSURE MANAGEMENT IN METABOLIC SYNDROME PATIENTS WITH 'STAGE 2' PRE-HYPERTENSION

Up to this point, evidence has been presented that patients with PHT2 and MS are at substantial absolute excess risk for CVD compared with age-matched individuals with normal BP. Moreover, these individuals are at high risk for progression to both established hypertension and diabetes, and they appear to be at high risk for microalbuminuria and CKD, which all confer substantial additional risk. After adjusting for multiple confounders including demographic factors, multiple comorbid cardiovascular risk factors and for progression to hypertension, PHT2 contributes significantly, positively, and independently to CVD. The absolute excess risk related to PHT2 is substantial and suggests that antihypertensive treatment would be beneficial. As noted, one fundamentally important clinical question that has not been fully resolved is the proportion of excess CVD, and especially coronary heart disease, risk that is prevented with antihypertensive therapy.

This review strongly suggests that a properly designed randomized, controlled clinical trial is needed to establish the effectiveness of antihypertensive therapy in MS patients with PHT2. In that regard, the recently released results of the TROPHY study are of interest [10, 69]. TROPHY demonstrates that treatment of individuals with PHT2 for 2 years is safe. During the first 2 years of the study, treatment with candesartan reduced the development of hypertension by a relative 66.3% and an absolute 26.8% compared to placebo. More than 60% of TROPHY participants had at least one other MS risk factor in addition to BP and 3/8 had two or more other risk factors and satisfied criteria for the MS. While TROPHY results provide important information regarding the safety and antihypertensive efficacy of angiotensin receptor blockade in patients with PHT2, this study was not designed to determine the benefit of these agents for reducing cardiovascular events in patients with PHT2.

In the absence of a definitive randomized, controlled trial, patients with the MS and PHT2 should be treated with BP-lowering medications if they have concomitant diabetes and/or nephropathy as defined in JNC7 (Table 2.4) [13]. Results from other trials suggest that MS patients with PHT2 who are obese, of African descent, or microalbuminuric or who have impaired fasting glucose or glucose tolerance are also at greater risk than patients without these additional risk factors [28, 30, 46]. Therefore, the risk:benefit ratio of antihypertensive therapy is more likely to be favourable for MS–PHT2 patients who meet these additional risk criteria than for those who are projected to be at lower absolute risk.

Antihypertensive therapy with an angiotensin-converting enzyme inhibitor or angiotensin receptor blocker is particularly attractive. In addition to lowering BP, these agents can reduce insulin resistance and inflammatory and coagulopathic markers and progression to diabetes mellitus and nephropathy, while improving endothelial function and target organ changes [60, 70–73]. However, assumptions of benefit are sometimes dead wrong [74–76], which further emphasizes the need for a well-designed clinical trial.

At a minimum, patients with the MS and PHT2 should receive lifestyle counselling to reduce both their excess CVD risk and to minimize their substantial likelihood of progression to hypertension, diabetes, and nephropathy. Aerobic exercise (fitness), the Dietary Approaches to Stop Hypertension (DASH) Eating Plan, and weight loss, combined with

Table 2.4 Recommendations for BP management in MS patients with PHT2

Risk group	*Lifestyle*	*Pharmacotherapy*
	Include DASH Eating Plan or Mediterranean Diet, walking 30 min daily or equivalent, 5–10% weight loss if overweight or obese	
'Low'	Yes	No, but follow at least every 6 months to reinforce lifestyle change and to detect progression to hypertension, type 2 diabetes or nephropathy and treat when any of these conditions develop
'Intermediate' One or more of: impaired fasting glucose, impaired glucose tolerance, microalbuminuria, obesity, African-American	Yes	Consider ACE-I or ARB monotherapy if BP remains in 'Stage 2' pre-hypertensive range after 3–6 months' lifestyle change to lower BP and reduce risk of progression to hypertension, type 2 diabetes and nephropathy. Add or switch to CCB if systolic BP decreases <10 mmHg on ACE-I or ARB monotherapy
'High' Type 2 diabetes Nephropathy –Stage 3 CKD –>300 mg albuminuria/day or >200 mg/g JNC7 compelling indication	Yes	Begin ACE-I or ARB immediately or after maximum of 3 months' lifestyle therapy if BP >130/80 mmHg with goal of reducing BP to <130/80 mmHg Titrate, add or change antihypertensive agents as required to achieve BP goal with preference to compounds that are evidence-based for concomitant compelling indications

smoking cessation and moderation of alcohol intake when appropriate, are especially attractive. These interventions can simultaneously reduce multiple risk factors, minimize progression to hypertension and diabetes, and possibly improve cardiovascular outcomes [77–82]. Regular clinical follow-up is required to reinforce the importance of lifestyle change, since the effectiveness even in rigorous and costly clinical trials is very limited. Moreover, regular follow-up is mandatory to promptly detect and institute appropriate pharmacotherapy for the many that progress to hypertension, diabetes or nephropathy.

REFERENCES

1. Wang Y, Wang QJ. The prevalence of prehypertension and hypertension among US adults according to the new Joint National Committee Guidelines. *Arch Intern Med* 2004; 164:2126–2134.
2. Greenlund KJ, Croft JB, Mensah GA. Prevalence of heart disease and stroke risk factors in persons with prehypertension in the United States, 1999–2000. *Arch Intern Med* 2004; 164:2113–2118.
3. Whelton PK, He J, Appel LJ *et al*. Primary prevention of hypertension: clinical and public health advisory from the National High Blood Pressure Education Program. *JAMA* 2002; 288:1881–1888.
4. Qureshi AI, Suri MF, Kirmani JF, Divani AA. Prevalence and trends of prehypertension and hypertension in United States: National Health and Nutrition Examination Surveys 1976 to 2000. *Med Sci Monit* 2005; 11:CR403–CR409.
5. NIH/NHLBI News Release. NHLBI issues new high blood pressure clinical practice guidelines. http://www.nhlbi.nih.bov/new/press/03-05-14.htm, February 8, 2006.

6. Fields LE, Burt VL, Cutler JA, Hughes J, Roccella EJ, Sorlie P. The burden of adult hypertension in the United States 1999 to 2000: a rising tide. *Hypertension* 2004; 44:398–404.
7. Neaton JD, Kuller L, Stamler J, Wentworth DN. Impact of systolic and diastolic blood pressure on cardiovascular mortality. In: Laragh JH, Brenner BM (eds). *Hypertension, Pathophysiology, Diagnosis, and Management*, 2nd edition. Raven Press Ltd., New York, 1995.
8. Robinson SC, Brucer M. Range of normal blood pressure: a statistical and clinical study of 11,383 persons. *Arch Intern Med* 1939; 64:409–444.
9. Levy RL, Hillman CC, Stoud WD *et al.* Transient tachycardia: prognostic significance alone and in association with transient hypertension. *JAMA* 1945; 129:585–588.
10. Julius S, Nesbitt S, Egan B *et al.*, The TROPHY study group. Trial of preventing hypertension: design and 2-year progress report. *Hypertension* 2004; 44:146–151.
11. Leitschuh M, Cuppies LA, Kannel W, Gagnon D, Chobanian A. High-normal blood pressure progression to hypertension in the Framingham Study. *Hypertension* 1991; 17:22–27.
12. Winegarden CR. From 'prehypertension' to hypertension? Additional evidence. *Ann Epidemiol* 2004; 15:720–725.
13. Chobanian AV, Bakris GL, Black HR *et al.*, The National High Blood Pressure Education Program Coordinating Committee. Seventh Report of the Joint National Committee on Prevention, Evaluation, and Treatment of High Blood Pressure. *Hypertension* 2003; 42:1206–1252.
14. Whelton PK, Perneger TV, Brancati FL, Klag MJ. Epidemiology and prevention of blood pressure-related renal disease. *J Hypertens* 1992; 10(suppl 7):S77–S84.
15. Kazumi T, Kawaguchi A, Sakai K, Hirano T, Yoshino G. Young men with high-normal blood pressure have lower serum adiponectin, smaller LDL size, and higher elevated heart rate than those with optimal blood pressure. *Diabetes Care* 2002; 25:971–976.
16. Julius S, Jamerson K, Mejia A, Krause L, Schcrk N, Jones K. The association of borderline hypertension with target organ changes and higher coronary risk. *JAMA* 1990; 264:354–358.
17. Lemne C, Hamsten A, Karpe F, Hilsson-Ehle P, de Faire U. Dyslipoproteinemic changes in borderline hypertension. *Hypertension* 1994; 24:605–610.
18. Nielsen JR, Oxhoj H, Fabricuis J. Left ventricular structural and functional changes in young men at increased risk of developing essential hypertension: assessment by echocardiography. *Ann Clin Res* 1988; 20(suppl 48):16–18.
19. Marabotti C, Genovesi-Ebert A, Palombo C, Giacona S, Michelassi C, Ghione S. Echo-Doppler assessment of left ventricular filling in borderline hypertension. *Am J Hypertens* 1989; 2:891–897.
20. Eliasson M, Jansson JH, Nilsson P, Asplund K. Increased levels of tissue plasminogen activator antigen in essential hypertension: a population-based study. *J Hypertens* 1997; 15:349–356.
21. Toikka JO, Laine H, Ahotupa M *et al.* Increased arterial intima-media thickness and in vivo LDL oxidation in young men with borderline hypertension. *Hypertension* 2000; 36:929–933.
22. Palombo C, Kozakova M, Magagna A *et al.* Early impairment of coronary flow reserve and increase in minimum coronary resistance in borderline hypertensive patients. *J Hypertens* 2000; 18:453–459.
23. Martinin G, Rabbia F, Gastaldi L *et al.* Heart rate variability and left ventricular diastolic function in patient with borderline hypertension with and without left ventricular hypertrophy. *Clin Exp Hypertension* 2001; 23:77–87.
24. Millgard J, Hagg A, Sarabi M, Lind L. Endothelium-dependent vasodilation in normotensive subjects with a familial history of essential hypertension and in young subjects with borderline hypertension. *Blood Press* 2002; 11:279–284.
25. Chrysohoou C, Pitsavos C, Panagiotakos DB, Skoumas J, Stefanadis C. Association between prehypertension status and inflammatory markers related to atherosclerotic disease. *Am J Hypertens* 2004; 17:568–573.
26. Vasan RS, Larson MG, Leip EP *et al.* Impact of high-normal blood pressure on the risk of cardiovascular disease. *N Engl J Med* 2001; 345:1291–1297.
27. Liszka HA, Mainous AG, King DE, Everett CJ, Egan BM. Prehypertension and cardiovascular morbidity. *Ann Fam Med* 2005; 3:294–299.
28. Kshirsagar AV, Carpenter M, Bang J, Wyatt SB, Colinders RE. Blood pressure usually considered normal is associated with an elevated risk of cardiovascular disease. *Am J Med* 2006; 119:133–141.
29. Nesbitt SN, Julius S, Leonard D, Egan BM, Grozinski M, The TROPHY Study Investigators. Is low-risk hypertension fact or fiction? Cardiovascular risk profile in the TROPHY Study. *Am J Hypertens* 2005; 18:979–984.

30. Zhang Y, Lee ET, Devereux RB *et al.* Prehypertension, diabetes, and cardiovascular disease risk in a population-based sample: the Strong Heart Study. *Hypertension* 2006; 47:410–414.
31. Alberti KGMM, Zimmett PF, The WHO Consuiltation. Definition, diagnosis and classification of diabetes mellitus and its complications. Part I. Diagnosis and classification of diabetes mellitus. Provisional report of a WHO consultation. *Diabet Med* 1998; 15:539–553.
32. WHO Consultation. Definition, diagnosis and classification of diabetes mellitus and its complications. Part I. Diagnosis and classification of diabetes mellitus. Non-communicable Disease Surveillance. World Health Organization, Geneva, 1999.
33. Executive Summary of the Third Report of the National Cholesterol Education Program (NCDEP) Expert panel on detection, evaluation, and treatment of high blood cholesterol in adults (Adult Treatment Panel III). *JAMA* 2001; 284:2486–2497.
34. Ford ES, Giles WH. A comparison of the prevalence of the metabolic syndrome using two proposed definitions. *Diabetes Care* 2003; 26:575–581.
35. Jorgensen ME, Bjerregaard P, Gyntelberg F, Borch-Johnsen K, The Greenland Population Study. Prevalence of the metabolic syndrome among the Inuit in Greenland. A comparison between two proposed definitions. *Diabetic Med* 2004; 21:1237–1242.
36. Hanley AJ, Wagenknecht LE, D'Agostino RB Jr, Zinman B, Haffner SM. Identification of subjects with insulin resistance and beta-cell dysfunction using alternative definitions of the metabolic syndrome. *Diabetes* 2003; 52:2740–2747.
37. Park Y-W, Zhu S, Palaniappan L *et al.* The metabolic syndrome: prevalence and associated risk factor findings in the US population from the Third National Health and Nutrition Examination Survey, 1988–1994. *Arch Intern Med* 2003; 163:427–436.
38. Egan BM, Greene EL, Goodfriend TL. The metabolic syndrome and the role of nonesterified fatty acids in blood pressure control and complications. *Curr Hypertens Rep* 2001; 3:107–116.
39. James PT, Rigby N, Leach R. International Obesity Task Force. The obesity epidemic, metabolic syndrome and future prevention strategies. *Eur J Cardiovasc Prev Rehabil* 2004; 11:3–8.
40. Ford ES, Giles WH. The prevalence of the metabolic syndrome by blood pressure status: findings from two national surveys. Abstract presented at the 20th Annual International Meeting of the International Society of Hypertension in Blacks (ISHIB), Puerto Rico, 2005.
41. Egan BM, Papademetriou V, Wofford M *et al.* Metabolic syndrome and insulin resistance: contrasting views in patients with high normal blood pressure. *Am J Hypertens* 2005; 18:3–12.
42. Lakka H-M, Laaksonen DE, Lakka TA *et al.* The metabolic syndrome and total and cardiovascular disease mortality in middle-aged men. *JAMA* 2002; 288:2709–2716.
43. Hu G, Qiao Q, Tuomilehto J, Balkau B, Borch-Johnsen K, Pyorala K, The DECODE Study Group. Prevalence of the metabolic syndrome and its relation to all-cause and cardiovascular mortality in nondiabetic European men and women. *Arch Intern Med* 2004; 165:1066–1076.
44. McNeill AM, Rosamond WD, Girman CJ *et al.* The metabolic syndrome and 11-year risk of incident cardiovascular disease in the Atherosclerosis Risk in Communities Study. *Diabetes Care* 2005; 28:385–390.
45. Wannamethee SG, Shaper AG, Lennon L, Morris RW. Metabolic syndrome vs Framingham risk score for prediction of coronary heart disease, stroke, and type 2 diabetes mellitus. *Arch Intern Med* 2005; 165:2644–2650.
46. Isomaa B, Almgren P, Tuomi T *et al.* Cardiovascular morbidity and mortality associated with the metabolic syndrome. *Diabetes Care* 2001; 24:683–689.
47. Borch-Johnsen K, Feldt-Rasmussen B, Strandgaard S, Schroll M, Jensen JS. Urinary albumin excretion: an independent predictor of ischemic heart disease. *Arterioscler Thromb Vasc Biol* 1999; 19:1992–1997.
48. Chen J, Muntner P, Hamm LL *et al.* The metabolic syndrome and chronic kidney disease in U.S. adults. *Ann Intern Med* 2004; 140:167–174.
49. Sowers JR, Haffner S. Treatment of cardiovascular and renal risk factors in the diabetic hypertensive. *Hypertension* 2002; 40:781–788.
50. Mokdad AH, Ford ES, Bowman BA *et al.* Prevalence of obesity, diabetes, and obesity-related health risk factors, 2001. *JAMA* 2001; 289:76–79.
51. Bosma RJ, van der Heide JJ, Oosterop EJ, de Jong PE, Navis G. Body mass index if associated with altered renal hemodynamics in non-obese healthy subjects. *Kidney Int* 2004; 65:259–265.
52. Chagnac A, Weinstein T, Korzets A, Ramadan E, Hirsch J, Gafter U. Glomerular hemodynamics in severe obesity. *Am J Physiol* 2000; 278:F817–F822.

53. de Jong PE, Verhave JC, Pinto-Sietsma JS, Hillege HL, The PREVEND Study Group. Obesity and target organ damage: the kidney. *Int J Obes Relat Metab Diord* 2002; 26(suppl 4):S21–S24.
54. Zheng R, Reisen E: Obesity-hypertension. The effects on cardiovascular and renal systems. *Am J Hypertens* 2000; 13:1308–1314.
55. Solerte SB, Rondanelli M, Giacchero R *et al.* Serum glucagon concentration and hyperinsulinemia influence renal hemodynamics and urinary protein loss in normotensive patients with central obesity. *Int J Obes Relat Metab Disord* 1999; 23:997–1003.
56. Pinto-Sietsma SJ, Navis G, Janssen WM, de Zeeuw D, Gans RO, de Jong PE, The PREVEND Study Group. A central body fat distribution is related to renal function impairment, even in lean subjects. *Am J Kidney Dis* 2003; 41:733–741.
57. Egan BM, Stepniakowski K, Goodfriend TL. Renin and aldosterone are higher and the hyperinsulinemic effects of salt restriction greater in subjects with risk factor clustering. *Am J Hypertens* 1994; 7:886–893.
58. Veterans Administration Cooperative Study Group on Antihypertensive Agents. Effects of treatment on morbidity in hypertension: II. Results in patients with diastolic blood pressure averaging 90 through 114 mmHg. *JAMA* 1970; 213:1143–1152.
59. Preston RA, Materson BJ, Reda DJ, Williams DW. Placebo-associated blood pressure response and adverse effects in the treatment of hypertension. *Arch Intern Med* 2000; 160:1449–1454.
60. Abuissa H, Jones PG, Marson SP, O-Keefe JH. Angiotensin-converting enzyme inhibitors or angiotensin receptor blockers for prevention of Type 2 diabetes. *J Am Coll Cardiol* 2005; 46:821–826.
61. Stamler J, Vaccaro O, Neaton JD, Wentworth D. Diabetes, other risk factors, and 12-yr cardiovascular mortality in men screened in the Multiple Risk Factor Intervention Trial. *Diabetes Care* 1993; 16:434–444.
62. Moser M. Diuretics and new onset diabetes: is it a problem? *J Hypertens* 2005; 23:666–668.
63. Aksnes TA, Reims HM, Kjeldsen SE, Mancia G. Antihypertensive treatment and new-onset diabetes. *Curr Hypertens Rep* 2005; 7:298–303.
64. Joint National Committee on Prevention, Detection, Evaluation, and Treatment of High Blood Pressure. The Sixth Report of the Joint National Committee on Prevention, Detection, Evaluation, and Treatment of High Blood Pressure. *Arch Intern Med* 1997; 157:2413–2446.
65. Ogden LG, He J, Lydick E, Whelton PK. Long-term absolute benefit of lowering blood pressure in hypertensive patients according to the JNC VI risk stratification. *Hypertension* 2000; 35:539–543.
66. Executive Summary of the Third Report of the National Cholesterol Education Program (NCEP). Expert Panel on Detection, Evaluation, and Treatment of High Blood Cholesterol in Adults (Adult Treatment Panel III). *JAMA* 2001; 285:2486–2497.
67. Materson BJ, Reda DJ, Preston RA *et al.*, The Department of Veterans Affairs Cooperative Study Group on Antihypertensive Drugs. Response to a second single antihypertensive agent used as monotherapy for hypertension after failure of the initial drug. *Arch Intern Med* 1995; 155:1757–1762.
68. Blumenfeld JD, Laragh JH. Renin system analysis. A rational method for the diagnosis and treatment of the individual patient with hypertension. *Am J Hypertens* 11:894–896.
69. Julius S, Nesbitt SD, Egan BM *et al.*, The Trial of Preventing Hypertension (TROPHY) investigators: feasibility of treating prehypertension with an angiotensin receptor blocker. *N Engl J Med* 2006; 354 (published online March 14, 2006).
70. Erdem Y, Usalan C, Haznedaroglu IC *et al.* Effects of angiotensin converting enzyme and angiotensin II receptor inhibition on impaired fibrinolysis in systemic hypertension. *Am J Hypertens* 1999; 12:1071–1076.
71. Yavuz D, Koc M, Toprak A *et al.* Effects of ACE inhibition and AT_1-receptor antagonism on endothelial function and insulin sensitivity in essential hypertensive patients. *J Renin Angiotensin Aldosterone Syst* 2003; 4:197–203.
72. Di Napoli M, Papa F. Angiotensin-converting enzyme inhibitor use is associated with reduced plasma concentration of C-reactive protein in patients with first-ever ischemic stroke. *Stroke* 2003; 34:2922–2929.
73. Rosei EA, Rizzoni D, Muiesan ML *et al.*, The CENTRO (Candeseartan on Athersoclerotic Risk Factors) Study Investigators. Effects of candesartan cilexetil and enalapril on inflammatory markers of atherosclerosis in hypertensive patients with non-insulin-dependent diabetes mellitus. *J Hypertens* 2005; 23:435–444.
74. Singh BN. Do antiarrhythmic drugs work? Some reflections on the implications of the Cardiac Arrhythmia Suppression Trial. *Clin Cardiol* 1990; 13:725–728.

75. Felker GM, O'Connor CM. Inotropic therapy for heart failure: an evidence-based approach. *Am Heart J* 2001; 142:393–401.
76. The Antihypertensive and Lipid-Lowering Treatment to Prevention Heart Attack Trial (ALLHAT). Major cardiovascular events in hypertensive patients randomized to doxazosin vs chlorthalidone. *JAMA* 2000; 283:1967–1975.
77. Hjermann I, Velve Byre K, Holme I, Leren P. Effect of diet and smoking intervention on the incidence of coronary heart disease. Report from the Oslo Study Group of a randomized trial in healthy men. *Lancet* 1981; 2:1303–1310.
78. The Trial of Hypertension Prevention Collaborative Research Group. Effects of weight loss and sodium restriction on blood pressure and hypertension incidence in overweight people with high-normal blood pressure. *Arch Intern Med* 1997; 157:657–667.
79. Appel LJ, Moore TJ, Obarzanek E *et al.*, The DASH Collaborative Research Group. A clinical trial of the effects of dietary patterns on blood pressure. *N Engl J Med* 1997; 336:1117–1124.
80. Esposito K, Marella R, Ciotaola M *et al.* Effect of a Mediterranean-style diet on endothelial dysfunction and markers of vascular inflammation in the metabolic syndrome. *JAMA* 2004; 292:1440–1446.
81. Katzmarzyk PT, Church TS, Blair SN. Cardiorespiratory fitness attenuates the effects of the metabolic syndrome on all-cause and cardiovascular disease mortality in men. *Arch Intern Med* 2004; 164:1092–1097.
82. The Diabetes Prevention Program Research Group. Reduction in the incidence of type 2 diabetes with lifestyle intervention or metformin. *N Engl J Med* 2002; 346:393–403.

3

The presence of proteinuria and antihypertensive therapy selection

N. Khosla, P. Sarafidis, G. L. Bakris

INTRODUCTION

A considerable number of recent clinical trials have focused on the role of microalbuminuria as a marker for increased renal injury and cardiovascular (CV) morbidity and mortality. This research has added greatly to the knowledge of maximizing risk reduction in patients previously unrecognized to be at high risk, but it should not divert attention away from those patients with frank proteinuria. Presence of proteinuria has a dual significance in patients with hypertension as it serves as a marker of considerable renal dysfunction and predictor of progression to end-stage kidney disease. Moreover, the presence of proteinuria is associated with increased risk for cardiovascular disease (CVD) [1]. This chapter reviews the role of proteinuria as a marker of increased renal and CV morbidity and mortality in hypertensive patients and discusses non-pharmacological and pharmacological therapy for reducing proteinuria.

DEFINITION AND PREVALENCE OF PROTEINURIA

A normally functioning kidney will excrete some protein in the urine. The composition of the protein excreted is 20% low molecular weight proteins, such as immunoglobulins, 40% Tamm-Horsfall mucoproteins secreted by the distal tubule, and 40% high molecular weight albumin. While the first two types of protein are not detectable using conventional dipsticks, albumin is measured routinely in the evaluation of abnormal urinary protein excretion. Microalbuminuria is defined as a urinary albumin excretion rate between the range of 20 and 200 μg/min or 30 and 299 mg/day. As widespread use of the urine albumin to creatinine ratio (UACR), is used to define the presence of microalbuminuria (>30 mg/g <300 mg/g) the utility of a spot UACR has increased. Any urinary protein excretion greater than these levels is defined as microalbuminuria or proteinuria [1]. The current guidelines recommend the use of UACR in lieu of other measures due to the inherent difficulties and patient inconvenience involved with a timed urine collection. However, the imprecise nature of albumin and creatinine measurement in the urine requires at least three measures of these parameters over a period of 2–3 months before determining the actual UACR for a particular patient (see Table 3.1). Ideally, these measures should be done on a fasting specimen that is collected from the first morning void [2].

Nitin Khosla, MD, Rush University Medical Center, Department of Preventive Medicine, Hypertension/Clinical Research Center, Chicago, Ilinois, USA

Pantelis Sarafidis, MD, Rush University Medical Center, Department of Preventive Medicine, Hypertension/Clinical Research Center, Chicago, Ilinois, USA

George L. Bakris, MD, Professor and Vice-Chairman, Department of Preventive Medicine, Director, Hypertension/Clinical Research Center, Rush University Medical Center, Chicago, Ilinois, USA

Table 3.1 Factors affecting the measurement of urine albumin: creatinine

Factors affecting albumin excretion
1. Blood pressure
2. Fasting vs. non-fasting sample
3. Time of day
4. Salt intake
5. Volume status
Factors affecting creatinine excretion
1. Gender
2. Muscle mass
3. Race

In the general population, the prevalence of proteinuria ranges from 1 to 10.1% [3]. The variation of this range can largely be explained by the different profiles of the patients in the various analyses. For example, the presence of diabetes mellitus can influence the prevalence of proteinuria that can be as high as 28% of Type 1 and 41% of Type 2 patients with diabetes [1]. It is important to note that the occurrence of hypertension in relation to abnormal urinary protein excretion is different in patients with Type 1 and Type 2 diabetes. Patients with Type 1 diabetes will have elevations in their systolic and diastolic blood pressures only after the development of nephropathy, manifested initially by microalbuminuria. Conversely, patients with Type 2 diabetes may have elevations in systolic blood pressure that precede the development of abnormal urinary protein excretion [4]. These data suggest that the mechanism of abnormal urinary protein excretion in Type 1 diabetes is a continuous spectrum beginning with microalbuminuria that relates to incipient nephropathy and ending with proteinuria, whereas in Type 2 diabetes abnormal urinary protein excretion relates primarily to atherosclerotic vascular damage.

The level of blood pressure also directly influences the development of proteinuria. In a clinical study of 387 hypertensive patients, the level of urinary protein excretion was found to be directly proportionate to the level of systolic, diastolic, and mean blood pressure measured at an office visit or with a 24-h ambulatory monitor [5]. A population study with 1567 participants revealed that there was an 18 mmHg higher systolic blood pressure in the group of non-diabetic individuals with microalbuminuria than in those without microalbuminuria [6]. Thus, it would appear that hypertension is the link explaining the higher prevalence of abnormal urinary protein excretion in older patients, as the prevalence of hypertension approaches 70% at the age 70 [7].

THE NATURAL HISTORY OF PROTEINURIA

When evaluating the natural history of proteinuria, a distinction must be made between those with and without diabetes mellitus. Since Kimmelstiel and Wilson first described proteinuria in a diabetic patient in 1936, much has been learned about the natural history of proteinuria in diabetes. Much of this knowledge comes from early studies involving Type 1 diabetic patients, which showed that the average time from diagnosis of diabetes to the development of proteinuria is 19 years. Further support for the concept that abnormal urinary protein excretion is a spectrum in patients with Type 1 diabetes comes from several studies that have shown that the strongest predictor of proteinuria development in such patients is the presence of microalbuminuria [8]. In fact, once microalbuminuria is present, 80% of Type 1 diabetic patients will go on to develop proteinuria and decline in glomerular filtration rate (GFR) [9].

The natural history of proteinuria in patients with Type 2 diabetes is more variable. Some evidence to relate microalbuminuria and proteinuria development does exist. In the Casale

Monferrato Study, 1253 Type 2 diabetic patients were followed for a median of 5.3 years. Approximately 4% of the patients with microalbuminuria would progress to proteinuria annually and the presence of microalbuminuria increases the risk of developing overt nephropathy by 42% [10]. However, this study also demonstrated that the level of glycaemic control, i.e. HbA1c level, was strongly predictive of proteinuria development. Another study of 224 Type 2 diabetic patients demonstrated that those with proteinuria had higher levels of systolic blood pressure than those with lower levels of urinary albumin excretion [11]. Thus, patients with either Type 1 or Type 2 diabetes will manifest proteinuria in relationship to a spectrum of atherosclerotic risk factors. The varying levels of glycaemic and blood pressure control among different patients with Type 2 diabetes help to explain the different courses in developing nephropathy seen among different patients.

The natural history of proteinuria in patients with non-diabetic renal disease is much less well defined. The most likely explanation for this is the varied causes of non-diabetic renal disease. However, it is clear that proteinuria correlates with impairment of renal function. This is demonstrated by a study of 7728 patients without diabetes which stratified patients into four different groups based on baseline albumin excretion: normal protein excretion (0–15 mg/day), high-normal (15–30), microalbuminuria (30–300), and macroalbuminuria (>300). The study showed that while the macroalbuminuria group had a decline in GFR, the high-normal and microalbuminuria groups actually had increased GFR [12]. The explanation for these findings relates to the pathophysiology of renal function loss in non-diabetic kidney disease. When an insult initiates renal injury and abnormal urinary protein excretion, the kidney responds to the ongoing damage by hypertrophying and hyperfiltering. Initially, this allows the kidney to meet the body's demands, but it leads to a vicious circle, as hyperfiltering will increase protein leakage and this will ultimately lead to increased renal damage and loss of more nephrons. The final result of this cascade is both proteinuria and decline in GFR.

ROLE OF PROTEINURIA IN SETTING BLOOD PRESSURE GOALS

All recent guidelines recommend a blood pressure goal of <130/80 mmHg for patients with diabetes or chronic kidney disease [1, 13, 14]. While data to support the goal of <130/80 mmHg in patients with diabetes are relatively robust they are almost exclusively derived from retrospective analyses of prospective studies that evaluated CV events. In the two studies of kidney disease progression that evaluated the lower blood pressure goal, neither showed a benefit at 5 years and the one study that did show benefit on kidney disease progression was largely comprised of patients with non-diabetic kidney disease and took 8 years of follow-up to demonstrate [15].

The Modification of Diet in Renal Disease Study (MDRD), which included patients with chronic kidney disease and proteinuria, provides the best evidence to support a lower blood pressure target in the appropriate chronic kidney disease patient population. The study found that, after 8 years of follow-up, those patients with baseline proteinuria >1 g/day that were randomized to a mean arterial pressure (MAP) of 92 mmHg had a slower decline in renal function and a lower incidence of renal failure compared to those randomized to a MAP of 107 mmHg [16]. It should also be noted that a meta-analysis of studies in non-diabetic kidney disease, systolic blood pressure of 110–129 mmHg was associated with the lowest risk of kidney disease progression in patients with urine protein excretion >1 g/day [17].

The results of the African-American Study of Kidney Disease (AASK), which included African-American patients with hypertensive kidney disease, add support to the notion that patients with significant proteinuria do benefit from a lower blood pressure target. The overall trial showed that patients randomized to a lower blood pressure target of a MAP <92 mmHg derived no benefit from this intervention in comparison to patients randomized to a usual target (MAP 102–107 mmHg) [18]. However, a further analysis showed that baseline proteinuria was the key factor that defined the results of the trial, as the lower blood pressure target did preserve renal function in the small subset of patients with proteinuria >1 g/day.

In contrast, in patients with non-diabetic kidney disease and lower levels of urine protein, the evidence for such a low blood pressure goal is not as strong. In the MDRD trial no significant benefit in renal protection was apparent in the subgroup of patients with urine protein excretion <1 g/day [16]. In the AASK trial, there was a non-significant trend towards a slower decline in GFR in the cohort of patients with proteinuria <1 g/day [18]. The meta-analysis by Jafar and co-workers [17] also provides further support for these findings, as it showed no significant association between the level of systolic blood pressure and the risk of kidney disease progression in patients with proteinuria <1 g/day.

The Ramipril Efficacy In Nephropathy trial (REIN-2) has been considered as evidence to contradict lower blood pressure targets in patients with proteinuria [19]. In this study, patients with non-diabetic nephropathy and urine protein excretion >1 g/day, already treated with the angiotensin-converting enzyme (ACE) inhibitor ramipril, were assigned to either conventional (diastolic blood pressure <90 mmHg) or intensified (systolic/diastolic blood pressure <130/80 mmHg) with the addition of the dihydropyridine (DHP) calcium antagonist felodipine. At the end of the treatment period, the cumulative incidence of end-stage renal disease (ESRD), rate of GFR decline, and residual proteinuria were similar in the two arms. However, this study was underpowered to detect a difference in decline in GFR between the two blood pressure groups as the median follow-up was only 1.6 years and there was only a 4.1/2.8 mmHg blood pressure difference between treatment groups throughout the study.

When all the evidence is pooled (Table 3.2), however, it is clear that a blood pressure target of <130/80 mmHg should definitely be sought, except for patients with diabetes or in those with non-diabetic chronic kidney disease and proteinuria >1 g/day. In patients without diabetes, whose proteinuria is between 300 mg and 1 g/day strong consideration should be given for this target as well, until specific trials clarify the best blood pressure targets in these types of patients.

TREATMENT OF HYPERTENSION AND PRESERVING RENAL FUNCTION IN PEOPLE WITH PROTEINURIA

NON-PHARMACOLOGICAL APPROACHES

Overall, managing hypertension in the United States has proved quite difficult as control rates are only 34% [13]. The addition of chronic kidney disease makes the management of

Table 3.2 Characteristics of studies evaluating the impact of different levels of blood pressure on renal outcomes

	MDRD	*AASK*	*REIN-2*
Mean follow-up (years)	6.2	3.8	1.6 (median)
Baseline GFR (ml/min)	32.0	46.0	35.0
Baseline level of protein excretion (g/day)	1.09	0.53	2.85
Difference in renal outcomes between higher and lower BP groups	No difference*	No difference*	No difference

*Subgroup analyses of these studies have demonstrated that patients with proteinuria >1 g/day do have slower declines in GFR when a mean arterial blood pressure of <125/75 mmHg is achieved.

hypertension even more difficult. Lifestyle changes such as weight loss, exercise, and alcohol moderation should play a central role in helping to manage hypertension in all patients, but low protein diets, low sodium intake, and smoking cessation have all been proposed to play a special role in patients with proteinuria. The MDRD is the largest trial to date to evaluate the role of a low protein diet in the presence of proteinuria [20]. The trial randomized patients with chronic kidney disease and proteinuria to two blood pressure groups as discussed previously and to either a low protein group (0.58 g/kg/day) or a very low protein group (0.28 g/kg/day). A 35% reduction (not significant) in the incidence of ESRD and/or serum creatinine was seen in the very low protein group at 3 years. These results are strengthened by a meta-analysis showing that a low protein diet reduces the decline in GFR by 0.53 ml/min/year [21]. These data suggest that recommending a low protein diet to patients with proteinuria and decreased GFR will help preserve renal function. However, physicians must balance this benefit with the difficulty that most patients have adhering to a strict diet restricting protein intake. Also, if choosing to use such a diet, physicians must be vigilant in monitoring patients for signs of malnutrition.

Hypertension in patients with chronic renal insufficiency manifested by either a decline in GFR or proteinuria has been shown to be mediated to a large extent by salt sensitivity. This was previously shown by Blythe in an elegant study comparing the response to salt loading in healthy patients to those with chronic kidney disease. Both groups were able to increase their fractional excretion of sodium after a salt load, but patients with chronic kidney disease showed elevations in their blood pressures [22]. Clearly, this was a response to the increase in extracellular volume resulting from the high salt intake and the impaired functioning kidneys were unable to deal with this volume expansion. High dietary sodium intake in patients with proteinuria is particularly deleterious for several other reasons. First, the presence of a high salt load itself will increase proteinuria by increasing the oncotic pressure of the glomerular filtrate which will lead to more protein being pulled into the urine [23]. Excessive dietary sodium intake, i.e. >6 g/day will also attenuate the protective effects of many antihypertensive medications on proteinuria reduction [24]. Thus, recommending a daily dietary sodium intake of 2–4 g in patients with chronic kidney disease will lead to lower levels of urinary protein excretion and will make it easier to control blood pressure.

Several population based studies have revealed a clear association between smoking and both an accelerated decline in renal function and increased risk of developing abnormal urine protein excretion [25, 26]. The Heart Outcomes and Prevention Evaluation (HOPE) trial confirmed this finding, showing that there was a 20% higher risk of developing microalbuminuria or proteinuria in current smokers when compared to non-smokers [27]. Though smoking has been demonstrated to be deleterious to renal function, no prospective trial has examined the impact that smoking cessation would have on those with already established renal disease or proteinuria. It is, however, reasonable to expect that the documented cardiovascular benefits seen with smoking cessation are enough to warrant physicians to recommend this intervention to patients with chronic kidney disease. Likely, this will also serve to preserve some renal function.

PHARMACOLOGIC THERAPY

Before choosing an antihypertensive agent, physicians must be aware of their overall goal in managing hypertension in patients with proteinuria. This goal involves not only lowering blood pressure to the target level of <130/80 mmHg, but also slowing the progression of kidney disease and reducing the CVD risk. Since all compounds that lower blood pressure are known to decrease CV risk, physicians must also be aware of the presence of proteinuria and use antihypertensive agents that reduce this as well since agents that reduce both blood pressure and proteinuria provide superior renal outcomes.

ANGIOTENSIN-CONVERTING ENZYME INHIBITORS

Early clinical trials demonstrated that ACE inhibitors have a blood pressure-independent renoprotective effect and it is presumed that this effect is related to reductions in proteinuria. This was first shown in the original trial of the Collaborative Study Group that randomized more than 400 Type 1 diabetics with a urinary protein excretion of >500 mg/day and serum creatinine <2.5 mg/dl to treatment with the ACE inhibitor captopril or placebo. After a median follow-up of 3 years, treatment with captopril led to a 43% risk reduction for doubling of serum creatinine and a 30% reduction in urinary protein excretion. Though there were small differences in the blood pressures achieved in the two groups, these effects were independent of level of blood pressure [28].

While several early trials involving Type 1 diabetics have supported the results of the Collaborative Study Group trial, more recent studies involving both Type 1 and Type 2 diabetics have suggested that the only benefit seen with ACE inhibitors is related to blood pressure reduction. The United Kingdom Prospective Diabetes Study (UKPDS) provides good evidence for this conclusion as captopril and atenolol had similar outcomes on micro- and macrovascular complications in hypertensive Type 2 diabetic patients [29]. *Post hoc* data from the Antihypertensive and Lipid Lowering Treatment to Prevent Heart Attack Trial (ALLHAT) and well-controlled animal studies have expanded the idea that ACE inhi bitors have no unique effects independent of blood pressure reduction in patients with non-diabetic kidney disease [30, 31]. The lack of benefit seen with ACE inhibitors in these later trials relates to several issues. Most importantly, all of the early trials included only patients with stage 3 nephropathy or worse and patients with more than 500 mg/day proteinuria. Since only proteinuria is clearly associated with increased risk of nephropathy progression, a reduction in urine albumin excretion in proteinuric patients should correlate with preservation of renal function. This has been recently confirmed in three post analyses of large renal outcome trials [32–34]. ALLHAT did not make any measure of proteinuria. As such, it is nearly impossible to interpret the lack of selective benefit of ACE inhibitor treatment in this trial.

The original captopril trial provides some of the strongest evidence to support the idea that proteinuria and advanced stage nephropathy are key factors in determining benefit from treatment with an ACE inhibitor. In this study, those whose serum creatinine values were >2.0 mg/dl derived the greatest benefit from adding ACE inhibition to a standard antihypertensive regimen in order to lower BP to <140/90 mmHg. The ACE inhibitor group had a 74% reduction in the risk of doubling serum creatinine compared with the placebo group. Only a 4% reduction in these endpoints was seen in patients with serum creatinine <1.0 mg/dl [28]. The REIN trial, which studied patients with non-diabetic renal disease, also showed that those with advanced nephropathy, i.e. serum creatinine values >2.0 mg/dl and >3.0 g/day proteinuria, had a 62% reduction in renal disease progression. This is in contrast to a 22% reduction in renal disease progression among those with microalbuminuria [35]. Similar findings have been noted by the ACE inhibition in Progressive Renal Insufficiency Study Group and in the meta-analysis of non-diabetic renal disease mentioned above [17, 36].

Lastly, in the AASK trial, where African-American patients with hypertensive kidney disease, mean serum creatinine of 2.2 mg/dl urine protein excretion of 0.6 g/day, were randomized to ramipril, amlodipine, or metoprolol, the ramipril group had a 36% reduction in the secondary composite outcome of 50% reduction of GFR, ESRD or death compared to amlodipine, and a 22% reduction compared to metoprolol. It should be noted that all the aforementioned trials had proteinuria at baseline in all participants except for the AASK trial where only 33% had proteinuria. Yet, even in AASK, reduction in proteinuria early in the disease course (6 months) predicted ESRD development at 5 years [32].

The sub-study of HOPE, the Microalbuminuria, Cardiovascular, and Renal Outcomes (MICRO)-HOPE, showed that adding ramipril to the antihypertensive regimen in patients at high risk for CV events, not only lowers the risk of developing overt nephropathy, but also decreases CV outcomes. Patients in the ramipril group had a 25% reduction in the primary outcome (myocardial infarction, stroke, or CV death) when compared to those treated with placebo [37]. Mann and Gerstein [38] discovered that the risk for CV events increases almost linearly as proteinuria increases and the risk reduction seen from using an ACE inhibitor is more pronounced the higher the level of proteinuria.

In summary, the data on ACE inhibitors indicate that they are quite effective in slowing the progression of advanced proteinuric nephropathy and decreasing CV events. However, the data only support this concept in patients with Stage 3 or higher nephropathy. This was also supported in a meta-analysis, although this meta-analysis demonstrated as well that patients with GFR >75 ml/min obtain benefit in slowing kidney disease progression only in relation to the blood pressure-lowering effect of ACE inhibitors [39]. While this meta-analysis has many problems, it further supports the notion that those with proteinuria do obtain unique benefits on diabetic kidney disease progression from ACE inhibitors.

ANGIOTENSIN RECEPTOR BLOCKERS

Angiotensin receptor blockers (ARBs) are one of the newest classes of antihypertensive medications. As such, data involving ARBs are less abundant than those relating to ACE inhibitors, but animal data suggest that the two classes provide similar renoprotection [31]. Two large renal outcome trials, the Reduction of Endpoints in Non-insulin dependent diabetes mellitus with the Angiotensin II Antagonist Losartan (RENAAL) trial [40] and the Irbesartan in Diabetic Nephropathy Trial (IDNT), have shown that this is also true in human populations. The RENAAL trial randomized 1513 Type 2 diabetic patients with mean creatinine 1.9 mg/dl and median UACR 1237 mg/g to the ARB losartan or placebo. After a mean follow-up of 3.4 years, losartan treatment was associated with a 16% reduction in the primary endpoint of doubling of baseline serum creatinine, progression to ESRD or death, a 35% reduction in UACR and a 15% decrease in the rate of reduction in estimated creatinine clearance [40]. It was also sought to determine whether there was a relationship between the amount of baseline proteinuria, initial reduction in proteinuria, or degree of residual proteinuria to the combined primary endpoint. As previously shown by other trials, RENAAL demonstrated that the level of baseline proteinuria had a nearly linear relationship with the risk for achieving the primary outcome. More importantly, the trial showed that for every 50% reduction in albuminuria in the first 6 months after initiating treatment with losartan, there was a 36% risk reduction of the primary endpoint and a 45% reduction for ESRD at trial end. The reduction in proteinuria in the first 6 months of therapy mirrored the nearly linear relationship between baseline albuminuria and renal risk [34]. Interestingly, it was estimated that losartan could delay the need for dialysis or transplantation for 2 years and the authors conclude that all of the renoprotection from the use of the losartan was attributed to the antiproteinuric effect of the ARB and was not related to the achieved blood pressure [34].

The IDNT randomized 1715 Type 2 diabetic patients with mean serum creatinine 1.7 mg/dl and median urinary protein excretion 2.9 g/day to irbesartan, amlodipine, or placebo and evaluated the same primary endpoint as RENAAL. Treatment with irbesartan resulted in a 20% reduction compared to placebo and 23% reduction compared to amlodipine in the primary composite outcome after a mean follow-up of 2.6 years, whereas proteinuria was decreased by 33% in the irbesartan group versus 6% in the amlodipine group and 10% in the placebo group [41]. This study also confirmed the relationship between baseline proteinuria and risk of renal disease progression, as it showed that for every 2-fold increase in the level of baseline proteinuria, the risk for reaching the primary endpoint doubled. Irrespective of treatment group, this risk was cut in half with every 50% reduction in proteinuria at 1 year. However, after 1 year of treatment, 40% of the patients in the irbesartan group had a greater than 50% reduction in proteinuria, compared to 20% in the amlodipine group and 25% in the placebo group. Once again, the authors of this trial attribute the superior renoprotective effect of irbesartan to its antiproteinuric properties [33].

A recent *post hoc* analysis of the data from the Losartan Intervention for Endpoint Reduction in Hypertension Study (LIFE) demonstrated that ARBs also reduce CV outcomes. Over 8000 patients with hypertension and left ventricular hypertrophy were followed for a mean of 4.8 years and were stratified into groups by baseline level of albumin excretion. It is important to note that while a small percentage of patients in this trial had overt proteinuria, the majority of participants had microalbuminuria. The analysis found that those with the highest baseline urinary protein excretion had a 3–4-fold greater risk of reaching the primary CV endpoint of first occurrence of CV death, non-fatal stroke, and non-fatal myocardial infarction when compared to those in the lowest group. The extent of proteinuria reduction at 5 years predicted the risk reduction for the primary endpoint [42]. A substudy of LIFE that looked at those with essential hypertension and no other documented signs of vascular disease demonstrated that losartan was superior to atenolol in reducing CV outcomes and this effect was independent of the blood pressure achieved.

In summary, it would appear that ACE inhibitors and ARBs provide similar CV and renal protection. This similarity was supported by the Diabetics Exposed to Telmisartan And Enalapril (DETAIL) study, which compared the effects of enalapril and telmisartan in a small number of patients with Type 2 diabetes, hypertension and urinary albumin excretion (UAE) between 11 and 999 μg/min (n = 250). It showed that the two agents had comparable effects on the change in GFR as assessed by iothalamate, UAE, and the rates of ESRD [43]. However, there are some that call for the use of ARBs in place of ACE inhibitors because they are generally better tolerated, have a lower incidence of hyperkalamia and cough, and are not associated with the life-threatening complication of angioedema [44]. The higher cost of ARBs does make this argument untenable for some. Overall, in clinical practice, it is reasonable to use the two classes interchangeably in patients with proteinuria.

CALCIUM CHANNEL BLOCKERS

The two different subtypes of calcium channel blockers (CCBs), non-dihydropyridine (non-DHP) and DHP have been shown to have divergent effects on proteinuria. This was best demonstrated by Smith and colleagues. A cohort of patients with diabetic nephropathy were followed for 2 years and changes in glomerular permeability were assessed. While patients randomized to a DHP CCB, nifedipine XL, had no change in proteinuria at 2 years, those receiving a non-DHP CCB had a 3-fold decrease in proteinuria [45]. Further evidence to support lack of proteinuria reduction with DHP CCBs comes from multicentre trials. In the IDNT trial in patients with diabetic nephropathy, amlodipine was associated with a 6% increase in proteinuria versus baseline and a 23% higher incidence of the primary endpoints of doubling of serum creatinine, onset of ESRD, or death. In the non-diabetic population of the AASK trial, the 58% increase in proteinuria seen at 6 months in those treated with amlodipine correlated with a greater incidence of the composite endpoint of a ≥50% reduction in GFR, ESRD, and/or death when compared to those treated with ramipril who had a 20% reduction in proteinuria [46]. An in-depth review of this entire subject further confirms the notion that there are clear differences between the effects of the subclasses of CCBs on the kidney but that these are only manifest in advanced disease with proteinuria [47]. This would be in keeping with the observation about ACE inhibitors, i.e. that in early kidney disease the focus should be on blood pressure control and in advanced disease it should be on both blood pressure and proteinuria reduction. This is exemplified by the data from the Bergamo Nephrologic Diabetes Complications Trial (BENEDICT). This study sought to compare the effect of a non-DHP CCB and an ACE inhibitor, alone or in combination, on development of MA in a group of hypertensive, normoalbuminuric Type 2 diabetics. No significant reduction in the incidence of MA development was seen in those treated with the non-DHP CCB alone. In fact, there was no difference in MA development in those treated with verapamil alone or with placebo [48]. The results of this trial are difficult to interpret for several reasons. First, had the trial achieved its target blood pressure of <120/80 mmHg, it is likely that MA development would have been greatly reduced in all of the subgroups. Secondly, the data from this trial cannot be applied to patients with proteinuria, since this trial studied a different stage of disease, one well known to respond well to blood pressure control alone. Thus, since BP was not a goal in this study it is difficult to extrapolate the findings. As previously discussed, proteinuria is a clear marker of renal dysfunction and non-DHP CCBs will affect the kidney differently in this population when compared to patients with normal renal function.

The mechanism for differences in CCB effects relates to DHP CCBs' effect on the kidney's ability to autoregulate blood flow [49, 50]. DHP CCBs' impairment of this ability gives the mistaken impression of preserved renal function. However, this perception is at the expense of increased intraglomerular pressures and increased levels of proteinuria, which in turn lead to poorer renal outcomes.

OTHER PHARMACOLOGIC APPROACHES TO BLOOD PRESSURE AND PROTEINURIA

The efficacy of the other classes of antihypertensives in decreasing proteinuria independently of blood pressure reduction is limited in comparison to the classes already discussed. Thiazide diuretics have not been shown to reduce urine protein excretion beyond the amount expected due to blood pressure reduction. However, as most patients with chronic kidney disease and proteinuria would need a combination of two or more antihypertensive by agents to reach the aforementioned blood pressure goals, and since renal function deterioration is accompanied by salt and water retention, a diuretic should be the first agent to add to an ACE inhibitor or ARB in patients with proteinuria if blood pressure is not controlled [1]. As thiazide diuretics become less effective when GFR falls below 40 ml/min/1.73 m^2, a loop diuretic is very likely to be needed in order to adequately control blood pressure in patients with a GFR below that level.

In general, β-blockers should be used in patients with proteinuria as third-line agents, in order again to achieve blood pressure control [1]. However, one of the newer β-blockers, carvedilol, has shown promise in reducing the incidence of MA and progression to proteinuria [51]. In the Glycemic Effects in Diabetes Mellitus Carvedilol–Metoprolol Comparison in Hypertensives (GEMINI) trial, carvedilol and metoprolol's effects on development and progression of microalbuminuria were evaluated. Patients receiving carvedilol had both a greater reduction in microalbuminuria and a lower risk of progressing from normoalbuminuria to microalbuminuria than those treated with metoprolol [51]. These results need confirmation in prospective trials examining patients with both renal insufficiency and proteinuria.

Perhaps the best prospective study to support the concept that proteinuria reduction in combination with blood pressure reduction is associated with better preservation of kidney function is the result of the Combination Treatment of Angiotensin-II Receptor Blocker and Angiotensin converting-enzyme Inhibitor in Non-diabetic Renal Disease (COOPERATE) trial. In this trial the impact on both blood pressure and proteinuria of an ACE inhibitor (trandolapril) and an ARB (losartan) or a combination of both in patients with non-diabetic kidney disease and mean urinary protein excretion of 2.5 g/day was evaluated. After 3 years of follow-up, the combination of the two agents led to no significant improvement in blood pressure when compared to either medication alone. However, the combination lead to a 75% reduction in proteinuria compared to a 42% reduction in those treated with trandolapril alone and a 44% reduction in those treated with losartan alone, as well as a 60–62% reduction in the primary endpoint of time to doubling of serum creatinine concentration or ESRD compared to either the trandolapril- or the losartan-treated group. Moreover, a substudy of the main trial using 24-h ambulatory monitoring demonstrated that

Table 3.3 Summary of important trials involving proteinuria reduction

Study	*Treatment groups*	*Follow-up (mean in years)*	*Achieved BP (mmHg)*	*Change in proteinuria*	*Relevant outcomes*
Captopril trial	Captopril or placebo	3 (median)	MAP 96 MAP 100	−30%	Captopril delays the the progression of diabetic nephropathy
AASK	Metoprolol, amipril, or amlodipine and conventional or intensive blood pressure targets	3.8	128/78 for lower group 141/85 for usual group	−14% for metoprolol −20% for ramipril +58% for amlodipine at 6 months	Ramipril slowed progression of renal disease when compared to the other groups
MICRO-HOPE	Ramipril or placebo		139.8 142.9	−20%	Ramipril reduces CV outcomes and slows the progression of renal disease when compared to placebo
RENAAL	Losartan or placebo	3.4	140/74 142/74	−35%	Losartan delayed the need for dialysis by 2 years when compared to placebo
IDNT	Irbesartan or amlodipine or placebo	2.6	140/77 141/77 144/80	−33% −6% −10%	Irbesartan reduced proteinuria to a greater extent and led to slower progression of renal disease when compared to the other groups
COOPERATE	Trandolapril or losartan, or combination of both	3	130/74.3 129.9/75.9 130.3/75.1	−42.1% −44.3% −75.6%	Combination of ACE inhibitor and ARB therapy led to profound reductions in proteinuria, but had little impact on blood pressure

those with the greatest reductions in proteinuria at 6 months had the slowest declines in GFR, an effect independent of blood pressure level achieved [52]. The notion that ACE inhibitors and ARBs should only be combined for proteinuria and NOT blood pressure reduction is confirmed by other clinical studies and a recent meta-analysis [53, 54].

Another useful combination could be the addition of an aldosterone receptor antagonist to patients already receiving an ACE inhibitor or an ARB. Plasma aldosterone levels are elevated in patients with chronic kidney disease and may contribute to renal injury [55], whereas blockade of the renin–angiotensin–aldosterone system (RAAS) with ACE inhibitors or ARBs does not necessarily result in a maintained decrease in plasma aldosterone levels in patients with renal insufficiency [56]. The addition of spironolactone in proteinuric patients already on an ACE inhibitor or an ARB has been shown to reduce proteinuria [57, 58]. Moreover, eplerenone, the newer aldosterone receptor antagonist, further reduced urine albumin excretion in patients with hypertension and left ventricular hypertrophy when added to an ACE inhibitor [59]. Larger future studies are needed to confirm these promising findings.

Combining an ACE inhibitor and a non-DHP CCB has also been demonstrated to reduce proteinuria. The first study to evaluate this combination included thirty patients with Type 2 diabetes. Patients were randomized to receive either lisinopril alone, verapamil alone, a combination of the two, or hydrochlorothiazide and guanfacine. Patients treated with the combination had a 78% reduction in albuminuria compared to a 59% reduction in those treated with lisinopril alone [60]. Also of note, patients receiving the combination therapy had the best side-effect profile of any of the groups. This was likely to have been because the combining the two drugs allowed for lower doses of each medication to be used. More recently, the Verapamil Versus Amlodipine in Non-diabetic Nephropathies Treated with Trandolapril (VVANNTT) study in non-diabetic kidney disease demonstrated improved glomerular permeability and an addition 40% reduction in proteinuria when a non-DHP CCB was combined with trandolapril as compared to a DHP CCB [61].

SUMMARY

Proteinuria is a well-known risk factor for the progression of renal disease and CV morbidity and mortality. In order to maximize risk reduction, physicians must focus on achieving a target blood pressure of <130/80 mmHg in those with urine albumin excretion >300 mg/day. Blockers of the renin–angiotensin–aldosterone system such as ACE inhibitors and ARBs should be used as first-line antihypertensive therapy in patients with proteinuria because these classes have a blood pressure-independent antiproteinuric effect and they have consistently been shown to improve renal and CV outcomes. Second-line approaches for proteinuria reduction include combining two classes of medications shown to reduce protein excretion. Table 3.3 summarizes the results of the clinical trials discussed in this paper and it helps to demonstrate the heightened risk associated with proteinuria. Physicians must recognize this and take aggressive measures to reduce proteinuria to give their patients maximal renal and CV protection.

REFERENCES

1. K/DOQI clinical practice guidelines on hypertension and antihypertensive agents in chronic kidney disease. *Am J Kidney Dis* 2004; 43(suppl 2):1–290.
2. Howey JE, Browning MC, Fraser CG. Biologic variation of urinary albumin: consequences for analysis, specimen collection, interpretation of results, and screening programs. *Am J Kidney Dis* 1989; 13:35–37.
3. Coresh J, Byrd-Holt D, Astor BC *et al.* Chronic kidney disease awareness, prevalence, and trends among U.S. adults, 1999 to 2000. *J Am Soc Nephrol* 2005; 16:180–188.
4. Schmitz A. Microalbuminuria, blood pressure, metabolic control, and renal involvement: longitudinal studies in white non-insulin-dependent diabetic patients. *Am J Hypertens* 1997; 10(Pt 2):189S–197S.
5. Bigazzi R, Bianchi S. Microalbuminuria as a marker of cardiovascular and renal disease in essential hypertension. *Nephrol Dial Transplant* 1995; 10(suppl 6):10–14.
6. Cirillo M, Senigalliesi L, Laurenzi M *et al.* Microalbuminuria in nondiabetic adults: relation of blood pressure, body mass index, plasma cholesterol levels, and smoking: The Gubbio Population Study. *Arch Intern Med* 1998; 158:1933–1939.
7. Jones CA, Francis ME, Eberhardt MS *et al.* Microalbuminuria in the US population: third National Health and Nutrition Examination Survey. *Am J Kidney Dis* 2002; 39:445–459.
8. Mathiesen ER, Oxenboll B, Johansen K, Svendsen PA, Deckert T. Incipient nephropathy in type 1 (insulin-dependent) diabetes. *Diabetologia* 1984; 26:406–410.
9. Mogensen CE, Christensen CK. Predicting diabetic nephropathy in insulin-dependent patients. *N Engl J Med* 1984; 311:89–93.
10. Bruno G, Merletti F, Biggeri A *et al.* Progression to overt nephropathy in type 2 diabetes: the Casale Monferrato Study. *Diabetes Care* 2003; 26:2150–2155.
11. Klein R, Klein BE, Moss SE, Cruickshanks KJ. Ten-year incidence of gross proteinuria in people with diabetes. *Diabetes* 1995; 44:916–923.

12. Pinto-Sietsma SJ, Janssen WM, Hillege HL, Navis G, de Zeeuw D, de Jong PE. Urinary albumin excretion is associated with renal functional abnormalities in a nondiabetic population. *J Am Soc Nephrol* 2000; 11:1882–1888.
13. Chobanian AV, Bakris GL, Black HR *et al.* The Seventh Report of the Joint National Committee on Prevention, Detection, Evaluation, and Treatment of High Blood Pressure: the JNC 7 report. *JAMA* 2003; 289:2560–2572.
14. 2003 European Society of Hypertension–European Society of Cardiology guidelines for the management of arterial hypertension. *J Hypertens* 2003; 21:1011–1053.
15. Sarnak MJ, Greene T, Wang X *et al.* The effect of a lower target blood pressure on the progression of kidney disease: long-term follow-up of the modification of diet in renal disease study. *Ann Intern Med* 2005; 142:342–351.
16. Peterson JC, Adler S, Burkart JM *et al.* Blood pressure control, proteinuria, and the progression of renal disease. The Modification of Diet in Renal Disease Study. *Ann Intern Med* 1995; 123:754–762.
17. Jafar TH, Stark PC, Schmid CH *et al.* Progression of chronic kidney disease: the role of blood pressure control, proteinuria, and angiotensin-converting enzyme inhibition: a patient-level meta-analysis. *Ann Intern Med* 2003; 139:244–252.
18. Wright JT Jr, Bakris G, Greene T *et al.* Effect of blood pressure lowering and antihypertensive drug class on progression of hypertensive kidney disease: results from the AASK trial. *JAMA* 2002; 288:2421–2431.
19. Ruggenenti P, Perna A, Loriga G *et al.* Blood-pressure control for renoprotection in patients with non-diabetic chronic renal disease (REIN-2): multicentre, randomised controlled trial. *Lancet* 2005; 365:939–946.
20. Klahr S, Levey AS, Beck GJ *et al.* The effects of dietary protein restriction and blood-pressure control on the progression of chronic renal disease. Modification of Diet in Renal Disease Study Group. *N Engl J Med* 1994; 330:877–884.
21. Kasiske BL, Lakatua JD, Ma JZ, Louis TA. A meta-analysis of the effects of dietary protein restriction on the rate of decline in renal function. *Am J Kidney Dis* 1998; 31:954–961.
22. Blythe WB. Natural history of hypertension in renal parenchymal disease. *Am J Kidney Dis* 1985; 5:A50–A56.
23. Bakris GL, Smith A. Effects of sodium intake on albumin excretion in patients with diabetic nephropathy treated with long-acting calcium antagonists. *Ann Intern Med* 1996;125:201–204.
24. Mishra SI, Jones-Burton C, Fink JC, Brown J, Bakris GL, Weir MR. Does dietary salt increase the risk for progression of kidney disease? *Curr Hypertens Rep* 2005; 7:385–391.
25. Halimi JM, Giraudeau B, Vol S *et al.* Effects of current smoking and smoking discontinuation on renal function and proteinuria in the general population. *Kidney Int* 2000; 58:1285–1292.
26. Briganti EM, Branley P, Chadban SJ *et al.* Smoking is associated with renal impairment and proteinuria in the normal population: the AusDiab kidney study. Australian Diabetes, Obesity and Lifestyle Study. *Am J Kidney Dis* 2002; 40:704–712.
27. Mann JF, Gerstein HC, Yi QL *et al.* Development of renal disease in people at high cardiovascular risk: results of the HOPE randomized study. *J Am Soc Nephrol* 2003; 14:641–647.
28. Lewis EJ, Hunsicker LG, Bain RP, Rohde RD. The effect of angiotensin-converting-enzyme inhibition on diabetic nephropathy. The Collaborative Study Group. *N Engl J Med* 1993; 329:1456–1462.
29. UK Prospective Diabetes Study Group. Efficacy of atenolol and captopril in reducing risk of macrovascular and microvascular complications in type 2 diabetes: UKPDS 39. *BMJ* 1998; 317:713–720.
30. Rahman M, Pressel S, Davis BR *et al.* Renal outcomes in high-risk hypertensive patients treated with an angiotensin-converting enzyme inhibitor or a calcium channel blocker vs a diuretic: a report from the Antihypertensive and Lipid-Lowering Treatment to Prevent Heart Attack Trial (ALLHAT). *Arch Intern Med* 2005; 165:936–946.
31. Griffin KA, bu-Amarah I, Picken M, Bidani AK. Renoprotection by ACE inhibition or aldosterone blockade is blood pressure-dependent. *Hypertension* 2003; 41:201–206.
32. Lea J, Greene T, Hebert L *et al.* The relationship between magnitude of proteinuria reduction and risk of end-stage renal disease: results of the African American study of kidney disease and hypertension. *Arch Intern Med* 2005; 165:947–953.
33. Atkins RC, Briganti EM, Lewis JB *et al.* Proteinuria reduction and progression to renal failure in patients with type 2 diabetes mellitus and overt nephropathy. *Am J Kidney Dis* 2005; 45:281–287.

34. De Zeeuw D, Remuzzi G, Parving HH *et al.* Proteinuria, a target for renoprotection in patients with type 2 diabetic nephropathy: lessons from RENAAL. *Kidney Int* 2004; 65:2309–2320.
35. The GISEN Group (Gruppo Italiano di Studi Epidemiologici in Nefrologia). Randomised placebo-controlled trial of effect of ramipril on decline in glomerular filtration rate and risk of terminal renal failure in proteinuric, non-diabetic nephropathy. *Lancet* 1997; 349:1857–1863.
36. Maschio G, Alberti D, Janin G *et al.*, The Angiotensin-Converting-Enzyme Inhibition in Progressive Renal Insufficiency Study Group. Effect of the angiotensin-converting-enzyme inhibitor benazepril on the progression of chronic renal insufficiency. *N Engl J Med* 1996; 334:939–945.
37. Heart Outcomes Prevention Evaluation Study Investigators. Effects of ramipril on cardiovascular and microvascular outcomes in people with diabetes mellitus: results of the HOPE study and MICRO-HOPE substudy. *Lancet* 2000; 355:253–259.
38. Mann JF, Yi QL, Gerstein HC. Albuminuria as a predictor of cardiovascular and renal outcomes in people with known atherosclerotic cardiovascular disease. *Kidney Int Suppl* 2004; 92:S59–S62.
39. Casas JP, Chua W, Loukogeorgakis S *et al.* Effect of inhibitors of the renin-angiotensin system and other antihypertensive drugs on renal outcomes: systematic review and meta-analysis. *Lancet* 2005; 366:2026–2033.
40. Brenner BM, Cooper ME, de Zeeuw D *et al.* Effects of losartan on renal and cardiovascular outcomes in patients with type 2 diabetes and nephropathy. *N Engl J Med* 2001; 345:861–869.
41. Lewis EJ, Hunsicker LG, Clarke WR *et al.* Renoprotective effect of the angiotensin-receptor antagonist irbesartan in patients with nephropathy due to type 2 diabetes. *N Engl J Med* 2001; 345:851–860.
42. Ibsen H, Olsen MH, Wachtell K *et al.* Reduction in albuminuria translates to reduction in cardiovascular events in hypertensive patients: losartan intervention for endpoint reduction in hypertension study. *Hypertension* 2005; 45:198–202.
43. Barnett AH, Bain SC, Bouter P *et al.* Angiotensin-receptor blockade versus converting-enzyme inhibition in type 2 diabetes and nephropathy. *N Engl J Med* 2004; 351:1952–1961.
44. Mangrum AJ, Bakris GL. Angiotensin-converting enzyme inhibitors and angiotensin receptor blockers in chronic renal disease: safety issues. *Semin Nephrol* 2004; 24:168–175.
45. Smith AC, Toto R, Bakris GL. Differential effects of calcium channel blockers on size selectivity of proteinuria in diabetic glomerulopathy. *Kidney Int* 1998; 54:889–896.
46. Wright JT Jr, Bakris G, Greene T *et al.* Effect of blood pressure lowering and antihypertensive drug class on progression of hypertensive kidney disease: results from the AASK trial. *JAMA* 2002; 288:2421–2431.
47. Nathan S, Pepine CJ, Bakris GL. Calcium antagonists: effects on cardio-renal risk in hypertensive patients. *Hypertension* 2005; 46:637–642.
48. Ruggenenti P, Fassi A, Ilieva AP *et al.* Preventing microalbuminuria in type 2 diabetes. *N Engl J Med* 2004; 351:1941–1951.
49. Griffin KA, Picken MM, Bakris GL, Bidani AK. Class differences in the effects of calcium channel blockers in the rat remnant kidney model. *Kidney Int* 1999; 55:1849–1860.
50. Griffin KA, Hacioglu R, bu-Amarah I, Loutzenhiser R, Williamson GA, Bidani AK. Effects of calcium channel blockers on 'dynamic' and 'steady-state step' renal autoregulation. *Am J Physiol Renal Physiol* 2004; 286:F1136–F1143.
51. Bakris GL, Fonseca V, Katholi RE *et al.* Differential effects of beta-blockers on albuminuria in patients with type 2 diabetes. *Hypertension* 2005; 46:1309–1315.
52. Nakao N, Seno H, Kasuga H, Toriyama T, Kawahara H, Fukagawa M. Effects of combination treatment with losartan and trandolapril on office and ambulatory blood pressures in non-diabetic renal disease: a COOPERATE-ABP substudy. *Am J Nephrol* 2004; 24:543–548.
53. Izzo JL Jr, Weinberg MS, Hainer JW, Kerkering J, Tou CK. Antihypertensive efficacy of candesartan-lisinopril in combination vs. up-titration of lisinopril: the AMAZE trials. *J Clin Hypertens (Greenwich)* 2004; 6:185–193.
54. Doulton TW, Macgregor GA. Combination renin-angiotensin system blockade in hypertension. *Kidney Int* 2005; 68:1898.
55. Hollenberg NK. Aldosterone in the development and progression of renal injury. *Kidney Int* 2004; 66:1–9.
56. Bakris GL, Siomos M, Richardson D *et al.* ACE inhibition or angiotensin receptor blockade: impact on potassium in renal failure. VAL-K Study Group. *Kidney Int* 2000; 58:2084–2092.
57. Rossing K, Schjoedt KJ, Smidt UM, Boomsma F, Parving HH. Beneficial effects of adding spironolactone to recommended antihypertensive treatment in diabetic nephropathy: a randomized, double-masked, cross-over study. *Diabetes Care* 2005; 28:2106–2112.

58. Chrysostomou A, Becker G. Spironolactone in addition to ACE inhibition to reduce proteinuria in patients with chronic renal disease. *N Engl J Med* 2001; 345:925–926.
59. Pitt B, Reichek N, Willenbrock R *et al.* Effects of eplerenone, enalapril, and eplerenone/enalapril in patients with essential hypertension and left ventricular hypertrophy: the 4E-left ventricular hypertrophy study. *Circulation* 2003; 108:1831–1838.
60. Bakris GL, Barnhill BW, Sadler R. Treatment of arterial hypertension in diabetic humans: importance of therapeutic selection. *Kidney Int* 1992; 41:912–919.
61. Boero R, Rollino C, Massara C *et al.* The verapamil versus amlodipine in non-diabetic nephropathies treated with trandolapril (VVANNTT) study. *Am J Kidney Dis* 2003; 42:67–75.

4

Cholesterol, blood pressure and statins

R. Ramamurthy, N. J. Stone

INTRODUCTION

Hypercholesterolaemia and hypertension are major risk factors for both coronary heart disease (CHD) and cerebrovascular disease (CD). Both of these risk factors have a substantial genetic component [1]. Yet, the vast majority of cases of CHD and CD are not seen in patients with single gene mutations of large effect. Thus, there is an important role for non-genetic factors that elevate lipid levels and blood pressure in the twin epidemics of CHD and CD seen in this country.

Of the non-genetic factors, weight gain is especially important. A prospective follow-up of 46 224 women who were subjects in the Nurses Health Study and free of hypertension at entry, showed that body mass index (BMI) and weight gain, but not weight cycles status, were independently associated with the development of hypertension [2]. The deleterious effect of weight gain is substantial. For each 10 Ib (4.5 kg) gain in weight between 1989 and 1993, the risk of hypertension increased 20% (odds ratio [OR] 1.20; 95% confidence interval [Cl] 1.15–1.24). Weight gain and subsequent obesity is also an important factor in the development of the metabolic syndrome [3]. This collection of easily measured metabolic variables (abdominal circumference, triglycerides, high-density lipoprotein cholesterol [HDL-c], blood pressure and fasting blood pressure) is common and associated with an increased risk for CHD and type 2 diabetes in both men and women [4].

Hypertension and high cholesterol have effects early in life on the process of atherosclerosis that underlies the clinical events that will occur decades later. A carefully done autopsy study in young trauma victims demonstrated that high-grade lesions in the proximal left anterior descending coronary artery were present in 2.4% of 15–19-year-old men and 20.3% of 30–34-year-old men as well as in 7–8% of 30–34-year-old women [5]. It was concerning that by age 30–34, 19% of men and 8% of women had atherosclerotic narrowing more than 40%. In this study, 43% had one and 35% had two or more risk factors underscoring the importance of risk factors in the development of atherosclerosis (Figure 4.1). Indeed, some risk factors such as hypertension are associated with an excess risk of CHD especially when present with other CHD risk factors or in patients with underlying target organ damage. Recent studies of CHD incidence in subjects chosen because of their risk status demonstrated that drug treatment of low-density lipoprotein cholesterol (LDL-c) reduces risk by a

Rekha Ramamurthy, MD, Fellow, Endocrinology Section, Department of Medicine, Feinberg School of Medicine, Northwestern University, Chicago, Ilinois, USA

Neil J. Stone, MD, FAHA, FACC, Professor of Clinical Medicine (Cardiology), Feinberg School of Medicine, Northwestern University, Consultant Cardiologist, Lipidologist Medical Director, Vascular Center of Bluhm Cardiovascular Institute, Northwestern Memorial Hospital, Chicago, Ilinois, USA

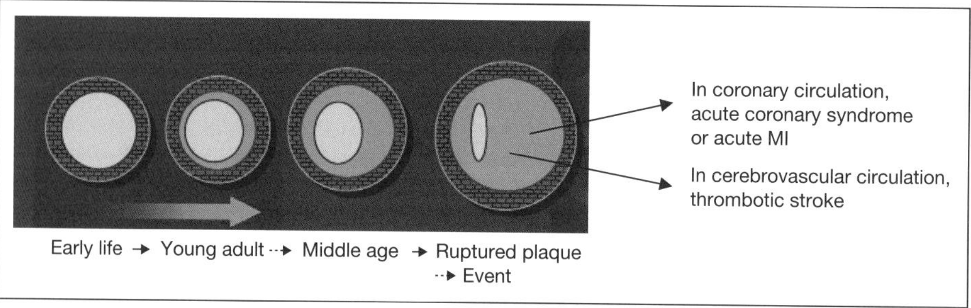

Figure 4.1 Risk factors and atherosclerosis: genetic susceptibility + age, cholesterol, blood pressure, tobacco usage, low HDL-c, central adiposity, diabetes (statins modify progression at every stage). Risk factors initiate and sustain the process of atherosclerosis, which is only minimally occlusive early on, but if and when the cholesterol-rich plaque ruptures, can eventually lead to clinical sequelae of CHD and stroke.

constant proportion of the existing risk irrespective of the starting level of the initial LDL-c or of the existing risk [6]. Thus, some argue that therapy to change risk factors such as high blood pressure or high cholesterol should therefore be determined by a person's level of risk, not by the level of the risk factors. Others point out that this dependence on absolute risk, instead of lifetime risk [7] misses the important opportunity to treat risk factors in a young individual before they have attained high risk status.

Thus, the risk of major cardiovascular events dramatically increases when hypercholesterolaemia and hypertension are coexistent. The Framingham Heart Study demonstrated that the prevalence of dyslipidaemia increased with increasing blood pressure levels. Indeed, approximately 40% of men and 33% of women in this study with blood pressure values >140/90 mmHg had coexistent hypercholesterolaemia. In this study, hypercholesterolaemia was broadly defined as a total cholesterol >240 mg/dl, HDL-c <35 mg/dl or being on current lipid-lowering treatment [8, 9]. Conversely, hypertension is a major risk factor in patients with elevated cholesterol levels. The Lipid Treatment Assessment Project showed that 47% of hypercholesterolaemic patients without clinically apparent coronary artery disease had two or more risk factors, with age (92%) being the most common followed closely by hypertension (70%) [10]. Moreover, the results of a large-scale primary prevention trial, the Multiple Risk Factor Intervention Trial (MRFIT) clearly demonstrated that the cardiovascular mortality associated with progressive increments in blood pressure is significantly higher in the group of patients with high cholesterol levels compared with those with low cholesterol levels [11]. Other studies have described that plasma cholesterol levels are elevated in hypertension-prone subjects compared with the normotensive population [12]. There is evidence that there is a significant increase in the 10-year relative risk (RR) 2.1 of developing stable hypertension in patients with baseline cholesterol levels above 200 mg/dl [13]. Thus, there is a strong synergistic relationship between the two major risk factors for the development of cardiovascular disease. This association may simply be explained by the casual coexistence of the two widely distributed cardiovascular risk factors or may reflect the presence of a common underlying metabolic abnormality, such as insulin resistance. Another possibility is that hypercholesterolaemia and hypertension have a primary pathogenic interaction.

The exact mechanism responsible for the relation between hypercholesterolaemia and blood pressure control is still under investigation. Several small studies have demonstrated a significant correlation between these two variables. These data beg the question whether cholesterol reduction can exert some of its benefits by improving blood pressure control. The possibility that cholesterol-lowering drugs would also treat hypertension would provide a rationale for therapeutic crossover that might result in highly effective management of the cardiovascular profile in high risk patients [14].

The 3-hydroxy-3-methylglutaryl (HMG-CoA) reductase inhibitors, more commonly known as 'statins', are potent cholesterol-lowering drugs and are the drugs of choice to lower LDL as well as triglyceride-rich remnants and intermediate density lipoproteins in those at risk [15]. The recent Cholesterol Treatment Trialists Collaborators' prospectively planned meta-analysis of 14 large-scale randomized, placebo-controlled clinical trials showed that in those with either CHD or in those at high 10-year risk of CHD, statins safely and effectively reduce cardiovascular risk. The magnitude of the effect is substantial. In over 90 000 subjects the 5-year incidence of major coronary events, coronary revascularization, and stroke in these trials was reduced by about one-fifth per mmol/l reduction in LDL-c (38.8 mg/dl). The absolute benefit seen with statin therapy related to both an individual's absolute risk of such events and to the absolute reduction in LDL-c achieved. Moreover, the significant benefits noted within the first year, were greater in subsequent years [16].

Despite these impressive effects, some physicians argue that statins have important effects that are separate from their LDL-c lowering effects. These have been termed 'pleiotrophic effects' and include beneficial effects on plaque stabilization, endothelial dysfunction, inflammation and coagulation [17]. Robinson and co-workers gathered data from five diet, three bile acid sequestrant, one surgery, and ten statin trials, with 81 859 participants to see if the regression lines for non-statin and statin trials were similar. They found a one-to-one relationship between LDL-c lowering and CHD and stroke reduction over 5 years of treatment and could not find evidence that pleiotropic effects of statins contributed to an additional cardiovascular risk reduction benefit beyond that expected [18].

THE HYPERTENSION-LIPID CONNECTION

The renin–angiotensin system or RAS may be a fundamental player in the evolution of hypertension and atherogenesis since antihypertensives such as angiotensin-converting enzyme inhibitors (ACE-I) and angiotensin receptor blockers (ARBs) are also antiatherogenic [19]. There is evidence that hypercholesterolaemia may activate the angiotensin II-(Ang II)-mediated endothelial injury and be the dominant factor in hyperlipidaemia-associated hypertension [20]. Ang II mediates its pro-atherogenic actions by activating AT_1 receptor which mediates the cardiovascular effects, including oxidative stress, vasoconstriction, aldosterone secretion, sodium absorption in the kidney, sympathetic stimulation, vasopressin release and vascular cell dysfunction. Ang II stimulates growth, migration and matrix production in vascular smooth muscle cells, increases expression of inflammatory adhesion molecules on the endothelium thereby activating monocytes and reduces endothelial nitric oxide (NO) synthase. Modifications of the vascular microenvironment toward increased oxidized products leads to generation of oxidized LDL particles and fatty streak formation, a precursor to atherogenesis. Endothelial dysfunction caused by oxidized LDL may lead to activation of RAS, which localized to the local endothelium and reduced expression of endothelial NO synthase (eNOS) [21]. These effects are thought to contribute to the impairment of endothelium-dependent vasodilatation and potentially adverse effects on blood pressure. Furthermore, there is an upregulation of the AT_1 receptor in hypercholesterolaemic men and this increase in expression in vascular smooth muscle cells, both *in vitro* and *in vivo*, has been attenuated with statin treatment [22]. Thus, this may explain in part why hypercholesterolaemia is frequently associated with hypertension.

ACTIONS OF STATINS

Currently available statins in the United States include lovastatin, fluvastatin, pravastatin, simvastatin, atorvastatin, and rosuvastatin. A class effect is the ability of statins to inhibit HMG-CoA reductase, the enzyme governing the rate-limiting step of cholesterol biosynthesis in the liver, upregulate LDL receptors, and consequently reduce plasma cholesterol levels.

In addition, statins appear, at least in part, to have a vasoprotective effect by modulating cell signalling pathways. Inhibition of HMG-CoA activity reduces isoprenylation of key G-proteins, such as p21 Rac, Ras, and Rho, which thereby reduce signal transduction via the AT_1 receptor [23, 24]. Statins are also known to increase both the expression and activity of endothelial NO [25, 26]. It is tempting to speculate that this combination of effects could explain the role of statins in improving endothelial function and potentially favourable effects on blood pressure.

The first clue for direct effects of statins on blood pressure regulation may be found in studies of animal models of hypertension. The advantage of these models is the ability to directly test haemodynamic effects of statins in the absence of any effect on plasma cholesterol levels as most of the rodent models routinely used either do not exhibit increased lipid levels or are resistant to the lipid-lowering effects of statins.

ANIMAL STUDIES

There is evidence that statins exert beneficial effects in part through direct effects on vascular cells independent of lowering of plasma cholesterol. Wassman and colleagues [27] characterized the effect of a 30-day treatment with atorvastatin in normocholesterolaemic, spontaneously hypertensive rats (SHR). Systolic blood pressure was significantly decreased in the rats treated with atorvastatin. In addition, they demonstrated that statin therapy improved endothelial function as assessed by carbachol-induced vasorelaxation in aortic segments and reduced Ang II-induced vasoconstriction. Expression levels of aortic AT_1 receptor and eNOS were determined. Atorvastatin not only downregulated AT_1 receptor expression compared to control but also upregulated expression of eNOS. Vascular production or reactive oxygen species was reduced in statin-treated SHR. This study shows that AT_1 receptor activation plays a pivotal role for induction of endothelial dysfunction and vasoconstriction and that statin treatment improves both these parameters.

Similar to the above study's findings, Zhou and co-workers [28] showed that the endothelial dysfunction in hypertensive Dahl salt-sensitive (DS) rats can be reversed with statin treatment. DS rats developed hypertension and impaired endothelial-dependent relaxation when given a high salt diet for 10 weeks. Treatment with atorvastatin prevented the impaired endothelial function, reduced left ventricular hypertrophy and proteinuria along with modest reduction in blood pressure and significant reduction in plasma cholesterol levels in this salt-sensitive animal model of hypertension.

Multiple studies in animal models of hypertension have shown a modest effect on blood pressure regulation and endothelial function setting the ground for further evaluation of these observations in the clinical setting.

SMALL-SCALE CLINICAL TRIALS

Epidemiological evidence for interaction between hypercholesterolaemia and hypertension is well documented. Data from older cardiovascular prevention trials such as the Lipid Research Clinics (LRC) Study that compared treatment of high cholesterol with cholestyramine vs. placebo showed that the incidence of new hypertension decreased by 25% over the course of the study [29]. This observation supported the notion that hypercholesterolaemia may be intimately related to hypertension.

Moreover, the therapeutic impact of statins seems to be enhanced in patients with coexistent high cholesterol and high blood pressure. The Scandinavian Simvastatin Survival Study (4S) reported an intriguing trend toward greater therapeutic efficacy in patients with elevated diastolic blood pressure [30]. In addition, in the past 4–5 years, multiple small-scale trials have emerged supporting the possibility that statins play a beneficial role in lowering blood pressure.

The Brisighella Heart Study performed in Italy is a prospective, population based, longitudinal clinical trial which was aimed at evaluating the effects of different lipid-lowering strategies on blood pressure control of subjects with hypercholesterolaemia [31]. A total of 1356 subjects with elevated serum cholesterol levels (i.e. ≥239 mg/dl) were randomized to one of three lipid-lowering regimens: low fat diet, cholestyramine, gemfibrozil or simvastatin. These subjects were treated for 5 years (1988–1993). Participants were divided at baseline into four quartiles according to systolic blood pressure level. Blood pressure measurements were evaluated at baseline and periodically during the 5 years of treatment. A significant decrease in blood pressure was observed in the upper two quartiles of systolic blood pressure (≥140 mmHg). The blood pressure reduction was enhanced in subjects treated with statins demonstrating that use of lipid-lowering agents could significantly improve blood pressure control in subjects with coexisting hypercholesterolaemia and hypertension.

A prospective double-blind, placebo-controlled, randomized crossover trial performed by Glorioso and colleagues [32] has shown additional evidence that statins have a modest effect on blood pressure. They specifically evaluated effect of pravastatin at 20–40 mg daily on resting systolic and diastolic blood pressure in 30 subjects aged 40–70 with untreated hypertension and with moderate hypercholesterolaemia. Pravastatin decreased LDL-c by 25%. The baseline systolic, diastolic, and pulse pressures were 149 ± 6, 97 ± 2, and 52 ± 6 mmHg, respectively and after 16 weeks of pravastatin treatment, blood pressures were decreased by 8, 5, and 3 mmHg, respectively. After 16 weeks, compared with placebo, pravastatin significantly decreased systolic, diastolic, and pulse pressures by 8, 5, and 3 mmHg, respectively ($P = 0.001$, 0.001, and 0.011). In this small, but carefully done study, the dose of pravastatin did not predict blood pressure response. Pravastatin therapy did result in a blunted cold pressor test response and reduced plasma endothelin-1 levels. The effects of pravastatin on blood pressure control were independent of age, gender, and baseline plasma LDL-c and HDL-c levels. The generalizability of these results was clearly limited by the selection of the trial subjects and by the limited duration of the trial. Nonetheless, it offered a useful hypothesis for testing.

Ferrier and co-workers [33] have further corroborated the above detailed blood pressure-lowering effects of statins, specifically with the use of high dose atorvastatin 80 mg/day, in normolipidaemic subjects with isolated systolic hypertension. After 3 months of therapy, they found that brachial systolic, diastolic and mean blood pressures were lower along with reduced large artery stiffness. Although the reduction in systolic and diastolic blood pressure by statins is small, the associated increase in peripheral vasodilatory capacity suggests an improvement in endothelial dysfunction.

The favourable effect of statins on blood pressure has also been confirmed in high risk groups. A study population of type 2 diabetes patients with hypercholesterolaemia and hypertension were treated with atorvastatin 10 mg/day and showed a significant reduction in diastolic blood pressure irrespective of any modifications to their antihypertensive treatment [34]. Prasad and colleagues [35] evaluated blood pressure reduction with HMG-CoA reductase inhibitors in renal transplant recipients which again confirmed the above observations. They identified 113 stable recipients with graft survival >1 year and were started on a statin (including atorvastatin, pravastatin, simvastatin, and fluvastatin) with no further adjustment of their existing antihypertensive regimen during the 12-month study period. At the end of this prospective, randomized, placebo-controlled study there was a significant reduction in the systolic (7 mmHg), diastolic (3 mmHg) and mean arterial blood pressure (4 mmHg) in the statin-treated group compared to control group.

Aside from the absolute blood pressure values, there is a growing body of evidence linking short-term or long-term variability of blood pressure to target organ damage. Sander and co-workers [36] established daytime blood pressure variability as the best predictor of intimal media thickness progression, a surrogate marker for subclinical atherosclerotic disease.

Indeed any antihypertensive treatment should not only lower absolute blood pressure values, but also correct blood pressure variability. Pelat and colleagues [37] studied a model of genetically dyslipidaemic mice and examined the effect of the most recent addition to the statin family, rosuvastatin, on different components of blood pressure and heart rate variability. Dyslipidaemic mice not only had significantly higher systolic and diastolic blood pressure values, but also showed an abolition of their normal circardian rhythm. Treatment of this mouse model with rosuvastatin for 2 weeks normalized both systolic and diastolic blood pressure values and corrected their circardian rhythm. Rosuvastatin-treated mice also recovered their sensitivity to NOS inhibition supporting the hypothesis that NO can be implicated in baroreflex sensitivity.

LARGE-SCALE CLINICAL TRIALS

As discussed earlier, there have been multiple other small-scale clinical trials which have confirmed the above finding that addition of statin therapy to an existing antihypertensive regimen improves blood pressure values modestly [25, 26, 38–45]. The effect seems to be enhanced in those receiving either an ACE inhibitor or calcium channel blocker containing regimen. Unfortunately, large-scale clinical trials have not been able to corroborate beneficial effects of statins on blood pressure reduction. Two primary prevention trials are informative. First, is the large prospective placebo-controlled, double-blinded study, the Anglo-Scandinavian Cardiac Outcomes Trial (ASCOT) that had 10 305 hypertensive subjects in its lipid-lowering arm (LLA) [46]. The primary objective of the LLA of ASCOT was to assess and compare the long-term effects of atorvastatin 10 mg/day on the combined endpoint of non-fatal MI and fatal CHD of a statin (plus antihypertensive treatment) compared with placebo (plus antihypertensive treatment) among subjects with total cholesterol of 254 mg/dl or less. The mean LDL-c in this population was about 130 mg/dl. Eligible subjects were men and women aged between 40 and 79 years at randomization with either untreated or treated hypertension. They had to have at least three other risk factors for CVD. Subjects in this trial received one of two randomized antihypertensive regimens consisting of amlodipine, perindoril or both and atenolol, chlorthalidone or both and were randomized to atorvastatin 10 mg daily or placebo. Participants were mainly white (95%) and male (81%) with a mean age of 63 years. The study was stopped prematurely after a median follow-up of 3.3 years owing to the significant clinical benefit seen in those assigned to atorvastatin. LDL-c lowering with atorvastatin conferred a 36% reduction in fatal CHD and non-fatal MI and a 27% reduction in the incidence of strokes compared with placebo. Blood pressure control throughout the trial was similar in the patients assigned to atorvastatin or placebo groups with mean values of 138.3/80.4 mmHg and 138.4/80.4 mmHg, respectively at the end of the study period. The results show that the benefits of statin treatment are additive to those of good blood pressure control. The study design prevented an answer to the question as to whether statins lower BP as antihypertensive medication was titrated upwards based on achieved blood pressure, thereby masking the impact of statin treatment on blood pressure.

A second major primary prevention study of cardiovascular disease with atorvastatin is the Collaborative Atorvastatin Diabetes Study (CARDS) [47]. This study was aimed to assess the effectiveness of statin therapy for prevention of major cardiovascular events in participants with type 2 diabetes without elevated concentrations of LDL-c. In CARDS, 2828 subjects aged 40–75 years were randomized to atorvastatin 10 mg daily or placebo and followed prospectively for a median duration of 3.9 years. Participants were again mainly white (94%) and male (68%). Study entrants had an LDL-c of 160 mg/dl, no previous documented history of cardiovascular disease, and at least one of the following: retinopathy, albuminuria, current smoking or hypertension. The trial was terminated 2 years earlier than expected. It showed that atorvastatin treatment had a 37% reduction of any major cardiovascular event, 47% reduction in stroke rate, and 27% reduction in death. At randomization,

Table 4.1 Trials of statins in chronic kidney disease (CKD)

Name	*Subjects*	*Trial design/duration*	*Results*
ALERT	2100 w/renal transplant	Fluvastatin 40 mg vs. placebo; mean follow-up 5.1 years	LDL-c lowered 32%; no significant reduction in primary endpoint of cardiac death, non-fatal MI or coronary intervention procedure. Fluvastatin associated with fewer cardiac deaths or non-fatal MI (70 vs. 104, 0.65 [0.48–0.88] $P = 0.005$)
4D	1300 diabetic subjects on haemodialysis	Atorvastatin 20 mg/day vs. placebo	Median LDL-c lowered 42% by atorvastatin. No statistically significant effect on the composite primary endpoint of cardiovascular death, non-fatal MI, stroke
AURORA	2700 haemodialysis subjects	Rosuvastatin vs. placebo	Expected in 2008
SHARP	9000 CKD subjects (pre-dialysis or dialysis)	Simvastatin 20 mg + ezetimibe 10 mg vs. placebo	Expected in 2009

two-thirds of patients in both treatment groups reported use of blood pressure-lowering drugs and at 4 years, 84% allocated placebo and 83% allocated atorvastatin were taking these drugs. Both mean systolic and diastolic blood pressures at the end of the study period were not statistically different (144/79 mmHg in the placebo group vs. 143/80 mmHg in the atorvastatin group).

Secondary prevention, large-scale trials do not offer support for a salutary effect of statins on blood pressure as well. Although a *post hoc* subgroup analysis, the effects of pravastatin on blood pressure were examined in the Cholesterol and Recurrent Events (CARE) study [48]. This randomized double-blind placebo-controlled trial of pravastatin 40 mg daily vs. placebo in 4159 survivors of myocardial infarction and cholesterol levels under 240 mg/dl collected blood pressure data over a median duration of follow-up of 57.8 months. The unadjusted and adjusted change in mean arterial, systolic, diastolic or pulse pressure from baseline was not significantly different for pravastatin or placebo recipients at 3, 6, 12 or 24 months after randomization.

A more intriguing hypothesis on how statins could benefit blood pressure has emerged from observations from three large-scale trials that contrasted pravastatin vs. placebo [49]. When all participants with moderate chronic kidney disease (CKD) at baseline were considered, pravastatin was associated with a 34% reduction in the adjusted rate of kidney function loss, although the absolute reduction in the rate of loss was clinically small. A letter to the editor noting this effect suggested that the benefit seen with statins in CKD could be related to their anti-inflammatory effects [50]. This is also a hypothesis worthy of further study.

Indeed, an examination of lipid therapy in CKD is a high priority. Table 4.1 shows the major trials that have been completed and are underway to examine this further [51–54]. The first two trials (ALERT and 4D) did not show a significant difference in the primary endpoint. This has created various hypotheses to explain the singular failure of statins in patients with advanced atherosclerosis. Fortunately, further studies are underway. The Aurora Study using rosuvastatin and the The Study of Heart and Renal Protection (SHARP) trial using combination therapy will lower LDL-c in more striking fashion and should allow us to see if LDL-c lowering therapy is effective in these patients.

The SHARP trial will compare in subjects 40 years and older receiving dialysis treatment and without a history of MI or coronary revascularization, ezetimibe 10 mg + simvastatin 20 mg daily vs. placebo in 8000 subjects with an elevated creatinine (≥1.5 mg/dl in women or ≥1.7 in men). All subjects would not normally be candidates for statin treatment. The primary endpoint will be major vascular events and the study is powered to detect a 20% reduction in major vascular events at the $P = 0.01$ level.

SUMMARY

Our review shows that hypercholesterolaemia and hypertension are commonly found together and are responsible for a substantial increase in global cardiovascular risk. Aggressive treatment of these two major risk factors provides proven benefit. Although in studies of chronic stable CHD it appears that statin lowering of LDL-c explains the benefit seen, there are important observations on the lipid-independent effects of statins that should be considered. These effects on endothelial function, inflammation, coagulation and plaque stability could include modest, but beneficial, effects on blood pressure. These cholesterol independent effects seem to be the result of inhibition of effects mediated by Ang II and stimulation of eNOS activity. Unfortunately, most of the data for blood pressure modification with statin therapy are from small-scale studies and have not been confirmed in large-scale, prospective, multicentre clinical trials. We believe that there is a need for further studies of statin effects on specific forms of hypertension. For example, we would suggest more studies on isolated systolic hypertension in older patients where a synergy between statins and antihypertensive agents would be greatly welcomed. Most important will be the trial data from SHARP and AURORA that will examine the utility of more powerful LDL-c lowering regimens on the sequelae of atherosclerosis in dialysis patients. These results are awaited eagerly.

REFERENCES

1. Glass KG, Witzum J. Atherosclerosis: the road ahead. *Cell* 2001; 104:503–516.
2. Field AE, Byers T, Hunter DJ *et al.* Weight cycling, weight gain, and risk of hypertension in women. *Am J Epidemiol* 1999; 150:1999; 573–579.
3. Grundy SM, Cleeman JI, Daniels SR *et al.* Diagnosis and management of the metabolic syndrome. An American Heart Association/National Heart, Lung, and Blood Institute Scientific Statement. *Circulation* 2005; 112:2735–2752.
4. Wilson PWF, D'Agostino RB, Parise H, Sullivan L, Meigs JB. Metabolic syndrome as a precursor of cardiovascular disease and type 2 diabetes mellitus. *Circulation* 2005; 112:3066–3072.
5. McGill HC, McMahan CA, Zieske AW *et al.* Association of coronary heart disease risk factors with microscopic qualities of coronary atherosclerosis in youth. *Circulation* 2000; 102:374–379.
6. Law MR, Wald NJ. Risk factor thresholds: their existence under scrutiny. *BMJ* 2002; 324:1570–1576.
7. Lloyd-Jones DM, Larson MG, Beiser A, Levy D. Lifetime risk of developing coronary heart disease. *Lancet* 1999; 353:89–92.
8. Kannel WB. Risk stratification in hypertension: new insights from the Framingham Study. *Am J Hypertens* 2000; 13(Pt 2):3S–10S.
9. Lloyd-Jones DM, Evans JC, Larson MC *et al.* Cross-classification of JNC VI blood pressure stages and risk groups in the Framingham Heart Study. *Arch Intern Med* 1999; 159:2206–2212.
10. Pearson TA, Laurora I, Chu H, Kajonek S. The lipid treatment assessment project (L-TAP): a multicenter survey to evaluate the percentages of dyslipidemic patients receiving lipid-lowering therapy and achieving low-density lipoprotein cholesterol goals. *Arch Intern Med* 2000; 160:459–467.
11. Neaton JD, Wentworth D. Serum cholesterol, blood pressure, cigarette smoking, and death from coronary heart disease. Overall findings and differences by age for 316,099 white men. Multiple Risk Factor Intervention Trial Research Group. *Arch Intern Med* 1992; 152:56–64.

12. Borghi C, Bacchelli S, Degli, Esposito D. Pressor and metabolic correlates to long-term development of stable hypertension in borderline hypertensive patients. *J Hypertens* 1997; 15:S111.
13. Veronesi M, Borghi C, Immordino V. Blood pressure reactivity and development of stable hypertension in borderline hypertensives. Role of plasma cholesterol [abstract]. *Am J Hypertens* 1998; 11:218A.
14. Borghi C, Veronesi M, Prandin MG, Dormi A, Ambrosioni E. Statins and blood pressure regulation. *Curr Hypertens Rep* 2001; 3:281–288.
15. Third report of the National Cholesterol Education Program (NCEP) Expert Panel on Detection, Evaluation, and Treatment of High Blood Cholesterol in Adults (Adult Treatment Panel III): final report. *Circulation* 2002; 106:3143–3421.
16. Baigent C, Keech A, Kearney PM *et al.* Cholesterol Treatment Trialists' (CTT) Collaborators. Efficacy and safety of cholesterol-lowering treatment: prospective meta-analysis of data from 90,056 participants in 14 randomised trials of statins. *Lancet* 2005; 366:1267–1278.
17. Davignon J. Beneficial cardiovascular pleitropic effects of statins. *Circulation* 2004; 109(suppl 1):III29–III43.
18. Robinson JG, Smith B, Maheshwari N, Schrott H. Pleiotropic effects of statins: benefit beyond cholesterol reduction? A meta-regression analysis. *J Am Coll Cardiol* 2005; 46:1855–1862.
19. Zanchetti A. The antiatherogenic effects of antihypertensive drugs: experimental and clinical evidence. *Clin Exp Hypertens A* 1992; 14:307–331.
20. Zanchetti A. Trials investigating the anti-atherosclerotic effects of antihypertensive drugs. *J Hypertens Suppl* 1996; 14:S77–S80; discussion S80–S81.
21. Kaesemeyer WH, Caldwell RB, Huang J, Caldwell RW. Pravastatin sodium activates endothelial nitric oxide synthase independent of its cholesterol-lowering actions. *J Am Coll Cardiol* 1999; 33:234–241.
22. Nickenig G, Baumer AT, Temur Y, Kebben D, Jockenhovel F, Bohm M. Statin-sensitive dysregulated AT1 receptor function and density in hypercholesterolemic men. *Circulation* 1999; 100:2131–2134.
23. Laufs U, Liao JK. Direct vascular effects of HMG-CoA reductase inhibitors. *Trends Cardiovasc Med* 2000; 10:143–148.
24. Guijarro C, Blanco-Coli LM, Ortego M *et al.* 3-Hydroxy-3-methylglutaryl coenzyme a reductase and isoprenylation inhibitors induce apoptosis of vascular smooth muscle cells in culture. *Circ Res* 1998; 83:490–500.
25. Hess DC, Fagan SC. Pharmacology and clinical experience with simvastatin. *Expert Opin Pharmacother* 2001; 2:153–163.
26. Sessa WC. Can modulation of endothelial nitric oxide synthase explain the vasculoprotective actions of statins? *Trends Mol Med* 2001; 7:189–191.
27. Wassmann S, Laufs U, Baumer AT *et al.* HMG-CoA reductase inhibitors improve endothelial dysfunction in normocholesterolemic hypertension via reduced production of reactive oxygen species. *Hypertension* 2001; 37:1450–1457.
28. Zhou MS, Jaimes EA, Raij L. Atorvastatin prevents end-organ injury in salt-sensitive hypertension: role of eNOS and oxidant stress. *Hypertension* 2004; 44:186–190.
29. Criqui MH, Cowan LD, Heiss G, Haskell WL, Laskarzewski PM, Chambless LE. Frequency and clustering of nonlipid coronary risk factors in dyslipoproteinemia. The Lipid Research Clinics Program Prevalence Study. *Circulation* 1986; 73(Pt 2):140–150.
30. Wilhelmsen L, Pyorala K, Wedel H, Cook T, Pedersen T, Kjekshus J. Risk factors for a major coronary event after myocardial infarction in the Scandinavian Simvastatin Survival Study (4S). Impact of predicted risk on the benefit of cholesterol-lowering treatment. *Eur Heart J* 2001; 22:1119–1127.
31. Borghi C, Dormi A, Veronesi M, Sangiorgi Z, Gaddi A. Association between different lipid-lowering treatment strategies and blood pressure control in the Brisighella Heart Study. *Am Heart J* 2004; 148:285–292.
32. Glorioso N, Troffa C, Filigheddu F *et al.* Effect of the HMG-CoA reductase inhibitors on blood pressure in patients with essential hypertension and primary hypercholesterolemia. *Hypertension* 1999; 34:1281–1286.
33. Ferrier KE, Muhlmann MH, Baguet JP *et al.* Intensive cholesterol reduction lowers blood pressure and large artery stiffness in isolated systolic hypertension. *J Am Coll Cardiol* 2002; 39:1020–1025.
34. Velussi M, Cernigoi AM, Tortul C, Merni C. Atorvastatin for the management of type 2 diabetic patients with dyslipidaemia. A mid-term (9 months) treatment experience. *Diabetes Nutr Metab* 1999; 12:407–412.
35. Prasad GV, Ahmed A, Nash MM, Zaltzman JS. Blood pressure reduction with HMG-CoA reductase inhibitors in renal transplant recipients. *Kidney Int* 2003; 63:360–364.
36. Sander D, Kukla C, Klingelhofer J, Winbeck K, Conrad B. Relationship between circadian blood pressure patterns and progression of early carotid atherosclerosis: a 3-year follow-up study. *Circulation* 2000; 102:1536–1541.

37. Pelat M, Dessy C, Massion P, Desager JP, Feron O, Balligand JL. Rosuvastatin decreases caveolin-1 and improves nitric oxide-dependent heart rate and blood pressure variability in apolipoprotein E−/− mice in vivo. *Circulation* 2003; 107:2480–2486.
38. Kanbay M, Yildiriv A, Bozbas H *et al*. Statin therapy helps to control blood pressure levels in hypertensive dyslipidemic patients. *Renal Failure* 2005; 27:297–303.
39. Danaoglu Z, Kultursay H, Kayikeioglu M, *et al*. Effect of statin therapy added to ACE-inhibitors on blood pressure control and endothelial functions in normolipidemic hypertensive patients [see comment]. *Anadolu Kardiyol Derg* 2003; 3:331–337.
40. Sposito AC, Mansur AP, Coelho OR, Nicolau JC, Ramires JA. Additional reduction in blood pressure after cholesterol-lowering treatment by statins (lovastatin or pravastatin) in hypercholesterolemic patients using angiotensin-converting enzyme inhibitors (enalapril or lisinopril). *Am J Cardiol* 1999; 83:1497–1499, A8.
41. Terzoli L, Mircoli L, Raco R, Ferrori AV. Lowering of elevated ambulatory blood pressure by HMG-CoA reductase inhibitors. *J Cardiovasc Pharmacol* 2005; 46:310–315.
42. Koh KK, Quon MJ, Han SH *et al*. Additive beneficial effects of losartan combined with simvastatin in the treatment of hypercholesterolemic, hypertensive patients. *Circulation* 2004; 110:3687–3692.
43. Koh KK, Quon MJ, Han SH *et al*. Vascular and metabolic effects of combined therapy with ramipril and simvastatin in patients with type 2 diabetes. *Hypertension* 2005; 45:1088–1093.
44. Ikeda T, Sakurai J, Nakayama D *et al*. Pravastatin has an additional depressor effect in patients undergoing long-term treatment with antihypertensive drugs. *Am J Hypertens* 2004; 17:502–506.
45. Leibovitz E, Beniashvili M, Zimlichman R, Freiman A, Shargorodsky M, Gavish D. Treatment with amlodipine and atorvastatin have additive effect in improvement of arterial compliance in hypertensive hyperlipidemic patients. *Am J Hypertens* 2003; 16(Pt 1):715–718.
46. Sever PS, Dahlof B, Poulter NR *et al*. Prevention of coronary and stroke events with atorvastatin in hypertensive patients who have average or lower-than-average cholesterol concentrations, in the Anglo-Scandinavian Cardiac Outcomes Trial–Lipid Lowering Arm (ASCOT–LLA): a multicentre randomised controlled trial. *Lancet* 2003; 361:1149–1158.
47. Colhoun HM, Betteridge DJ, Durrington PN *et al*. Primary prevention of cardiovascular disease with atorvastatin in type 2 diabetes in the Collaborative Atorvastatin Diabetes Study (CARDS): multicentre randomised placebo-controlled trial. *Lancet* 2004; 364:685–696.
48. Tonelli M, Sacks F, Pfeffer M, Lopez-Jimenez F, Jhangri GS, Curhan G. Effect of pravastatin on blood pressure in people with cardiovascular disease. *J Hum Hypertens* 2006 April 20.
49. Tonelli M, Isles C, Craven T *et al*. Effect of pravastatin on rate of kidney function loss in people with or at risk for coronary disease. *Circulation* 2005; 112:171–178.
50. Rashidi A, Rahman M, Tonelli M *et al*. Letter regarding article by Tonelli *et al*. 'Effect of Pravastatin on Rate of Kidney Function Loss in People With or at Risk for Coronary Disease' Response. *Circulation* 2006; 113:e59–e60.
51. Holdaas H, Fellstrom B, Jardine AG *et al*. Assessment of LEscol in Renal Transplantation (ALERT) Study Investigators. Effect of fluvastatin on cardiac outcomes in renal transplant recipients: a multicentre, randomised, placebo-controlled trial. *Lancet* 2003; 361:2024–2031.
52. Wanner C, Krane V, Marz W *et al*. German Diabetes and Dialysis Study Investigators. Atorvastatin in patients with type 2 diabetes mellitus undergoing hemodialysis. *N Engl J Med* 2005; 353:238–248.
53. Fellstrom BC, Holdaas H, Jardine AG. Why do we need a statin trial in hemodialysis patients? *Kidney Int Suppl* 2003; 84:S204–S206.
54. Landray M, Baigent C, Leaper C *et al*. The second United Kingdom Heart and Renal Protection (UK-HARP-II) Study: a randomized controlled study of the biochemical safety and efficacy of adding ezetimibe to simvastatin as initial therapy among patients with CKD. *Am J Kidney Dis* 2006; 47:385–395.

5

Do antihypertensive agents influence lipid profiles and lipid therapy?

S. K. Arora, S. I. McFarlane

Hypertension is a major public health problem of epidemic proportions. In the United States alone, up to 60 million adults have high blood pressure [1, 2]. Hypertension is an important modifiable risk factor for cardiovascular disease (CVD) [1]. Furthermore, control of hypertension is a key strategy for primary and secondary prevention of CVD [1]. Evidence from several randomized controlled trials indicates that reduction of blood pressure by 5–10 mmHg reduces stroke and coronary heart disease (CHD) by nearly 35–40% and 15–25% respectively [1, 3–6]. Although reduction in blood pressure, both systolic and diastolic, has been shown to decrease the CV events with stronger tendencies towards particularly stroke, many of the patients treated for high blood pressure still suffer CHD events despite blood pressure control [7, 8]. This suboptimal CHD reduction with antihypertensive medications compared to significant reduction in stroke incidence has been thought to be, in part, due to adverse metabolic and lipid effects of these medications [7, 8]. Therefore, addressing the effect of antihypertensive medications on conventional and non-conventional CVD risk factors is of utmost importance to further reduce such a risk in this patient population. Among the adverse metabolic effects of antihypertensive medications, dyslipidaemia, which is thought to be a stronger predictor of CHD than stroke, is particularly common. These antihypertensive medications, including β-blockers and diuretics, have also been shown to have other adverse metabolic effects as well such as impaired glucose tolerance and increased insulin resistance [8].

In this review, we will discuss the metabolic effects of various classes of antihypertensive medications, with a particular emphasis on dyslipidaemia, a potentially modifiable major risk factor in this high risk population.

HYPERTENSION AND DYSLIPIDAEMIA: COMMONLY COEXISTING CARDIOVASCULAR RISK FACTORS

Epidemiologic studies have demonstrated positive association between hypertension and dyslipidaemia [9, 10]. The Framingham Heart Study demonstrated that prevalence of dyslipidaemia increases with increasing blood pressure level [9]. More than 40% men and 33% women in this population with blood pressure 140/90 mmHg or higher had dyslipidaemia, defined as total cholesterol >240 mg/dl, high density lipoprotein (HDL) ≤35 mg/dl or treatment with lipid-lowering agents [9]. A study from Australia also reported significantly higher

Surender K. Arora, MD, Assistant Instructor, Division of Endocrinology, Diabetes and Hypertension, SUNY-Downstate and Kings County Hospital, Brooklyn, New York, USA

Samy I. McFarlane, MD, MPH, Associate Professor, Chief, Division of Endocrinology, Diabetes and Hypertension, SUNY-Downstate and Kings County Hospital, Brooklyn, New York, USA

levels of serum cholesterol and serum triglycerides (TGs) in subjects with hypertension compared with normotensive subjects [10]. In a study involving more than 41 000 subjects, significant correlation between hypertension and lipid fractions was demonstrated [11]. Furthermore, Williams and colleagues [12] reported high prevalence of lipid abnormalities in siblings of hypertensive subjects. These findings were further described as *familial dyslipidaemic hypertension syndrome,* highlighting the frequent coexistence of these two major risk factors [12]. Subjects with dyslipidaemic hypertension show a nearly 4-fold increase in coronary mortality rate compared to those with either dyslipidaemia or hypertension alone, suggesting more than simple additive effects of these factors on CVD events [13].

A similar increase in coronary events was also demonstrated in the Prospective Cardiovascular Munster Study where 4-year incidence of myocardial infarction was twice as high in hypertensive subjects compared with the normotensive population but much higher in the presence of both hypertension and dyslipidaemia [14]. Flesch and co-workers [15] studied lipid distribution in 105 patients with mild to moderate hypertension without any clinically or ultrasonographically detected atherosclerosis compared to 65 age-matched healthy subjects. A significant positive association was observed between arterial hypertension and serum low density lipoprotein (LDL), Apo B, TGs and very low density lipoprotein (VLDL) levels. No significant differences in serum total cholesterol and HDL levels were detected between the hypertensive and normotensive group [15]. Catalano and colleagues [16] also reported significantly higher TGs and VLDL levels in hypertensive subjects compared with the control group. Significant differences in serum levels of Apo AI, AII, CII and Apo E were also observed but there were no significant differences in total, HDL and LDL cholesterol between the two groups. The authors concluded that alteration in apolipoprotein profile might contribute to increased CVD risk in the hypertensive population [16].

In animal studies of spontaneously hypertensive rats, an augmentation of lipid metabolism in the liver with moderate hyperlipidaemia, primarily an increase in TG fraction, has been reported [17]. High prevalence of hypertension among hyperlipidaemic subjects has also been reported from the Lipid Treatment Assessment Project [18].

Collectively, these data indicate that both hypertension and dyslipidaemia are closely inter-related with lipid abnormalities present in the majority of hypertensive subjects and *vice versa*. This association may be further explained by insulin resistance and endothelial dysfunction as follows:

INSULIN RESISTANCE

Both hypertension and hyperlipidaemia are key components of 'cardiometabolic syndrome' and are linked through insulin resistance which is central to the pathogenesis of this syndrome [19, 20]. Mechanisms for the development of hypertension in insulin resistance include renal sodium retention, activation of the sympathetic nervous system, altered membrane cation transport, growth-promoting effects on vascular smooth muscle cells and enhanced vascular reactivity [21] (Figure 5.1). Insulin resistance is also associated with visceral fat resistance to metabolic effects of insulin while retaining increased sensitivity to lipolytic hormones [21]. This results in increased release of free fatty acids (FFA) into the portal system and provides excess substrate for hepatic VLDL and TG synthesis [21]. As a result, dyslipidaemia associated with insulin resistance has elevated TGs and oxidized LDL with low HDL. Because of clustering of various CVD risk factors including hypertension and dyslipidaemia, insulin resistance confers a markedly increased risk of CVD [21].

ENDOTHELIAL DYSFUNCTION

Another factor linking hypertension and hyperlipidaemia is endothelial dysfunction (Figure 5.2). Endothelium is a source for several vasoactive factors including nitric oxide (NO),

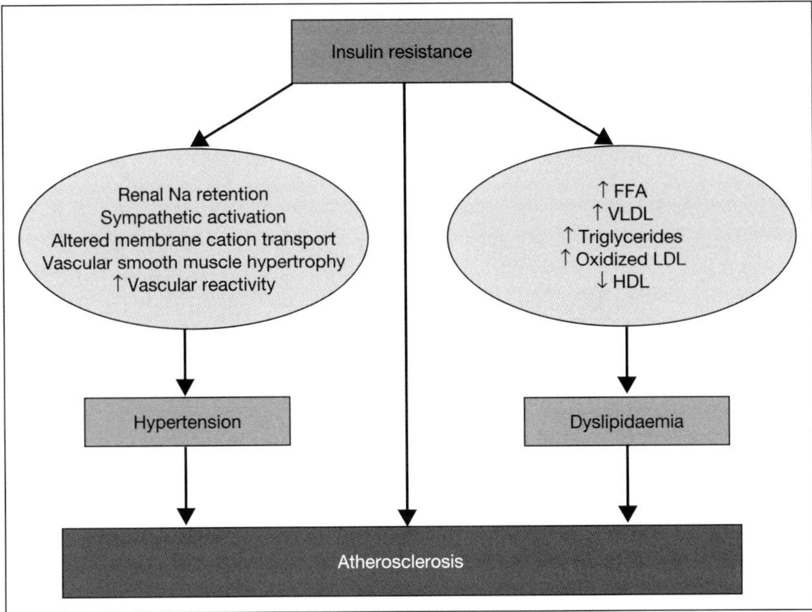

Figure 5.1 Insulin resistance mediates hypertension through several mechanisms including renal sodium retention, activation of the sympathetic system, altered membrane cation transport, and by promoting vascular smooth muscle hypertrophy and reactivity. Insulin resistance also leads to dyslipidaemia by increasing lipolysis, resulting in increased FFA availability to the liver resulting in increased synthesis of VLDL and TGs and reduction in HDL cholesterol. Insulin resistance also causes atherogenesis by causing alteration in LDL phenotype to small, dense particles which are more atherogenic.

prostacyclin and endothelin-1 which play an important role in the regulation of vascular tone [22, 23]. Both hypertension and hyperlipidaemia are associated with decreased basal and stimulated release of endothelium-derived NO [24]. Incubation of endothelial cells with human LDL has been demonstrated to cause upregulation of caveolin 1, a negative modulator of endothelial enzyme NO synthase (eNOS) [22]. This results in tonic inhibition of eNOS and prevents its activation by various stimuli, leading to decreased ability to produce NO which is a potent vasodilator and antitrophic agent [22]. Therefore, endothelial dysfunction may result in vascular smooth muscle hypertrophy leading to increased vascular stiffness and decreased vascular reactivity [23]. Oxidized LDL particles selectively reduce NO-mediated endothelium-dependent relaxations to various stimuli including aggregating platelets, serotonin and thrombin and increase the risk of coronary atherogenesis [24]. High TGs have also been implicated in endothelial dysfunction which may further worsen in the presence of elevated LDL cholesterol [22, 25]. Furthermore, LDL cholesterol has also been demonstrated to upregulate the AT_1 subtype of angiotensin II receptors as well as endothelin 1, leading to increase in blood pressure [23, 26]. Statins inhibit the enzyme hydroxyl–methyl–glutaryl coenzyme A (HMG CoA) reductase and have also been reported to decrease AT_1 receptor expression and activation [23, 26, 27]. Treatment of hypercholesterolaemia with statins has been demonstrated to reduce not only LDL cholesterol but blood pressure as well [27]. Angiotensin II is a major prooxidant mediator in vessel walls leading to increased oxidized LDL in the subendothelium, which in turn promotes atherogenesis by initiation and propagation of an inflammatory response [22, 23]. On the other hand, treatment of hypertension with agents such as angiotensin-converting enzyme inhibitors (ACE-I) has been demonstrated to reduce serum cholesterol [23]. Ageing is associated with increased

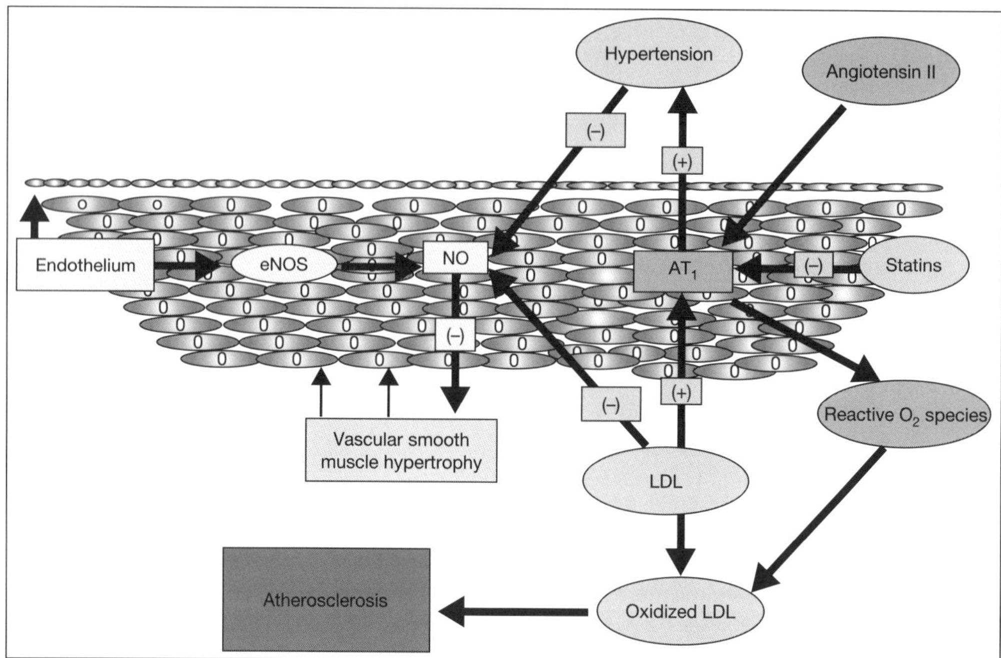

Figure 5.2 Endothelium synthesizes eNOS, the NO synthase enzyme, leading to production of NO. This NO synthesis is blunted by hypertension and in the presence of LDL cholesterol. The NO has an antitrophic effect on vascular smooth muscle cells and reduction in endothelial NO production causes vascular smooth muscle hypertrophy. LDL cholesterol upregulates the AT_1 subtype of angiotensin II receptor and may worsen hypertension whereas statins may reduce the expression of vascular AT_1 receptor and may help reduce blood pressure. Angiotensin II mediates production of reactive oxygen species through the AT_1 receptors and increases oxidation of subendothelial LDL particles to a smaller, denser, more atherogenic form, thereby promoting atherosclerosis.

levels of endothelin-1, a potent vasoconstrictor, which may explain the increased risk of hypertension with advanced age [22].

ANTIHYPERTENSIVE AGENTS AND LIPIDS

A number of studies have shown that antihypertensive medications may have significant metabolic effects and influence carbohydrate metabolism and lipids [7, 8, 28, 29]. This is particularly the case for thiazide diuretics and β-blockers which have been known to adversely affect serum lipids and glucose levels and may be associated with increased risk of developing diabetes [30, 31]. Since both dyslipidaemia and diabetes are risk factors for CVD, the utility of these agents for control of hypertension as primary and secondary prevention strategies for CVD has raised concerns in literature [31].

In a large cross-section study of more than 15 000 subjects, total cholesterol was 4.0 mg/dl higher in those taking antihypertensive medications after adjustment for age, sex, weight, smoking, alcohol, blood pressure and exercise compared to those not on antihypertensive medications [32]. In this study, HDL cholesterol was also 2.5 mg/dl lower in the treated group [32]. In another large cross-sectional survey of more than 14 000 women screened for CVD risk factors in the United Kingdom, untreated hypertensives and those taking antihypertensive medications with BP $> 140/90$ mmHg had the most atherogenic risk factor profile with higher total and LDL cholesterol and lower HDL values [33]. In the Helsinki Heart

Study, data from the placebo arm of the linked antihypertensive therapy including diuretics and β-blockers with increase in serum TGs and low HDL cholesterol [7]. Though a number of studies have examined the effects of various antihypertensive agents on serum lipids, it is a Herculean task to compare and contrast the relative effects of different agents due to the large number of studies conducted with different agents and under different clinical settings. Detailed and valuable information regarding effects of antihypertensive agents on serum lipids was provided in a large meta-analysis of 474 controlled and uncontrolled clinical trials examining 85 antihypertensive agents in more than 65 000 subjects [8, 28]. Effects of various antihypertensive agents on serum lipid profile are summarized in Table 5.1.

Diuretics unfavourably alter the lipid profile leading to increase in total, LDL cholesterol and TGs together with decrease in HDL cholesterol. The effects on total cholesterol are dose and race dependent to some extent and tend to be greater in blacks, whereas effects on TGs were gender related leading to a more pronounced elevation in men. This effect, however, was seen only in short-term studies [28]. Similarly, the increase in LDL cholesterol was more pronounced in men and correlated with baseline LDL levels. Interestingly, the decrease in HDL was seen only in diabetic patients [28].

Among thiazide diuretics, chlorthalidone was particularly associated with greater elevation in LDL cholesterol whereas indapamide, another thiazide agent, did not show any significant alteration of TGs [28]. While most studies agree about the effects of thiazide diuretics on total cholesterol and TGs, results are not consistent in regard to the effects on LDL and HDL cholesterol. Overall, these effects could potentially worsen the dyslipidaemia of diabetes, especially at higher doses and particularly in black males [28].

In the Antihypertensive and Lipid Lowering Treatment to Prevent Heart Attack Trial (ALLHAT), the serum cholesterol at 2 years and 4 years was significantly higher in the chlorthalidone group than in the lisinopril group [30]. The serum cholesterol was also higher compared to the amlodipine group at 2 years but not at 4 years. In a randomized placebo-controlled trial examining the effect of six different antihypertensive agents, hydrochlorthiazide caused a short- term increase in TGs, cholesterol and Apo B levels at the end of titration but the changes were not significantly different from placebo at the end of 1 year [29]. In this study, a significant reduction in HDL subfraction 2 (HDL_2) was also observed at the end of 1 year.

Collectively, these data suggest that the deleterious effects of thiazide-type diuretics on lipid profile might be short-term and may disappear with long-term use of these agents. Furthermore, these adverse effects on lipids have been primarily shown with the use of higher dosages of the thiazide agents [8, 28]. Moreover, alteration of lipid metabolism with the thiazide diuretics has not been shown, to date, to adversely affect the CVD endpoints such as strokes and myocardial infarctions. In fact, these agents have been shown to reduce CVD events as demonstrated in the ALLHAT trial, the largest hypertension trial ever conducted [30].

β-Blockers, in general, are associated with increase in serum TGs and decrease in serum HDL levels [8, 28]. These effects tend to be smaller with cardioselective β-blocking agents and in those with intrinsic sympathomimetic activity (ISA) (Table 5.1). Agents with combined cardioselectivity and ISA may decrease total and LDL cholesterol in addition to a net increase in HDL cholesterol [8, 28]. Pindolol, a selective β-1 receptor blocker with ISA, was specifically associated with lower TGs and higher HDL cholesterol [28]. On the other hand, atenolol, a selective β-1 blocker without ISA, was shown to reduce HDL cholesterol albeit without effects on TGs, total and LDL cholesterol [29].

α-Blockers have the most favourable effects of all antihypertensive agents on serum lipids and are associated with improvement in all the components with decreases in TGs, total and LDL cholesterol accompanied by increase in HDL cholesterol [8, 28]. These effects correlate with baseline levels and can be blunted by combining β-blockade with α-blockers. Prazosin was associated with greater reduction in LDL cholesterol compared to other agents in the same class [28]. Although most studies are consistent regarding the

Table 5.1 Effect of different classes of antihypertensive agents of plasma lipoproteins

Drugs	*Total cholesterol*	*Triglycerides*	*HDL cholesterol*	*LDL cholesterol*	*Comments*
Diuretics	↑	↑*	↓**	↑	*In short studies, in men only **In diabetes
β-blockers	NS	↑	↓	NS	
β-1 selective	NS	↑*	↓*	NS	*Less prominent than non-selective β-blockers
ISA	↓	↑*	↓*		*Less prominent than non-selective β-blockers
β-1 + ISA	↓	NS	NS	↓	
α-blockers	↓*	↓	↑	↓*	*Not seen with combined α- + β-blockers
ACE inhibitors	↓	↓			
Vasodilators	↓		↑	↓	
Calcium channel blockers	–	–	–	–	Lipid neutral

HDL = high density lipoprotein; ISA = intrinsic sympathomimetic activity; LDL = low density lipoprotein; NS = not significant.

effects of α-blockers on TGs, the data are not consistent, regarding the effects on other lipid parameters. Lakshman and co-workers reported significant decreases in total cholesterol and Apo B with prazosin in the short term but no significant difference from other antihypertensive groups at 1 year [29]. No change in HDL_2 was observed with prazosin at the end of 1 year.

Vasodilators also had beneficial effects on lipid profile with reduction in total and LDL cholesterol and increases in serum HDL cholesterol [8, 28]. These agents also blunted the increase in TGs with use of β-blockers and selectively decreased TGs in black populations [28]. Many studies, however, reported vasodilators to be lipid neutral rather than beneficial [28].

CENTRAL α-2 AGONISTS

The effects of central sympatholytics strongly correlated with the use of two drugs (guanafacine and guanabenz) and were limited to decrease in total cholesterol and, to some extent, HDL cholesterol. No significant effects on lipids were seen with other agents of this class [28]. However, in one study, clonidine was associated with decrease in HDL_2 at 1 year [29].

Angiotensin-converting enzyme inhibitors were associated with decreases in total cholesterol, particularly in the diabetic population [8, 28]. There is also a reduction in TGs. This reduction in TG correlated with baseline levels and was more pronounced in younger subjects. Most other studies, however, report ACE-I as having a neutral effect on serum lipids [8, 28, 29].

Calcium channel blockers were also reported as lipid neutral in the meta-analysis by Kasiske and colleagues as well as many other studies [8, 28, 29].

Although effect on lipid profile was demonstrated with use of the various antihypertensive medications, blood pressure correlated weakly with total cholesterol and LDL cholesterol and there was no correlation observed with TGs and HDL cholesterol values [7, 28].

INTENSIVE BEHAVIOURAL MODIFICATION

An important factor which can modify the adverse lipid effects of antihypertensive agents is intensive behavioural modification. In the Treatment of Mild Hypertension Study (TOMHS), the long-term plasma lipid changes with antihypertensive treatment including six different agents in combination with intensive behavioural therapy were examined [6]. In subjects with mild hypertension, the degree of weight loss was significantly related to favourable lipid changes. Doxazosin, an α-blocker, was associated with significant decreases in total and LDL cholesterol and TGs, and increase in HDL cholesterol. Acebutalol was associated with decreases in total and LDL cholesterol though the reduction in TGs and increase in HDL was not as significant as with other agents [6]. In this study, enalapril, an ACE inhibitor, was associated with significant decrease in TGs and increase in HDL cholesterol. Chlorthalidone, a thiazide diuretic, was associated with significantly high plasma cholesterol compared with placebo at 12 months but the difference was not significant at 24 months. Many of these beneficial effects could be potentially related to weight loss and behavioural modification. Overall, α-blocker therapy was associated with maximum metabolic benefits [6]. Therefore, behavioural modifications with diet and weight loss appear to significantly influence the lipid modifying effects of antihypertensive agents.

MAGNITUDE OF CHANGE IN LIPID PROFILES WITH THE USE OF VARIOUS ANTIHYPERTENSIVE AGENTS

Although the effect of various antihypertensive medications on lipid metabolism has been shown in several studies, the magnitude of such an effect has only been demonstrated in a few analyses [8, 28]. In the meta-analysis by Kasiske and colleagues the effects of antihypertensive agents were class dependent [28]. Adverse effects on lipids were observed with use of diuretics and β-blockers, particularly those with non-selective β-blocking properties compared to the agents with cardioselectivity and ISA [8, 28]. On the other hand, beneficial lipid effects were reported with the use of α-blockers, ACE inhibitors and vasodilators. Calcium channel blockers and central sympatholytics (other than guanfacine and guanabenz) were mostly lipid neutral [8, 28] (Table 5.2).

In the Systolic Hypertension in Elderly Program (SHEP) study including 4736 men and women above 59 years, active therapy with chlorthalidone with or without atenolol/reserpine was compared to placebo and effects on lipids were examined after 3 years [34]. Only mild lipid effects were observed with increases of 0.09 mmol/l and 0.9 mmol/l in total cholesterol and TGs respectively. In this study, HDL cholesterol also decreased by 0.03 mmol/l after 3 years of active treatment [34]. Although the effect on various lipid parameters appears small, the significance of these observations is not. It has been estimated that a 0.03 mmol/l (1 mg/dl) increase in HDL is associated with a significant 4–5% reduction in the number of deaths from CVD. Similarly, reduction in LDL cholesterol by 1 mg/dl is estimated to reduce CHD risk by 1% [35]. Conversely, small increases in total or LDL cholesterol and TGs may translate into significant increase in adverse CVD outcomes [36]. Therefore, these small changes in lipids associated with antihypertensive agents are potentially clinically relevant and have to be considered in terms of overall effects of antihypertensive agents on CVD outcomes. In contrast, another recent study did not show any significant effects on lipids with antihypertensive therapy except for reductions in HDL_2 with diuretics, β-blockers and clonidine [29]. However, validity of the results of this study is limited by potential selection bias and hence, their findings cannot be generalized [37].

Table 5.2 Magnitude of effect of different antihypertensive agents on serum lipids (based on analysis by Kasiske and colleagues [28])

Medication	*Change in total cholesterol mmol/l (mg/dl)*	*Change in LDL cholesterol mmol/dl (mg/dl)*	*Change in TGs mmol/l (mg/dl)*	*Change in HDL cholesterol mmol/l (mg/dl)*	**Comments**
Diuretics	0.13 (5)	0.15–0.19* (5.8–7.35)*	0.10 (8.88)	−0.02 (−0.77)	*In blacks and at high dose
β-blockers					
Non-selective	NS	NS	0.35 (31)	−0.10 (−3.87)	
β-1-selective	NS	NS	0.11 (9.8)	−0.07 (−2.7)	
ISA	−0.14 (−5.4)	−0.17 (−6.6)	NS	NS	
α-blockers	−0.23 (−8.9)	−0.20 (−7.7)	−0.07 (−6.2)	0.02 (0.77)	
ACE-I	−0.22 (−8.5)*	NS	−0.07 (−6.2)**	NS	*In diabetes **With high baseline TG level
Vasodilators	−0.22 (−8.5)	−0.22 (−8.5)	NS	0.06 (2.32)	
Central sympatholytics	−0.21 (−8.1)*	NS	NS	−0.04 (−1.5)*	*Seen with guanfacine and guanabenz only

ACE-I = angiotensin-converting enzyme inhibitor; HDL = high density lipoprotein; ISA = intrinsic sympathomimetic activity; LDL = low density lipoprotein; NS = not significant; TG = triglycerides.

MECHANISTIC INSIGHTS INTO THE EFFECTS OF ANTIHYPERTENSIVE THERAPY ON LIPID METABOLISM

Evidence evolving from recently conducted trials along with basic science experiments have helped shed some light on the mechanistic insights of the metabolic effects of various antihypertensive agents. Among these metabolic changes are effects on lipid profile, at least in part. Several general mechanisms have been proposed to explain the effects of antihypertensive agents on plasma lipids (Table 5.3). These include, but are not limited to, effects on insulin sensitivity, alteration of α and β receptor mediated autonomic activity and effects on haemodynamics and body composition.

EFFECTS ON INSULIN SENSITIVITY

Insulin sensitivity is an important determinant of lipoprotein metabolism and alteration in tissue insulin sensitivity may result in significant changes in plasma lipoprotein profile [21]. Antihypertensive agents that improve insulin sensitivity such as α-adrenergic-blockers, vasodilators and ACE inhibitors tend to have beneficial effects on plasma lipoproteins whereas diuretics and β-blockers which are associated with decrease in insulin sensitivity may cause worsening of plasma lipoproteins [8]. Resistance of adipocytes to insulin action results in increased FFA flux to the liver as well as suppression of post-prandial adipocyte FFA sequestration [8]. This increase in FFA availability to the liver results in increased VLDL and TG synthesis [8, 21]. Furthermore, insulin resistance is associated with reduced

Table 5.3 Mechanism of lipid modifying effects of various antihypertensive agents

Antihypertensive class	*Metabolic effect*
Diuretics	■ Hypokalaemia-mediated blunting of pancreatic insulin secretion ■ Worsening of insulin resistance and increased risk of new diabetes ■ Hypovolaemia-mediated sympathetic system stimulation ■ Altered sodium balance with reflex stimulation of renin–angiotensin–aldosterone system
β-blockers	■ ↓ First phase insulin secretion with ↑ second phase insulin secretion ■ Weight gain with worsening insulin resistance ■ Increased risk of new diabetes ■ ↓ Basal energy expenditure and thermogenic response to food ■ ↓ Skeletal LPL activity and LCAT activity ■ ↓ LDL particle size to smaller, denser more atherogenic type
α-blockers	■ ↑ Insulin sensitivity ■ ↑ Capillary recruitment and preferential shunting of blood flow to insulin sensitive skeletal muscle fibres ■ ↑ LPL & LCAT activity ■ ↑ TG clearance mediated by hepatic α-receptors
Central α-2 agonists	Central modulation of adrenergic activity
ACE inhibitors	↑ Insulin sensitivity/metabolically neutral
Vasodilators	■ ↑ Capillary recruitment and preferential shunting of blood flow to insulin sensitive skeletal muscle fibres
Calcium channel blockers	■ Metabolically neutral

ACE = angiotensin-converting enzyme; LCAT = lecithin cholesterol acyltransferase; LDL = low density lipoprotein; LPL = lipoprotein lipase; TG = triglycerides.

lipoprotein lipase (LPL) activity in skeletal muscles and adipocytes resulting in decreased clearance of TG-rich lipoprotein (TL) [8]. Moreover, blunting of insulin-mediated vasodilatation further reduces the clearance of TL by decreasing the delivery of post-prandial nutrient-rich plasma to target tissues for LPL action [8]. In the meta-analysis by Kasiske and colleagues positive correlation was observed between changes in fasting blood sugar as well as glycated haemoglobin (HbA1c) and various lipid fractions including total cholesterol, LDL cholesterol, HDL cholesterol and TGs. In general, the changes in lipids paralleled changes in fasting glucose [28].

ALTERATION OF AUTONOMIC ACTIVITY

Increase in α-adrenergic tone is associated with altered nutrient blood flow and reduced hepatic clearance of TL [8]. α-Blockers may favourably improve the microcirculatory haemodynamics and insulin sensitivity with increased clearance of TL [8]. α-blocking agents are also associated with increased lecithin cholesterol acyltransferase activity (LCAT) and elevated HDL cholesterol whereas β-blockers decrease LCAT activity resulting in reduction in HDL cholesterol [8]. Blockade of β-adrenergic receptors is further associated with reduced skeletal muscle LPL activity and inhibition of adipocyte lipolysis with reduction in FFA levels and hepatic VLDL secretion [8].

HAEMODYNAMIC CHANGES AND BODY HABITUS

β-blocker therapy is associated with weight gain and may increase abdominal adiposity with worsening of insulin resistance and dyslipidaemia [8]. Diuretics may be associated with hypovolaemia with reflex stimulation of the renin–angiotensin–aldosterone and sympathetic systems which could also cause decrease in insulin sensitivity and worsen plasma lipoproteins [8].

Diuretics: Diuretics have been reported to decrease insulin sensitivity and are associated with increased risk of development of new diabetes [30]. Low HDL with diuretic use is seen in patients with diabetes, thereby suggesting a role for insulin resistance [28]. Furthermore, hypokalaemia associated with diuretic use is known to cause blunting of pancreatic insulin secretion and impaired glucose tolerance. However, lipid abnormalities with diuretic use have also been reported despite maintenance of normal potassium levels [8].

Diuretics can also influence the sympathetic adrenergic system to cause alterations in lipid metabolism [8]. It is likely that altered sodium balance and hypovolaemia associated with diuretic use may cause activation of the sympathetic nervous system with increased β-adrenergic-mediated lipolysis and α-adrenergic-mediated microcirculatory changes with resultant hyperlipidaemia [8, 38]. This hypothesis is further supported by the fact that adverse lipid effects are seen primarily with higher doses of diuretics which are more likely to cause altered sodium balance and reflex sympathetic activity [8, 28].

β-blockers: Like diuretics, antihypertensive agents with β-adrenergic receptor blocking properties have also been demonstrated to increase the risk of new diabetes [8, 31]. The hyperlipidaemia associated with β-blockers (↑TG, ↓HDL) has a similar pattern to that seen in insulin resistance suggesting a possible link between these conditions.

β-blockers have been demonstrated to reduce first phase insulin secretion as well as insulin clearance, while increasing second phase insulin secretion resulting in hyperinsulinaemia and insulin resistance [8]. Furthermore, weight gain associated with β-blocker therapy may also contribute to lipid abnormalities by promoting visceral fat accumulation and insulin resistance [39]. This effect is likely mediated by reductions in basal energy expenditure and thermogenic response to food [39]. β-blockers can also reduce skeletal LPL and LCAT activity resulting in low HDL levels [8]. Moreover, β-blocker therapy has also been reported to shift the LDL particle size to a more atherogenic smaller, denser phenotype which increases the risk of CVD [8]. One study reported increased HDL cholesterol and decreased TGs with carvedilol, a non-selective β- and α-1 receptor blocker compared with a cardioselective agent, atenolol [40]. Therefore, agents with ISA or those with combined β- and α-receptor blocking activity may have relatively beneficial effects as compared with non-selective β-blockers [28].

α-blockers: α-adrenergic receptor blockers are associated with beneficial effects on plasma lipoproteins with reduction in TGs and increase in HDL cholesterol by increasing insulin sensitivity [8]. These effects may be mediated by blockade of α-adrenergic receptors with increase in capillary recruitment and shunting of blood flow towards skeletal muscle fibres with higher insulin sensitivity and LPL activity [8]. α-adrenergic blockade may also increase HDL by stimulating LCAT activity. Alteration of α-receptors in hepatic vessels may increase catabolism of TL. This improves insulin-mediated glucose disposal and TL clearance with resultant decreases in TG and other lipoprotein parameters [8]. One study reported improvement in insulin sensitivity, increase in LPL activity and decrease in serum TG levels with doxazosin [41]. The authors of this study also observed a strong correlation between increase in LPL activity and decrease in serum TG, thereby suggesting that increase in LPL activity could explain increase in TG catabolism [41].

CENTRAL SYMPATHOLYTICS

Central α-2 receptor agonists have sympatholytic activity and may be associated with beneficial effects on lipids by modulating α-adrenergic tone [8].

ACE INHIBITORS

In the Heart Outcomes Prevention Evaluation (HOPE) study, incidence of new diabetes was lower in the ramipril group compared to placebo, suggesting a possible role for ACE inhibitors in diabetes prevention [42]. This is being further studied in the ongoing Diabetes Reduction with Ramipril and Rosiglitazone Medications (DREAM) study to ascertain the role of ramipril and rosiglitazone, a thiazolidinedione, in diabetes prevention [43]. In general, ACE inhibitors tend to be lipid neutral and are not associated with significant adverse effects on lipids although captopril has been reported to increase insulin sensitivity [8, 28].

CALCIUM CHANNEL BLOCKERS (CCB)

In general, CCBs are metabolically neutral and are not associated with any significant effects on insulin sensitivity or lipid profile [8, 28]. The lack of beneficial lipids effects with CCB and ACE inhibitors despite vasodilating properties may be related to more generalized vascular effects without preferential shunting of blood flow to more insulin sensitive tissues [8].

CLINICAL IMPLICATIONS OF THE LIPID ABNORMALITIES ASSOCIATED WITH USE OF ANTIHYPERTENSIVE AGENTS

After examining the effects of various antihypertensive agents on plasma lipoproteins, an important question that remains to be answered is 'Are these effects clinically relevant?' Evidence from the Framingham study indicates that, for the same amount of blood pressure reduction, agents that adversely affect lipids may cause less reduction in CVD [7]. As mentioned previously, the improvement in CHD mortality with antihypertensive agents, mostly including diuretics and β-blockers, was less than expected from the level of blood pressure reduction, thereby suggesting that adverse metabolic effects of these agents could be responsible for this apparent discrepancy [7, 44]. Many studies have reported a lack of significant benefits in terms of CVD outcome with β-blockers [45, 46]. In a meta-analysis of several trials including >16 000 patients above the age of 60 years, no significant reduction in cardiovascular and all-cause mortality with β-blocker therapy compared with placebo was observed [46]. In the MRC trial in the elderly, β-blocker therapy was associated with no significant benefit over placebo and a paradoxical increase in CVD outcomes was observed after adding β-blockers to diuretic therapy [47]. In the Helsinki Businessmen Study, increased CHD mortality in the active treatment group with use of β-blocker (pindolol) was observed [7]. A recent meta-analysis indicated that treatment of primary hypertension with β-blockers is associated with substantially higher risk of stroke than treatment with other antihypertensive agents [45]. In fact, long-term therapy with β-blockers has been linked with increased risk of diabetes [31]. This, combined with β-blocker-induced weight gain as well as worsening of insulin resistance and serum lipids, puts the utility of β-blockers in preventing CVD into question [46, 48]. Similarly, diuretic therapy has been associated with a significant increase in CHD mortality compared to placebo in subjects with minor abnormalities in baseline ECG in the Multiple Risk Factor Intervention Trial (MRFIT) [49]. To what extent these metabolic effects of the diuretics and β-blocker therapy on serum lipids are responsible for adverse CVD outcomes is largely unknown. On the other hand, treatment with antihypertensive agents with beneficial effects on lipids (α-blockers) or lipid neutral agents as CCB has not been shown to be significantly advantageous compared to treatment with diuretics or β-blockers. In the ALLHAT trial, a large randomized, double-blind, active-controlled clinical trial comparing conventional treatment with diuretics (chlorthalidone) with ACE inhibitor (lisinopril), CCB (amlodipine) and α-blocker (doxazosin), chlorthalidone was superior to doxazosin in reducing BP and preventing CVD events, particularly heart failure [30]. Neither lisinopril nor amlodipine was superior to chlorthalidone in preventing major coronary events or in increasing survival. This was despite an increase in cholesterol and higher incidence of new diabetes in the chlorthalidone group compared to the lisinopril and amlodipine groups [30]. Chlorthalidone was superior to amlodipine in preventing heart failure and to lisinopril in lowering BP and preventing aggregate CVD events including stroke, heart failure, angina and coronary revascularization [30]. Therefore, despite adverse effects on lipids and higher risk of diabetes, a diuretic based therapy was equivalent in terms of CVD prevention and superior in terms of heart failure prevention compared to ACE inhibitors and CCB. Furthermore, α-blocker therapy was not as effective and was actually detrimental compared to diuretic therapy in spite of having significant beneficial effects on lipids in many studies [30].

The STOP Hypertension-2 study, a prospective randomized trial, compared effects of older antihypertensive agents (β-blockers and diuretics) to the newer agents (CCB – isradipine and felodipine and ACE inhibitors – enalapril and lisinopril) on CVD mortality in elderly patients with hypertension [50]. The ACE inhibitors and CCB had efficacy similar to conventional therapy in preventing CVD outcomes [50]. In the SHEP and the Systolic Hypertension in Europe (Syst Eur) trials comparing chlorthalidone and dihydropyridine-CCB with placebo respectively, similar reductions in major CHD outcomes were observed [3, 5]. Therefore, it is apparent that despite absence of significant lipid effects, treatment with CCB and ACE inhibitors is not superior to conventional treatment with diuretics and β-blockers.

SUMMARY

The authors conclude that adverse effects on lipid metabolism associated with the use of β-blocker and diuretics do not seem to translate into measurable cardiovascular endpoints. Furthermore, beneficial effects of α-blockade on lipid profile did not afford any benefits in terms of cardiovascular risk reduction. In fact, in the largest hypertension trial ever conducted, the α-blocker arm was terminated prematurely due to increased cardiovascular events compared to chlorthalidone which decreased cardiovascular events despite adverse effects [30].

We further conclude that unless long-term trials with cardiovascular endpoints are conducted to specifically examine the effects of the antihypertensive agents on lipid metabolism, the current evidence does not suggest adverse long-term cardiovascular effects with the use of these agents in the recommended dosages. Importantly, the clinicians should focus more on achieving the target blood pressure recommended for different groups of patients according to their risk profile [1]. Blood pressure control has been shown to be largely suboptimal despite clear evidence to the CVD benefits achieved with blood pressure reduction [51].

ACKNOWLEDGMENT

This work is supported by grants from the National Institute of Health (USA) # K12HD043428, BIRCWH and also by grant support from the American Diabetes Association, 7-05-RA-89, to SIM.

REFERENCES

1. Chobanian AV, Bakris GL, Black HR *et al.* The seventh report of the joint national committee on prevention, detection, evaluation, and treatment of high blood pressure: the JNC 7 report. *JAMA* 2003; 289:2560–2572.
2. Hyman DJ, Pavlik VN. Characteristics of patients with uncontrolled hypertension in the United States. *N Engl J Med* 2001; 345:479–486.
3. SCR Group. Prevention of stroke by antihypertensive drug treatment in older persons with isolated systolic hypertension. Final results of the systolic hypertension in the elderly program (SHEP). SHEP Cooperative Research Group. *JAMA* 1991; 265:3255–3264.
4. Curb JD, Pressel SL, Cutler JA *et al.* Effect of diuretic-based antihypertensive treatment on cardiovascular disease risk in older diabetic patients with isolated systolic hypertension. Systolic Hypertension in the Elderly Program Cooperative Research Group. *JAMA* 1996; 276:1886–1892.

5. Staessen JA, Fagard R, Thijs L *et al.* Randomised double-blind comparison of placebo and active treatment for older patients with isolated systolic hypertension. The Systolic Hypertension in Europe (Syst-Eur) Trial Investigators. *Lancet* 1997; 350:757–764.
6. Neaton JD, Grimm RH Jr, Prineas RJ *et al.* Treatment of Mild Hypertension Study. Final results. Treatment of Mild Hypertension Study Research Group. *JAMA* 1993; 270:713–724.
7. Manttari M, Tenkanen L, Manninen V, Alikoski T, Frick MH. Antihypertensive therapy in dyslipidemic men. Effects on coronary heart disease incidence and total mortality. *Hypertension* 1995; 25:47–52.
8. Brook RD. Mechanism of differential effects of antihypertensive agents on serum lipids. *Curr Hypertens Rep* 2000; 2:370–377.
9. Lloyd-Jones DM, Evans JC, Larson MG, O'Donnell CJ, Wilson PW, Levy D. Cross-classification of JNC VI blood pressure stages and risk groups in the Framingham Heart Study. *Arch Intern Med* 1999; 159:2206–2212.
10. MacMahon SW, Macdonald GJ, Blacket RB. Plasma lipoprotein levels in treated and untreated hypertensive men and women. The National Heart Foundation of Australia Risk Factor Prevalence Study. *Arteriosclerosis* 1985; 5:391–396.
11. Goode GK, Miller JP, Heagerty AM. Hyperlipidaemia, hypertension, and coronary heart disease. *Lancet* 1995; 345:362–364.
12. Williams RR, Hunt SC, Hopkins PN *et al.* Familial dyslipidemic hypertension. Evidence from 58 Utah families for a syndrome present in approximately 12% of patients with essential hypertension. *JAMA* 1988; 259:3579–3586.
13. Selby JV, Newman B, Quiroga J, Christian JC, Austin MA, Fabsitz RR. Concordance for dyslipidemic hypertension in male twins. *JAMA* 1991; 265:2079–2084.
14. Assmann G, Schulte H. The Prospective Cardiovascular Munster Study: prevalence and prognostic significance of hyperlipidaemia in men with systemic hypertension. *Am J Cardiol* 1987; 59:9G–17G.
15. Flesch M, Sachinidis A, Ko YD, Kraft K, Vetter H. Plasma lipids and lipoproteins and essential hypertension. *Clin Investig* 1994; 72:944–950.
16. Catalano M, Aronica A, Carzaniga G, Seregni R, Libretti A. Serum lipids and apolipoproteins in patients with essential hypertension. *Atherosclerosis* 1991; 87:17–22.
17. Orbetzova V, Kiprov D, Puchlev A. The action of arterial hypertension on lipid and lipoprotein metabolism. II. Qualitative and quantitative alterations of blood serum, liver and aortic lipids and lipoproteins in Okamoto-Aoki rats with spontaneous hypertension. *Cor Vasa* 1976; 18:221–232.
18. Pearson TA, Laurora I, Chu H, Kafonek S. The lipid treatment assessment project (L-TAP): a multicenter survey to evaluate the percentages of dyslipidemic patients receiving lipid-lowering therapy and achieving low-density lipoprotein cholesterol goals. *Arch Intern Med* 2000; 160: 459–467.
19. Sowers JR. Update on the cardiometabolic syndrome. *Clin Cornerstone* 2001; 4:17–23.
20. Castro JP, El-Atat FA, McFarlane SI, Aneja A, Sowers JR. Cardiometabolic syndrome: pathophysiology and treatment. *Curr Hypertens Rep* 2003; 5:393–401.
21. McFarlane SI, Banerji M, Sowers JR. Insulin resistance and cardiovascular disease. *J Clin Endocrinol Metab* 2001; 86:713–718.
22. Pelat M, Balligand JL. Statins and hypertension. *Semin Vasc Med* 2004; 4:367–375.
23. McFarlane SI, Kumar A, Sowers JR. Mechanisms by which angiotensin-converting enzyme inhibitors prevent diabetes and cardiovascular disease. *Am J Cardiol* 2003; 91:30H–37H.
24. Luscher TF, Dohi Y, Tanner FC, Boulanger C. Endothelium-dependent control of vascular tone: effects of age, hypertension and lipids. *Basic Res Cardiol* 1991; 86(suppl 2):143–158.
25. Jagla A, Schrezenmeir J. Postprandial triglycerides and endothelial function. *Exp Clin Endocrinol Diabetes* 2001; 109:S533–S547.
26. Sander GE, Giles TD. Hypertension and lipids: lipid factors in the hypertension syndrome. *Curr Hypertens Rep* 2002; 4:458–463.
27. McFarlane SI, Muniyappa R, Francisco R, Sowers JR. Clinical review 145: pleiotropic effects of statins: lipid reduction and beyond. *J Clin Endocrinol Metab* 2002; 87:1451–1458.
28. Kasiske BL, Ma JZ, Kalil RS, Louis TA. Effects of antihypertensive therapy on serum lipids. *Ann Intern Med* 1995; 122:133–141.
29. Lakshman MR, Reda DJ, Materson BJ, Cushman WC, Freis ED. Department of Veterans Affairs Cooperative Study Group on Antihypertensive Agents. Diuretics and beta-blockers do not have adverse effects at 1 year on plasma lipid and lipoprotein profiles in men with hypertension. *Arch Intern Med* 1999; 159:551–558.

30. ALLHAT. Major outcomes in high-risk hypertensive patients randomized to angiotensin-converting enzyme inhibitor or calcium channel blocker vs diuretic: The Antihypertensive and Lipid-Lowering Treatment to Prevent Heart Attack Trial (ALLHAT). *JAMA* 2002; 288:2981–2997.
31. Gress TW, Nieto FJ, Shahar E, Wofford MR, Brancati FL. Hypertension and antihypertensive therapy as risk factors for type 2 diabetes mellitus. Atherosclerosis risk in communities study. *N Engl J Med* 2000; 342:905–912.
32. Strickland D, Sprafka JM, Luepker RV, Grimm RH Jr. Association of antihypertensive agents and blood lipids in a population-based survey. *Epidemiology* 1994; 5:96–101.
33. Nanchahal K, Ashton WD, Wood DA: Association between blood pressure, the treatment of hypertension, and cardiovascular risk factors in women. *J Hypertens* 2000; 18:833–841.
34. Savage PJ, Pressel SL, Curb JD *et al.* SHEP Cooperative Research Group. Influence of long-term, low-dose, diuretic-based, antihypertensive therapy on glucose, lipid, uric acid, and potassium levels in older men and women with isolated systolic hypertension: the systolic hypertension in the elderly program. *Arch Intern Med* 1998; 158:741–751.
35. TNCE Program: Executive Summary of The Third Report of The National Cholesterol Education Program (NCEP) Expert Panel on Detection, Evaluation, And Treatment of High Blood Cholesterol In Adults (Adult Treatment Panel III). *JAMA* 2001; 285:2486–2497.
36. Peters AL, Hsueh W. Antihypertensive agents in diabetic patients: great benefits, special risks. *Arch Intern Med* 1999; 159:541–542.
37. Golomb BA, Criqui MH. Antihypertensives: much ado about lipids. *Arch Intern Med* 1999; 159:535–537.
38. Weidmann P, de Courten M, Ferrari P. Effect of diuretics on the plasma lipid profile. *Eur Heart J* 1992; 13(suppl G):61–67.
39. Sharma AM, Pischon T, Hardt S, Kunz I, Luft FC. Hypothesis: Beta-adrenergic receptor blockers and weight gain: a systematic analysis. *Hypertension* 2001; 37:250–254.
40. Giugliano D, Acampora R, Marfella R *et al.* Metabolic and cardiovascular effects of carvedilol and atenolol in non-insulin-dependent diabetes mellitus and hypertension. A randomized, controlled trial. *Ann Intern Med* 1997; 126:955–959.
41. Andersson PE, Lithell H. Metabolic effects of doxazosin and enalapril in hypertriglyceridemic, hypertensive men. Relationship to changes in skeletal muscle blood flow. *Am J Hypertens* 1996; 9:323–333.
42. Yusuf S, Sleight P, Pogue J, Bosch J, Davies R, Dagenais G. The Heart Outcomes Prevention Evaluation Study Investigators. Effects of an angiotensin-converting-enzyme inhibitor, ramipril, on cardiovascular events in high-risk patients. *N Engl J Med* 2000; 342:145–153.
43. Gerstein HC, Yusuf S, Holman R, Bosch J, Pogue J. Rationale, design and recruitment characteristics of a large, simple international trial of diabetes prevention: the DREAM trial. *Diabetologia* 2004; 47:1519–1527.
44. Collins R, Peto R, MacMahon S *et al.* Blood pressure, stroke, and coronary heart disease. Part 2, Short-term reductions in blood pressure: overview of randomised drug trials in their epidemiological context. *Lancet* 1990; 335:827–838.
45. Lindholm LH, Carlberg B, Samuelsson O. Should beta blockers remain first choice in the treatment of primary hypertension? A meta-analysis. *Lancet* 2005; 366:1545–1553.
46. Messerli FH, Grossman E, Goldbourt U. Are beta-blockers efficacious as first-line therapy for hypertension in the elderly? A systematic review. *JAMA* 1998; 279:1903–1907.
47. MRC Working Party. Medical Research Council trial of treatment of hypertension in older adults: principal results. *BMJ* 1992; 304:405–412.
48. Messerli FH. The LIFE study: the straw that should break the camel's back. *Eur Heart J* 2003; 24:487–489.
49. MRFIT: Multiple Risk Factor Intervention Trial Research Group. Baseline rest electrocardiographic abnormalities, antihypertensive treatment, and mortality in the Multiple Risk Factor Intervention Trial. *Am J Cardiol* 1985; 55:1–15.
50. Hansson L, Lindholm LH, Ekbom T *et al.* Randomised trial of old and new antihypertensive drugs in elderly patients: cardiovascular mortality and morbidity in the Swedish Trial in Old Patients with Hypertension-2 study. *Lancet* 1999; 354:1751–1756.
51. Staessen JA, Wang JG, Thijs L. Cardiovascular protection and blood pressure reduction: a meta-analysis. *Lancet* 2001; 358:1305–1315.

6

How strong is the evidence for a blood pressure goal of less than 130/80 mmHg for the high-risk patient?

A. Rashidi, M. Rahman

Hypertension is the most important preventable cause of premature death [1]. The benefits of antihypertensive therapy for prevention of cardiovascular and renal mortality and morbidity are well known [2, 3]. Blood pressure values of less than 140/90 mmHg have been the traditional goals in the management of hypertension. These thresholds are best supported by data from the Multiple Risk Factor Intervention Trial (MRFIT) 10-year follow-up report; although cardiovascular disease (CVD) risk was continuous across the spectrum of blood pressure levels, relatively clear changes in the slope of the lines depicting CVD risk in treated hypertensives were evident around the 140 and 90 mmHg points [4]. However, there are selected populations of hypertensive patients who are high risk, and may benefit from a lower blood pressure goal. Diabetic patients and patients with chronic kidney disease are two such groups identified by several national guidelines to target for lower blood pressure goals (<130/80 mmHg, Table 6.1) [5–7]. These guidelines are based on epidemiologic data showing the relationship between hypertension and renal/cardiovascular outcomes, and clinical trial data showing a beneficial effect of lower blood pressure levels on prevention of renal disease and CVD. The purpose of this review is to critically examine the epidemiologic and clinical trial evidence supporting the benefit of lower blood pressure goals in these high risk patients.

CHRONIC KIDNEY DISEASE

Chronic kidney disease is a very common condition; it is estimated that in the US there are over 10 million individuals with chronic kidney disease [8]. This population is at high risk for progression to end-stage renal disease, and also, as is being increasingly recognized, for development of CVD [8]. Hypertension is a well known risk factor for progression of renal disease, and for CVD. Therefore, treatment of hypertension is an integral component of the care of the patient with chronic kidney disease. Most guidelines recommend the use of angiotensin-converting enzyme (ACE) inhibitors and blood pressure goals of <130/80 mmHg in these patients. We will review the evidence supporting the efficacy of a low blood pressure goal for preventing renal and cardiovascular outcomes in patients with chronic kidney disease.

Arash Rashidi, MD, Fellow, Division of Nephrology and Hypertension, Case Western Reserve University, University Hospitals of Cleveland, Cleveland VA Medical Center, Cleveland, Ohio, USA

Mahboob Rahman, MD, MS, Associate Professor of Medicine, Division of Nephrology and Hypertension, Case Western Reserve University, University Hospitals of Cleveland, Cleveland VA Medical Center, Cleveland, Ohio, USA

Table 6.1 Current national guideline recommendations for target blood pressure in patients with diabetes and chronic kidney disease

Guideline	*Blood pressure treatment goal in diabetic patients*	*Blood pressure treatment goal in chronic kidney disease patients*
Australian Hypertension Management Guide [37]	<130/85 mmHg	<130/85 mmHg and if proteinuria is more than 1 g/day the BP goal is <125/75 mmHg
Canadian recommendations for the management of hypertension [38]	<130/80 mmHg	130/80 mmHg and if proteinuria is more than 1 g/day the BP goal is <125/75 mmHg
European Society of Hypertension–European Society of Cardiology [34]	<130/80 mmHg	Not mentioned
The British Hypertension Society Guidelines [7]	<130/80 mmHg	Not mentioned
The Seventh Report of the Joint National Committee (JNC7) [5]	<130/80 mmHg	<130/80 mmHg
World Health Organization (WHO)/International Society of Hypertension (ISH) statement on management of hypertension [6]	<130/80 mmHg	<130/80 mmHg

RENAL OUTCOMES

The relationship between hypertension and progression of kidney disease is well established [9]. In addition, the presence of hypertension accelerates decline in renal function regardless of the primary aetiology of renal disease. Epidemiologic data suggest that the increased risk of renal dysfunction starts in the 'high normal' range of blood pressure. In a long-term follow-up of participants screened for the MRFIT study, patients with a systolic blood pressure (SBP) in the 130–139 range were almost twice as likely to develop end-stage renal disease compared to those with a SBP <120 mmHg [10]. Given the strong epidemiologic data suggesting a renoprotective effect of lower levels of blood pressure, several prospective clinical trials directly comparing a low to usual blood pressure group have been conducted. The African American Study of Kidney Disease and Hypertension (AASK) Study was a randomized, double-blind multicentre study that enrolled 1194 hypertensive African-American patients with a glomerular filtration rate (GFR) between 20 and 65 ml/min/1.73 m^2, and no other known cause of renal disease [11]. Patients with diabetes, urinary protein to creatinine ratio greater than 2.5, clinical congestive heart failure, or serious systemic disease were excluded. In a factorial design, participants were randomized to a usual mean arterial pressure goal of 102–107 mmHg ($n = 554$) or to a lower mean arterial pressure goal of 92 mmHg or lower ($n = 540$), and to treatment with one of three antihypertensive drugs (a sustained-release β-blocker, metoprolol, 50–200 mg/day; an ACE inhibitor, ramipril, 2.5–10 mg/day; or a dihydropyridine calcium channel blocker, amlodipine, 5–10 mg/day). The mean age of the study population was 54 years, and 38% were female with a mean baseline GFR of 46 ml/min/1.73 m^2. There were no significant differences in clinical characteristics between the usual and low blood pressure groups at baseline. After randomization, blood pressure decreased from 152/96 to 128/78 mmHg in the lower blood pressure group and from 149/95 to 141/85 mmHg in the usual blood pressure goal group resulting in a mean separation of approximately 10 mmHg mean arterial pressure throughout most of the follow-up period. Despite this degree of separation of blood pressure, the mean rate of decline in GFR did not differ significantly between the lower and usual blood pressure groups over the total follow-up period from baseline to 4 years (2.21 [0.17] vs. 1.95 [0.17] ml/min/1.73 m^2/year; $P = 0.24$). Similarly, there was no difference in the incidence of end-stage renal disease, 50% decline in GFR, death, or a composite of these events between the two blood pressure groups. There was a trend for greater benefit of the lower blood pressure goal in patients with higher baseline proteinuria, but this did not reach statistical significance. The only beneficial effect of the lower blood pressure goal that could be demonstrated was that proteinuria increased by 7% in the usual blood pressure group and decreased by 17% in the lower blood pressure group during the first 6 months; these differences between treatment groups persisted throughout the study. There were no differences in adverse effects or cardiovascular outcomes between the two blood pressure arms. In summary, the AASK study demonstrated that despite a 10 mmHg lower mean arterial pressure, the low blood pressure group did not benefit with regard to decline in GFR, end-stage renal disease, or death during the 4-year follow-up period. However, patients assigned to the lower blood pressure goal had lower levels of proteinuria during the course of the study. This finding is important in the context of recent data implicating proteinuria not only as a marker, but as a mediator of progressive renal injury [12]. Another aspect of the AASK study that may have influenced the blood pressure comparison is the fact that the rate of decline in GFR in the study as a whole was relatively low (−2 ml/min/1.73 m^2/year). It is possible that patients with a more rapid decline in GFR may see a greater benefit of lower blood pressure. On the other hand, epidemiologic studies may overestimate the effect of blood pressure on decline in GFR compared with that seen in clinical trials.

It is possible that the beneficial effects of the lower blood pressure manifest initially as lower levels of proteinuria, raising speculation that with a longer duration of follow-up, clinically apparent benefits may be derived. The need for a longer duration of follow-up is supported by the Modification of Diet in Renal Disease (MDRD) study and its long-term follow-up; participants with predominantly non-diabetic renal disease assigned to the low blood pressure goal (mean arterial pressure <92 mmHg) did not benefit with regard to decline in GFR or clinical renal events over the course of the 3-year follow-up compared with those assigned to the usual blood pressure goal (mean arterial pressure 107) [13]. However, the difference in mean blood pressure between the usual-pressure and the low-pressure groups during the study was relatively small (4.7 mmHg), and a beneficial effect of low blood pressure on decline in GFR could be demonstrated only in the subset of patients with proteinuria greater than 1 g/day at baseline. The recent report of the long-term follow-up of the MDRD participants suggests that the low blood pressure goal may be associated with clinical benefit after several years of follow-up [14]. After the conclusion of the study in 1993, participants returned to their usual providers with no specific recommendations for a level of blood pressure or choice of antihypertensive drug therapy. No information about the blood pressure control or antihypertensive drug therapy was available after the conclusion of the study. Kidney failure outcomes were ascertained through the United States Renal Data System in 2000, allowing median follow-up of 10.7 years. At this point in follow-up, participants assigned to the low target blood pressure had a 32% lower risk for kidney failure (95% confidence internal [CI] 0.57–0.82) and 23% lower risk for a composite of kidney failure or death (95% CI 0.65–0.91). These data suggest that lower blood pressure targets may result in improved clinical outcomes that are demonstrable after several years of follow-up, and that the relatively short follow-up in most clinical trials may not be adequate to fully see the beneficial effects of lower blood pressure levels on renal outcomes. However, the lack of information comparing the two groups with regard to blood pressure levels and antihypertensive medication use after the end of the study is a serious concern in the interpretation of these results.

The second Ramipril Efficacy in Nephropathy study (REIN-2) also examined the effect of level of blood pressure on decline in renal function; an important difference from the other studies was that all patients were prescribed ACE inhibitors, thereby removing a potential confounding factor influencing rate of decline in renal function [15]. Patients with non-diabetic renal disease and proteinuria were assigned to a conventional blood pressure group (diastolic blood pressure less than 90 mmHg) and intensified blood pressure control (BP $<$ 130/80 mmHg). After a median follow-up of 19 months, the mean difference in blood pressure between the two groups was 4.1/2.8 mmHg. There was no difference in incidence of end-stage renal disease, rate of decline in GFR, or change in proteinuria between the conventional and intensified blood pressure control groups. In fact, the study was stopped prematurely because the data safety and monitoring board recommended that it was futile to continue. These data suggest that in patients with non-diabetic proteinuric nephropathy who are treated with ACE inhibition, further reduction in blood pressure may not improve renal outcomes.

Jafar *et al.* [16] addressed the issue of level of blood pressure control in a patient-level meta-analyses of 11 studies. In this analysis, the lowest risk for kidney disease progression was at a SBP of 110–129 mmHg. Risk for progression was elevated in patients with a SBP in the 130–139 mmHg range (relative risk [RR] 1.83; 95% CI 0.97–3.44) and markedly elevated in patients with a SBP at or above 160 mmHg (RR 3.14; 95% CI 1.64–5.99). However, these results were strongly influenced by baseline proteinuria; low blood pressure had minimal impact on patients with less than 1 g proteinuria/day. Conversely, patients with greater than 1 g proteinuria had a striking elevation in risk for progression at higher blood pressures. In a slightly different patient population – patients with polycystic kidney disease – a prospective, randomized, 7-year study was performed to examine the effect of rigorous ($<$120/80 mmHg) vs. standard (135–140/85–90 mmHg) blood pressure control on left ventricular mass index and kidney function in 75 hypertensive polycystic kidney disease patients [17]. During the study, average mean arterial pressure was 90 $\pm$ 5 mmHg for the rigorous group and 101 $\pm$ 4 mmHg for the standard group ($P < 0.0001$). Although the left ventricular mass index decreased by 21% in the standard group and by 35% in the rigorous group, there was no statistically significant difference in rate of decline in renal function between the two groups.

CARDIOVASCULAR OUTCOMES

Another important consideration in defining a target blood pressure is risk of CVD. The relationship between blood pressure and risk of cardiovascular events is continuous, consistent, and independent of other risk factors [18]. For example, beginning at 115/75 mmHg, cardiovascular risk doubles for each increment of 20/10 mmHg. Data from observational studies involving more than 1 million individuals have indicated that death from both ischaemic heart disease and stroke increases progressively and linearly from blood pressure levels as low as 115 mmHg systolic and 75 mmHg diastolic upward [19].

Patients with chronic kidney disease are at very high risk for CVD [20, 21]. Though there are limited data specifically in patients with chronic kidney disease, data in the general population strongly support a continuous relationship between blood pressure and CVD outcomes. Similarly, there are few clinical trial data specifically in chronic kidney disease patients evaluating the beneficial effects of a lower than usual blood pressure goal on cardiovascular outcomes. A subgroup analysis of the Hypertension Optimal Treatment (HOT) study showed that there was no difference in risk of CVD in the three target blood pressure groups in patients with chronic kidney disease [22]. However, the number of patients in this subgroup was relatively small and not powered to study this issue. More recently, a *post hoc* analysis of the Irbesatan Diabetic Nephropathy Trial (IDNT) showed that, in patients with diabetic nephropathy, progressively lower achieved SBP to 120 mmHg was associated with a decrease in cardiovascular mortality and congestive heart failure, but not myocardial infarctions [23]. A SBP below this threshold was associated with increased risk for cardiovascular deaths and congestive heart failure events. Achieved diastolic blood pressure <85 mmHg was associated with a trend to increase in all-cause mortality significant increase in myocardial infarction, but decreased risk for strokes.

Many, but not all current guidelines, recommend a blood pressure goal of less 130/80 mmHg in patients with chronic kidney disease. The epidemiologic association between blood pressure and renal outcomes, the clinical trial evidence showing benefit of a low blood pressure goal in proteinuric patients, and the meta-analyses of these trials strongly support the beneficial effect of a lower than usual blood pressure goal in these patients. However, it is not clear if patients without significant proteinuria, and/or patients on adequate doses of inhibitors of the renin–angiotensin axis will derive additional benefit from lowering of blood pressure beyond the usual targets. In addition, while the association between tight blood pressure and CVD is well established in the general population, its extrapolation to patients with chronic kidney disease needs to be confirmed by studies in these patients. In addition, prospective clinical trials, or at a minimum, *post hoc* analyses of other existing clinical trials are needed to confirm that lower levels of blood pressure, compared to conventional targets do reduce risk of CVD in patients with chronic kidney disease. These may be best accomplished by meta-analyses of large clinical trials.

DIABETES

High blood pressure is a major risk factor for CVD and kidney dysfunction in diabetic patients. Appropriate treatment of hypertension in diabetic patients can both prevent CVD and minimise progression of chronic kidney disease [24]. We will review the evidence that supports a 'tight' blood pressure goal in diabetic patients to prevent renal and CVD.

RENAL OUTCOMES

Several clinical trials have, either directly or indirectly, addressed the issue of defining the optimal level of blood pressure in diabetic patients to slow decline in renal function. Most of these studies were evaluating the now proven beneficial effect of inhibition of the renin-angiotensin axis in diabetic nephropathy, but also demonstrated the benefit of aggressive lowering of blood pressure. The Reduction of Endpoints in Non-Insulin Dependent Diabetes Mellitus with the Angiotensin II Antagonist Losaitan (RENAAL) study was a randomized, placebo-controlled study of losartan vs. placebo, with other agents added to achieve the goal of a trough BP below 140/90 mmHg, and had a mean follow-up of 3.4 years [25]. The study comprised 1513 participants with established nephropathy and hypertension associated with type 2 diabetes. Analyses from this study showed that a baseline SBP range of 140–159 mmHg increased risk for end-stage renal disease or death by 38% (P = 0.05) compared with those below 130 mmHg. In a multivariate model, every 10 mmHg rise in baseline SBP increased the risk for end-stage renal disease or death by 6.7% ($P = 0.007$) when adjusting for urinary albumin–creatinine ratio, serum-creatinine, serum-albumin, haemoglobin, and haemoglobin A1c [25].

The IDNT had patients with established diabetic nephropathy with overt proteinuria and mild to moderate renal insufficiency [26]. Patients were randomized to irbesartan 300 mg/day, amlodipine 10 mg/day, or placebo. The SBP target was either ≥135 mmHg when baseline SBP was 145 mmHg or less, or 10 mmHg below the baseline SBP when baseline SBP was between 146 and 170 mmHg. The patients who achieved a SBP less than 134 mmHg had the best renal outcome; 17% reached a renal endpoint (doubling of their serum–creatinine or end-stage renal disease) during the course of follow-up compared to 38% of patients who had a follow-up SBP more than 149 mmHg (RR 2.2; $P < 0.05$). A decrease of 20 mmHg in achieved SBP was associated with a 47% decrease in the risk for developing a renal endpoint. Renal outcomes in patients with a follow-up SBP less than 120 mmHg were not associated with better outcome; in fact the patients with this lower follow-up SBP had higher cardiovascular mortality. Within each treatment group, regardless of treatment type, renal outcomes improved progressively at lower follow-up SBP levels. This study clearly defines that lower blood pressure in patients with diabetic nephropathy leads to better renal outcomes, independent of baseline renal function and suggests that the best target SBP in patients with diabetic nephropathy may be between 120 and 130 mmHg.

Somewhat different results were seen in the Appropriate Blood Pressure Control in Diabetes (ABCD) trial which compared the effects of intensive vs. moderate blood pressure control on the incidence and progression of type 2 diabetic complications [27]. After 5.3 years of follow-up of 470 patients, the mean blood pressure achieved was 132/78 mmHg in the intensive group and 138/86 mmHg in the moderate control group. During the 5-year follow-up period, no difference was observed between intensive vs. moderate blood pressure control with regard to the change in creatinine clearance (5–6 ml/min/1.73 m^2/year throughout the follow-up period whether they were on intensive or moderate therapy). There was also no difference between the interventions with regard to individuals progressing from normoalbuminuria to microalbuminuria (25% intensive therapy vs. 18% moderate therapy; $P = 0.20$) or microalbuminuria to overt albuminuria (16% intensive therapy vs. 23% moderate therapy; $P = 0.28$). In normotensive patients in the ABCD study, although no difference was demonstrated in creatinine clearance between the moderate blood pressure control group (mean blood pressure 137/81 mmHg) and the intensive blood pressure control group (mean blood pressure 128/75 mmHg), a lower percentage of patients in the intensive group progressed from normoalbuminuria to microalbuminuria and microalbuminuria to overt albuminuria [28].

A similar benefit of lower blood pressure levels on proteinuria in diabetic patients was shown by Lewis *et al.* [29] who studied 129 patients with type 1 diabetes and diabetic nephropathy who had previously participated in the Angiotensin-Converting Enzyme Inhibition in Diabetic Nephropathy study. They were randomly assigned to a mean arterial blood pressure (MAP) goal of 92 mmHg or less (group I) or 100–107 mmHg (group II). The average difference in MAP between groups was 6 mmHg over the 24-month follow-up. While there was no statistically significant differences in the rate of decline in renal function between groups, there was a significant difference in follow-up total urinary protein excretion between group I (535 mg/24 h) and group II (1723 mg/24 h; $P = 0.02$). Similar beneficial effects of aggressive blood pressure reduction on diabetic nephropathy have been shown in the UK prospective diabetes studies (UKPDS) [30].

In summary, a consistent body of evidence supports the concept that aggressively lowering blood pressure slows decline in renal function and/or lowers proteinuria in diabetic patients.

CARDIOVASCULAR OUTCOMES

Epidemiologic studies have consistently shown that a SBP of <130 mmHg is associated with lower cardiovascular outcomes in diabetic patients [19, 31]. Many clinical trials also support this concept. The HOT trial was designed to assess the association between major cardiovascular events (non-fatal myocardial infarction, non-fatal stroke, and cardiovascular death) in three target blood pressure groups (≤90, ≤85 and ≤80 diastolic mmHg) [32]. Felodipine with a dose of 5 mg once a day was given as baseline therapy with the addition of other agents, according to a five-step regimen. In 1501 patients with diabetes mellitus at baseline, the risk of major cardiovascular events in the ≤80 mmHg group was halved in comparison with that of the target group ≤90 mmHg. This change was attenuated but remained significant when silent myocardial infarctions were included. Stroke also showed a declining rate with lower target blood pressure groups, with a risk reduction of about 30% in the ≤80 mmHg target group vs. ≤90 mmHg target group. Cardiovascular mortality was also significantly lower in the ≤80 mmHg target group than in each of the other target groups. Overall, the results of the HOT trial suggests that a lower target diastolic pressure has a cardioprotective effect in diabetics and that 80 rather than 85 mmHg should be the preferred goal diastolic pressure in these patients.

Tight blood pressure control also resulted in improved micro- and macrovascular outcomes in the UKPDS [8]. One thousand one hundred and forty-eight patients with type 2 diabetes were randomly assigned to a tight blood pressure control group (achieved blood pressures 144/82 mmHg) or a conventional blood pressure control group (achieved BP 154/87 mmHg). Patients in the lower blood pressure group had a 24% reduction in diabetes-related endpoints (including microvascular disease) (37 vs. 49%), a 32% reduction in deaths related to diabetes (24 vs. 35%), 44% fewer strokes, and a 34 and 47% reduction in significant deterioration in retinopathy and visual acuity, respectively. There was a significant relation between follow-up SBP and incidence of macro- and microvascular complications in diabetic patients, with a continuous increment of complications for values greater than 120 mmHg.

In the hypertensive component of the ABCD trial, the overall mortality was lower (5.5%) in the intensive treatment group (mean BP 132/78) compared to 10.7% in the moderate control group (mean BP 138/86) ($P = 0.037$) [27]. In the normotensive component of the ABCD study, achieved blood pressures for the moderate and intensive control groups were 137/81 and 128/75 mmHg respectively. After 5 years of follow-up, lower incidence of stroke and progression of diabetic retinopathy was observed in the intensive control group.

In a prospective meta-analysis by the Blood Pressure Lowering Treatment Trialists' Collaboration, twenty-seven randomized trials with 33 395 patients with diabetes were reviewed [33]. Patients with diabetes who had been targeted to lower BP goal, achieved greater reductions in the risk of total cardiovascular events ($P = 0.03$) and cardiovascular deaths ($P = 0.02$) than those without diabetes.

SUMMARY

In summary, the totality of the evidence supporting the benefit of aggressive blood pressure lowering in diabetic patients appears convincing to justify a lower blood pressure goal in diabetic patients. Data from the HOT study clearly define the diastolic blood pressure goal to be less than 80 mmHg in diabetic patients. The systolic goal of 130 mmHg appears to be based mostly on epidemiologic and observational data, which is clearly very impressive, and shows a linear relationship between SBP and outcomes starting at a SBP greater than 120 mmHg. However, in most clinical trials that showed cardiovascular benefit with 'aggressive' blood pressure lowering in diabetic patients, mean SBP was still over 130 (144 in UKPDS, 144 in HOT, and 132 mmHg in ABCD-HT) [34]. The ongoing Action to Control Cardiovascular Risk in Diabetes (ACCORD) study may provide the definitive answer whether lowering blood pressure to normal (<120 mmHg systolic) will reduce CVD risk better compared to a target of <140 mmHg systolic in diabetic patients.

Despite the broad endorsement of these treatment goals by guideline committees, achievement of these targets remains less than optimal in most populations. The additional lowering of blood pressure often requires multiple drug therapy, increases costs of care and healthcare utilization, and requires patient compliance. Formal cost–benefit analyses have shown that cost-effectiveness ratio of tight blood pressure control compares favourably with other accepted healthcare programmes [35]. In the setting of clinical trials, with additional resources and staff, the majority of patients are controlled to goal [36]. Efforts to achieve goal blood pressure in these high risk populations, therefore, have to be multidisciplinary to include patient education, improving access and availability of heathcare and medications, and minimization of 'physician inertia' with suitable reimbursement for the care of these complex patients. It is clear that the public health benefits that can be potentially derived from achieving target blood pressure in high risk patients are substantial; allocation of adequate resources at various levels in the healthcare system are essential to reach these goals.

REFERENCES

1. Ezzati M, Lopez AD, Rodgers A, Vander HS, Murray CJ. Selected major risk factors and global and regional burden of disease. *Lancet* 2002; 360:1347–1360.
2. Turnbull F. Effects of different blood-pressure-lowering regimens on major cardiovascular events: results of prospectively-designed overviews of randomized trials. *Lancet* 2003; 362:1527–1535.
3. Agodoa LY, Appel L, Bakris GL *et al*. Effect of ramipril vs amlodipine on renal outcomes in hypertensive nephrosclerosis: a randomized controlled trial. *JAMA* 2001; 285:2719–2728.
4. The Multiple Risk Factor Intervention Trial Research Group. Mortality rates after 10.5 years for participants in the Multiple Risk Factor Intervention Trial. Findings related to a priori hypotheses of the trial. *JAMA* 1990; 263:1795–1801.
5. Chobanian AV, Bakris GL, Black HR *et al*. The Seventh Report of the Joint National Committee on Prevention, Detection, Evaluation, and Treatment of High Blood Pressure: the JNC 7 report. *JAMA* 2003; 289:2560–2572.
6. Whitworth JA. 2003 World Health Organization (WHO)/International Society of Hypertension (ISH) statement on management of hypertension. *J Hypertens* 2003; 21:1983–1992.
7. Williams B, Poulter NR, Brown MJ *et al*. British Hypertension Society guidelines for hypertension management 2004 (BHS-IV): summary. *Br Med J* 2004; 328:634–640.
8. K/DOQI clinical practice guidelines for chronic kidney disease: evaluation, classification, and stratification. Kidney Disease Outcome Quality Initiative. *Am J Kidney Dis* 2002; 39(suppl 2):S1–S246.
9. K/DOQI clinical practice guidelines on hypertension and antihypertensive agents in chronic kidney disease. *Am J Kidney Dis* 2004; 43(suppl 1):S1-S290.
10. Klag MJ, Whelton PK, Randall BL *et al*. Blood pressure and end-stage renal disease in men. *N Engl J Med* 1996; 334:13–18.
11. Wright JT Jr, Bakris G, Greene T *et al*. Effect of blood pressure lowering and antihypertensive drug class on progression of hypertensive kidney disease: results from the AASK trial. *JAMA* 2002; 288:2421–2431.
12. Hirschberg R, Wang S. Proteinuria and growth factors in the development of tubulointerstitial injury and scarring in kidney disease. *Curr Opin Nephrol Hypertens* 2005; 14:43–52.
13. Klahr S, Levey AS, Beck GJ *et al*. Modification of Diet in Renal Disease Study Group. The effects of dietary protein restriction and blood-pressure control on the progression of chronic renal disease. *N Engl J Med* 1994; 330:877–884.
14. Sarnak MJ, Greene T, Wang X *et al*. The effect of a lower target blood pressure on the progression of kidney disease: long-term follow-up of the modification of diet in renal disease study. *Ann Intern Med* 2005; 142:342–351.
15. Ruggenenti P, Perna A, Loriga G *et al*. Blood-pressure control for renoprotection in patients with non-diabetic chronic renal disease (REIN-2): multicentre, randomized controlled trial. *Lancet* 2005; 365:939–946.
16. Jafar TH, Stark PC, Schmid CH *et al*. Progression of chronic kidney disease: the role of blood pressure control, proteinuria, and angiotensin-converting enzyme inhibition: a patient-level meta-analysis. *Ann Intern Med* 2003; 139:244–252.
17. Schrier R, McFann K, Johnson A *et al*. Cardiac and renal effects of standard versus rigorous blood pressure control in autosomal-dominant polycystic kidney disease: results of a seven-year prospective randomized study. *J Am Soc Nephrol* 2002; 13:1733–1739.
18. Chobanian AV, Bakris GL, Black HR *et al*. Seventh Report of the Joint National Committee on Prevention, Detection, Evaluation, and Treatment of High Blood Pressure. *Hypertension* 2003; 42:1206–1252.
19. Lewington S, Clarke R, Qizilbash N, Peto R, Collins R. Age-specific relevance of usual blood pressure to vascular mortality: a meta-analysis of individual data for one million adults in 61 prospective studies. *Lancet* 2002; 360:1903–1913.

20. Rahman M, Brown CD, Coresh J *et al.* The prevalence of reduced glomerular filtration rate in older hypertensive patients and its association with cardiovascular disease: a report from the Antihypertensive and Lipid-Lowering Treatment to Prevent Heart Attack Trial. *Arch Intern Med* 2004; 164:969–976.
21. Sarnak MJ, Levey AS, Schoolwerth AC *et al.* Kidney disease as a risk factor for development of cardiovascular disease: a statement from the American Heart Association Councils on Kidney in Cardiovascular Disease, High Blood Pressure Research, Clinical Cardiology, and Epidemiology and Prevention. *Hypertension* 2003; 42:1050–1065.
22. Ruilope LM, Salvetti A, Jamerson K *et al.* Renal function and intensive lowering of blood pressure in hypertensive participants of the hypertension optimal treatment (HOT) study. *J Am Soc Nephrol* 2001; 12:218–225.
23. Berl T, Hunsicker LG, Lewis JB *et al.* Impact of achieved blood pressure on cardiovascular outcomes in the Irbesartan Diabetic Nephropathy Trial. *J Am Soc Nephrol* 2005; 16:2170–2179.
24. Standards of medical care in diabetes. *Diabetes Care* 2005; 28(suppl 1):S4–S36.
25. Bakris GL, Weir MR, Shanifar S *et al.* Effects of blood pressure level on progression of diabetic nephropathy: results from the RENAAL study. *Arch Intern Med* 2003; 163:1555–1565.
26. Pohl MA, Blumenthal S, Cordonnier DJ *et al.* Independent and additive impact of blood pressure control and angiotensin II receptor blockade on renal outcomes in the irbesartan diabetic nephropathy trial: clinical implications and limitations. *J Am Soc Nephrol* 2005; 16:3027–3037.
27. Estacio RO, Jeffers BW, Gifford N, Schrier RW. Effect of blood pressure control on diabetic microvascular complications in patients with hypertension and type 2 diabetes. *Diabetes Care* 2000; 23(suppl 2):B54–B64.
28. Schrier RW, Estacio RO, Esler A, Mehler P. Effects of aggressive blood pressure control in normotensive type 2 diabetic patients on albuminuria, retinopathy and strokes. *Kidney Int* 2002; 61:1086–1097.
29. Lewis JB, Berl T, Bain RP, Rohde RD, Lewis EJ. Collaborative Study Group. Effect of intensive blood pressure control on the course of type 1 diabetic nephropathy. *Am J Kidney Dis* 1999; 34:809–817.
30. UK Prospective Diabetes Study Group. Tight blood pressure control and risk of macrovascular and microvascular complications in type 2 diabetes: UKPDS 38. *Br Med J* 1998; 317:703–713.
31. Stamler J, Stamler R, Neaton JD. Blood pressure, systolic and diastolic, and cardiovascular risks. US population data. *Arch Intern Med* 1993; 153:598–615.
32. Hansson L, Zanchetti A, Carruthers SG *et al.* HOT Study Group. Effects of intensive blood-pressure lowering and low-dose aspirin in patients with hypertension: principal results of the Hypertension Optimal Treatment (HOT) randomized trial. *Lancet* 1998; 351:1755–1762.
33. Turnbull F, Neal B, Algert C *et al.* Effects of different blood pressure-lowering regimens on major cardiovascular events in individuals with and without diabetes mellitus: results of prospectively designed overviews of randomized trials. *Arch Intern Med* 2005; 165:1410–1419.
34. 2003 European Society of Hypertension–European Society of Cardiology guidelines for the management of arterial hypertension. *J Hypertens* 2003; 21:1011–1053.
35. UK Prospective Diabetes Study Group. Cost effectiveness analysis of improved blood pressure control in hypertensive patients with type 2 diabetes: UKPDS 40. *Br Med J* 1998; 317:720–726.
36. Wright JT Jr, Agodoa L, Contreras G *et al.* Successful blood pressure control in the African American Study of Kidney Disease and Hypertension. *Arch Intern Med* 2002; 162:1636–1643.
37. Hypertension Management Guide for Doctors 2004. National Heart Foundation; 2004. www.heartfoundation.com.au/downloads/hypertension_management_guide_2004.pdf. 2005.
38. 2005 Canadian recommendations for the management of hypertension. http://www.hypertension.ca/Documentation/Recommandation05_va.pdf. 2005.

7

Approaches to cardiovascular risk reduction in patients with cardio–metabolic–renal risk

W. A. Hsueh, G. L. Bakris

INTRODUCTION

Modifiable cardiovascular (CV) risk factors often occur together in the same individual. An increasingly common example is the metabolic syndrome, generally associated with being overweight and with increased visceral adiposity [1–3]. It is currently estimated that about 55 million Americans (about 25% of the population) have the metabolic syndrome using Adult Treatment Panel III (ATP III) criteria (Table 7.1). This epidemic is driven to a large extent by the production of cytokines and hormones through endocrine action of the visceral adipocyte (Figure 7.1). Moreover, the prevalence of coronary heart disease (CHD) events is increased in the presence of the metabolic syndrome (Figure 7.2).

Increased production of adipocyte-derived factors such as tumor necrosis factor α (TNFα), leptin, free fatty acids (FFA), and possibly angiotensinogen combined with decreased production of adiponectin contribute to insulin resistance at the level of both the skeletal muscle and liver, ultimately resulting in type 2 diabetes [4–7]. The elevated FFA and insulin resistance contribute to the dyslipidaemia of metabolic syndrome, low high-density lipoprotein cholesterol (HDL-c) and elevated triglycerides, while increased angiotensinogen and leptin appear to explain, at least in part, the increased prevalence of hypertension in obesity [7–10]. There is debate as to whether components of the metabolic have synergetic or only additive effects to enhance CV disease, but there is agreement that components should be treated aggressively for CV protection [2, 11–13].

Recent studies have addressed the presence of CV risk factors in patients with documented CV disease. In 122 458 patients enrolled in randomized clinical trials of CHD performed over the past decade, it was identified that 85% of women and 81% of men had at least 1 of 4 conventional risk factors (Table 7.2), including smoking, diabetes and hypertension, while only 10–15% lacked any of these [14]. Premature coronary artery disease was related to cigarette smoking in men and both cigarette smoking and diabetes in women. Over 50% of patients had 2–4 risk factors particularly in age groups less than 65 years old. Similar data were reported for a US based analyses of nearly 75 000 subjects with CHD [15]. In reality, these data may be underestimates of the presence of CV risk factors because many patients are unaware of their disease. For example, a third of patients with hypertension are unaware that they have hypertension, and nearly 50% of patients with diabetes or hypercholesterolaemia do not know that they have these risk factors [16]. Furthermore, it is reported that physicians generally

Willa A. Hsueh, MD, Professor of Medicine, Chief, Endocrine Division, Department of Medicine, UCLA Medical Center, Los Angeles, California, USA

George L. Bakris, MD, Professor and Vice-Chairman, Department of Preventive Medicine, Director, Hypertension/ Clinical Research Center, Rush University Medical Center, Chicago, Ilinois, USA

Table 7.1 Metabolic syndrome diagnosis: ATP III emphasizes clinical practice

Risk factor	*Defining level*
Abdominal obesity (in)	Waist:
Men	>40
Women	>35
Triglycerides (mg/dl)	≥150
HDL-c (mg/dl)	
Men	<40
Women	<50
BP (mmHg)	≥130/≥85
Fasting glucose (mg/dl)	≥110 (ADA ≥100)

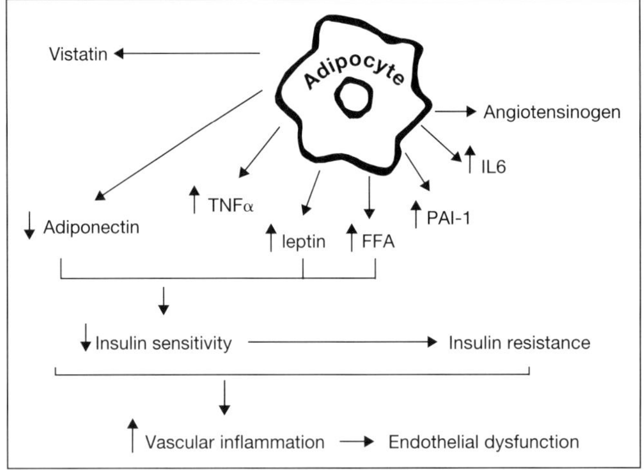

Figure 7.1 Adipokines mediate insulin resistance and inflammation.

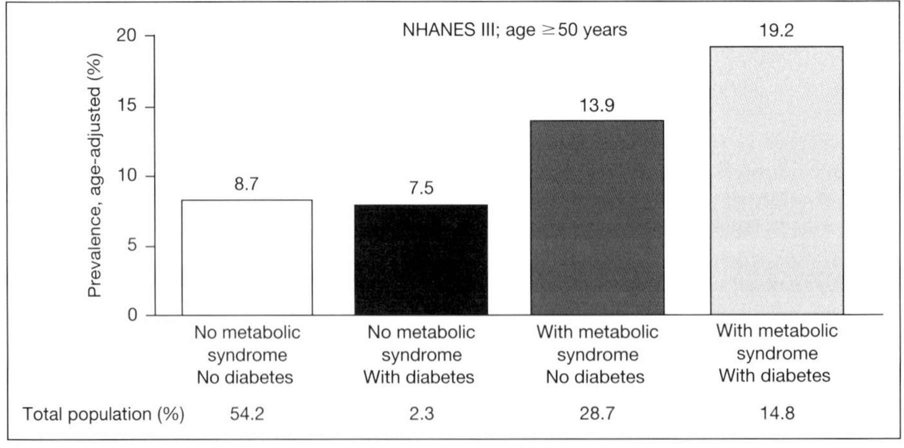

Figure 7.2 Prevalence of CHD is increased with the metabolic syndrome. NHANES = National Health and Nutrition Examination Survey. With permission [14].

Table 7.2 Prevalence of conventional risk factors by age and sex*

	Age (years)									
	≤45		46–55		56–65		66–75		>75	
	Women	*Men*	*Women*	*Men*	*Women*	*Men*	*Women*	*Men*	*Women*	*Men*
Individual risk factors										
No.	1623	10 531	4608	21 632	8858	25 666	12 285	22 215	7215	7825
Current smoking	72.0	71.7**	57.9	58.7**	38.9	39.8**	19.1	23.3	7.9	11.8
Diabetes	17.8	7.4	19.7	12.1	24.1	16.9	25.2	19.2	22.0	18.4
Hyperlipidaemia	33.2	37.0***	41.0	38.5***	45.0	36.3	42.2	30.7	29.1	20.4
Hypertension	37.1	25.3	46.8	33.6	54.6	40.5	60.1	45.1	60.2	43.1
Total no. of risk factors										
No. with complete data	1569	10 251	4453	20 996	8524	24 817	11 807	21 411	6885	7485
No. of risk factors										
0	9.4	11.4	10.7	13.3	12.0	18.4	15.8	24.6	23.3	35.5
1	41.9	48.0	35.5	44.4	34.5	41.8	36.4	41.5	41.7	40.7
2	30.8	29.8	35.1	30.1	34.7	29.2	34.6	26.0	28.1	19.3
3	15.2	9.9	16.3	10.8	16.7	9.5	12.4	7.4	6.7	4.2
4	2.7	0.9	2.5	1.3	2.0	1.1	0.8	0.6	0.2	0.2

*All data are expressed as percentages unless otherwise specified. Risk factor prevalence differences between women and men are statistically significant at $P < 0.001$ unless otherwise noted.

**Risk factor prevalence differences between women and men are non-significant.

***Risk factor prevalence differences between women and men are statistically significant at $P < 0.01$.

under diagnose these conventional risk factors [17, 18]. Because of these important issues and the fact that cardiovascular disease (CVD) remains the number one cause of death nearly worldwide, there is increased emphasis in diagnosis and treatment of 'global' CV risk.

GOALS FOR CV RISK REDUCTION: BE AGGRESSIVE

As more clinical trial results emerge, recommended goals for CV risk factor reduction have become more stringent and are based on the presence of both other risk factors and disease itself. For example, diabetes is considered a coronary artery disease risk equivalent [19]. Therefore, recommended goals are lower for patients with diabetes compared to those without diabetes [20] (Table 7.3). A HbA1c of 6.5–7% is recommended to prevent microvascular complications (retinopathy, nephropathy and neuropathy), but there is increasing evidence that tight glucose control impacts on atherosclerosis [21, 22]. Low density lipoprotein cholesterol (LDL-c) is recommended at 100 mg/dl, but if CHD is present a level of 70 mg/dl is suggested.

Studies are currently being conducted to determine if even lower LDL-c levels are indicated. HDL-c levels are recommended to be >40 mg/dl and triglycerides <150 mg/dl, and are commonly abnormal in diabetes and constitute the dyslipidaemia of the metabolic syndrome. A blood pressure (BP) goal of <130/80 mmHg rather than the usual goal of <140/90 mmHg is recommended because the Hypertension Optimal Treatment (HOT) trial clearly demonstrated a linear relationship between CV protection and diastolic BP treated to

Table 7.3 Target goals for CV risk factor reduction recommended for patients with diabetes mellitus

HbA1c	<65%
LDL-c	100 mg/dl, if CHD present 70 mg/dl
HDL-c	>40 mg/dl
Triglyceride	<150 mg/dl
BP	<130/80 mmHg, if proteinuria present <125/75 mmHg

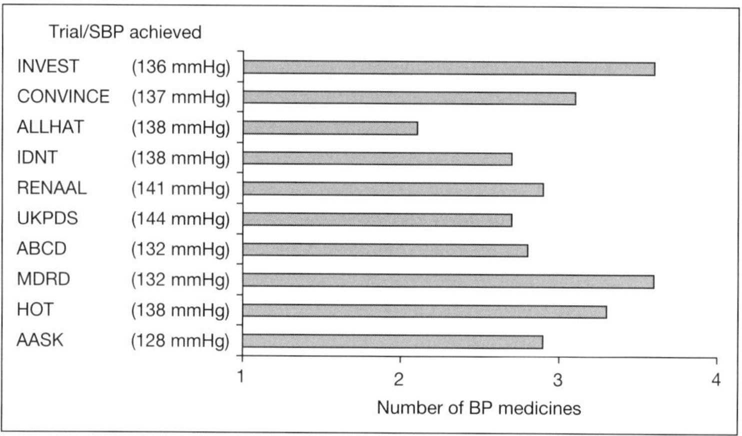

Figure 7.3 Average number of antihypertensive agents needed per patient to achieve target BP goals.

80 mmHg among those with diabetes. For renal protection, BP levels of 125/75 mmHg have been shown to be more effective than higher BP, in those with proteinuric advanced kidney disease [23].

In nearly all cholesterol-lowering or anti-hypertensive clinical trials, patients with diabetes have as much and often more relative risk reduction with treatment compared to patients without diabetes. Moreover, Gaede and colleagues [24] demonstrated that aggressive lowering of global CV risk in patients with diabetes lowered CV disease by 80%. An important issue, therefore, in patients with diabetes is the number of pharmacological agents needed to achieve the recommended goals for CV risk reduction. A general estimate of the number of agents that may be required includes two agents for glucose reduction, and approximately 3.2 for hypertension (Figure 7.3), one to two for lipids, and aspirin for the enhanced thrombotic tendency in diabetes, i.e. nearly eight drugs just for prevention of sequelae of diabetes. Combination therapies are needed for many reasons including patient compliance, economics, decreasing physician burden, etc.

COMBINATIONS THAT MAKE SENSE

Combination agents to treat a single CV risk factor are rational and necessary. Knowledge of the physiology and mechanisms of injury to CV, renal and cerebral systems is expanding and multiple pathophysiological pathways leading to disease and tissue damage have been identified. The following focuses on control of BP, lipids and glucose.

Table 7.4 Classification and management of BP for adults

BP classification	SBP* (mmHg)	DBP* (mmHg)	Lifestyle modification	Initial drug therapy: Without compelling indication	Initial drug therapy: With compelling indications
Normal	<120 and	<80	Encourage		
Pre-hypertension	120–139	or 80–89	Yes	Non anti-hypertensive drug indicated	Drug(s) for compelling indications***
Stage 1 hypertension	140–159	or 90–99	Yes	Thiazide-type diuretics for most. May consider ACE-I, ARB, BB, CCB, or **combination*****	Drug(s) for the compelling indications***
Stage 2 hypertension	≥160	or ≥100	Yes	Two-drug **combination** for most** (usually thiazide-type diuretic and ACE-I or ARB or BB or CCB)	Other antihypertensive drugs (diuretics, ACE-I, ARB, BB, CCB) as needed

*Treatment determined by highest BP category.
**Initial combined therapy should be used cautiously in those at risk for orthostatic hypotension.
***Treat patients with chronic kidney disease or diabetes to BP goal of <130/80 mmHg.

Table 7.5 Compelling indications for individual drug classes

Compelling indication	*Initial therapy options*	*Clinical trial basis*
Diabetes	THIAZ, BB, ACE, ARB, CCB	NKF-ADA Guideline, UKPDS, ALLHAT
Chronic kidney disease	ACE-I, ARB	NKF Guideline, Captopril Trial, RENAAL, IDNT, REIN, AASK
Recurrent stroke prevention	THIAZ, ACE-I	PROGRESS

BLOOD PRESSURE

Multiple mechanisms primarily involving the kidney, vasculature, heart and central nervous system work in concert to elevate BP. Clinical trials have taught us that (1) using moderate doses of two different antihypertensive agents is more effective than using higher doses of a single agent, since inhibition of several pathways may have synergistic effects associated with less side-effects; (2) certain agents may also be 'indicated' for diseases associated with hypertension, e.g. nephropathy, or that lower BP, e.g. heart failure, post-myocardial infarction, as noted in the Joint National Committee 7 (JNC7) report [16] (Tables 7.4 and 7.5) and, thus, should be considered in patients with those associated disease states; and (3) therapy should be individualized, e.g. diabetes, elderly, etc. As such, it is difficult to propose combinations that apply to all hypertensives, which now number about 65 million

Table 7.6 Changes in proteinuria at 6 months to 1 year following treatment predicts long-term renal outcomes

*Increased time to dialysis** *(30–35% proteinuria reduction)*	*No change in time to dialysis* *(no proteinuria reduction)*
AASK Trial (non-diabetic) RENAAL (diabetes) IDNT (diabetes) COOPERATE (non-diabetic)	DHPCCB arm-IDNT (diabetes) DHPCCB arm-AASK (non-diabetic)

*>30% reduction in proteinuria at 6 months to a year following anti-hypertensive therapy. Effect independent of magnitude of BP reduction.

people in the USA. Nevertheless, some recommendations can be considered. The JNC7 report recommended chlorthalidone or hydrochlorothiazide as initial antihypertensive therapy. However, in moderate to high doses these diuretics can aggravate glucose and lipid control, but their combination at low doses with agents that inhibit the renin–angiotensin–aldosterone system such as angiotensin-converting enzyme inhibitors (ACE-Is) or angiotensin AT1 receptor blockers (ARBs), increases their BP-lowering efficacy and reduces the risk of worsening metabolic parameters. Furthermore, since ACE-Is and ARBs are indicated for a wide variety of diseases that accompany hypertension (Table 7.5), the combination of ACE-I or ARB with low-dose diuretic makes therapeutic sense.

A recent meta-analysis of clinical trials in diabetes that evaluated progression of nephropathy noted that ACE-Is and ARBs offered no unique benefits on disease progression apart from BP lowering [25]. Unfortunately, this observation needs to be tempered by the following facts. In their analysis, Casas and colleagues evaluated a variety of studies that included those with very good kidney function and some with advanced disease with proteinuria. It should be noted that all the studies that support the use of agents that block the renin–angiotensin system as unique agents for protecting the kidney have been done in people with advanced nephropathy, i.e. GFR <50 ml/min, who also have substantive proteinuria, i.e. >500 mg/day. In all these studies, the unique nature of ACE-Is and ARBs is clear (Table 7.6). However, in those with better levels of kidney function without proteinuria there is no obvious unique benefit of these agents apart from BP reduction. This was also noted in the Casas analysis where the mean GFR was 74 ml/min and the majority of the studies they evaluated did not have proteinuria. Moreover, the sub-analysis of the studies that did have proteinuria clearly favoured the blockade of the renin–angiotensin system over conventional treatment.

It should also be noted that for optimal protection of renal function there must be a reduction in proteinuria along with a reduction in BP (Table 7.6). It is now clear from four different outcome trials, two in diabetes, two in non-diabetic kidney disease, that a reduction of more than 35% at 6 months predicts progression to dialysis at 3–5 years [26–29].

LIPIDS

LDL-c lowering is indicated for anyone with CV risk with more aggressive lowering for higher risk. Statins are first-line therapy for cholesterol lowering and work by inhibiting liver cholesterol production which also results in increased expression of LDL receptors in the liver and enhanced clearance of LDL-c from the circulation. Recently, ezetimibe was approved for cholesterol lowering by inhibiting intestinal cholesterol absorption, while it also increases liver expression of LDL receptors to further enhance LCL-c clearance [30, 31].

Table 7.7 Oral therapies for type 2 diabetes

Insulin sensitizers
PPARγ ligands: Skeletal muscle, liver
Metformin: Liver
Stimulate islet cell insulin release
Sulfonylurea
Metaglitanides
Slow gut carbohydrate absorption
Acarbose
GLP-1
Exenatide
DPP-4 inhibitor
Weight loss
Rimonabant
Xenical
Meridian

Both statins and ezetimibe have additive, perhaps even synergistic action to lower LDL-c. In addition, ezetimibe enhances the HDL-c-raising and triglyceride-lowering effects of statins and may even enhance the anti-inflammatory effect of statins [32, 33]. Because ezetimibe has few side-effects, its combination with statins makes therapeutic sense. Statins can also be used in combination with niacin and inhibitors of bile acid resorption, but the latter two agents often have difficult-to-handle side-effects. Fibrates increase HDL-c and decrease triglycerides, but must be used cautiously in combination with statins because of the potential for myopathy.

GLUCOSE

The pathogenesis of hyperglycaemia includes insulin resistance increased hepatic glucose production with inadequate suppression by insulin, inadequate insulin production to overcome the insulin resistance because of the islet cell damage and apoptosis, and excess visceral adiposity which is a major contributor to insulin resistance and liver and islet cell abnormalities. Therapeutic strategies have been designed to correct all of these defects (Table 7.7). Importantly, these strategies can be used in combination, similar to the approach using antihypertensive therapies, with additive and possibly synergistic actions to lower glucose.

The newer agents may have important actions in addition to glucose lowering. These actions may dictate, in part, the choice of these agents. For example, ligands to the nuclear receptor peroxisome proliferator activated receptor γ (PPARγ) are insulin sensitizers but also inhibit inflammatory signals from the adipocyte and monocyte and increase adiponectin which not only helps to correct metabolic defects of the metabolic syndrome, but may protect from CV risk [34, 35]. Although the results of recent clinical trials using such agents to assess CV outcome have fallen short of the mark in clearly showing a benefit, an effect (that was in part related to a patient population that may not have been of sufficient size to show a benefit over the short follow-up period of the study) [36] has been observed.

A major side-effect of thiazolidinediones, however, is weight gain related to adipocyte differentiation and fluid retention. Data from a recent study from Viberti's group eluicidate the mechanism of this fluid retention, which is related to the activation of the epithelial sodium channel (ENaC) in the distal tubule. Agents that block this channel, including amiloride and spironolactone, indirectly, markedly reduce pre-existing oedema and attenuate increases in oedema.

Metformin, which promotes weight loss and suppresses hepatic glucose production is a rational combination for PPARγ ligands. Exenatide, one of the newest agents approved for glucose control in diabetes, restores first phase insulin secretion, slows gastric emptying and suppresses appetite and when added to metformin or sulfonylurea, further reduces plasma glucose, both fasting and post-prandial. It also induces weight loss and, hence, may be useful to administer in combination with PPARγ ligands. Exenatide may also provide long-term islet cell protection resulting in durable glycaemic control and perhaps even prevention of diabetes [37, 38]. Clinical trials are currently underway, and if positive, would underscore earlier use of these agents in both pre-diabetes and diabetes.

SUMMARY

The earlier the intervention after lifestyle modification has been tried and found to be inadequate for whatever reason, the better the results. The use of combination therapy is now available for all three major risk factors: cholesterol, glucose and blood pressure. The next decade will be marked by studies that will help us evaluate the best way to use such medications to effect CV risk factor reduction. Trials such as DREAM, ACCORD, NAVIGATOR and ACCOMPLISH, all due to be completed between now and 2009, will help in these goals as well as defining the optimal BP and other risk factor reductions that can be achieved. However, we already know from the Steno diabetes group that intensive intervention of all risk factors reduces absolute risk by 20% for CV events [24].

REFERENCES

1. de Ferranti SD, Gauvreau K, Ludwig DS, Newburger JW, Rifai N. Inflammation and changes in metabolic syndrome abnormalities in US adolescents: findings from the 1988–1994 and 1999–2000 National Health and Nutrition Examination Surveys. *Clin Chem* 2006 (in press).
2. Drown DJ. Metabolic syndrome: a constellation of risk factors for vascular disease and diabetes with deadly consequences. *Prog Cardiovasc Nurs* 2002; 17:151.
3. Haffner SM. Obesity and the metabolic syndrome: the San Antonio Heart Study. *Br J Nutr* 2000; 83(suppl 1):S67–S70.
4. Bergman RN, Van Citters GW, Mittelman SD *et al*. Central role of the adipocyte in the metabolic syndrome. *J Investig Med* 2001; 49:119–126.
5. Steppan CM, Bailey ST, Bhat S *et al*. The hormone resistin links obesity to diabetes. *Nature* 2001; 409:307–312.
6. Kougias P, Chai H, Lin PH, Yao Q, Lumsden AB, Chen C. Effects of adipocyte-derived cytokines on endothelial functions: implication of vascular disease. *J Surg Res* 2005; 126:121–129.
7. Rondinone CM. Adipocyte-derived hormones, cytokines, and mediators. *Endocrine* 2006; 29:81–90.
8. Haffner SM, Mykkanen L, Rainwater DL, Karhapaa P, Laakso M. Is leptin concentration associated with the insulin resistance syndrome in nondiabetic men? *Obes Res* 1999; 7:164–169.
9. Hall JE, Crook ED, Jones DW, Wofford MR, Dubbert PM. Mechanisms of obesity-associated cardiovascular and renal disease. *Am J Med Sci* 2002; 324:127–137.
10. Karhunen LJ, Lappalainen RI, Haffner SM *et al*. Serum leptin, food intake and preferences for sugar and fat in obese women. *Int J Obes Relat Metab Disord* 1998; 22:819–821.
11. Saely CH, Koch L, Schmid F *et al*. Adult Treatment Panel III 2001 but not International Diabetes Federation 2005 criteria of the metabolic syndrome predict clinical cardiovascular events in subjects who underwent coronary angiography. *Diabetes Care* 2006; 29:901–907.
12. Tuomilehto J. Cardiovascular risk: prevention and treatment of the metabolic syndrome. *Diabetes Res Clin Pract* 2005; 68(suppl 2):S28–S35.
13. Greenberg AS. The expanding scope of the metabolic syndrome and implications for the management of cardiovascular risk in type 2 diabetes with particular focus on the emerging role of the thiazolidinediones. *J Diabetes Complications* 2003; 17:218–228.
14. Alexander CM, Landsman PB, Teutsch SM, Haffner SM. NCEP-defined metabolic syndrome, diabetes, and prevalence of coronary heart disease among NHANES III participants age 50 years and older. *Diabetes* 2003; 52:1210–1214.

15. Muntner P, He J, Chen J, Fonseca V, Whelton PK. Prevalence of non-traditional cardiovascular disease risk factors among persons with impaired fasting glucose, impaired glucose tolerance, diabetes, and the metabolic syndrome: analysis of the Third National Health and Nutrition Examination Survey (NHANES III). *Ann Epidemiol* 2004; 14:686–695.
16. Chobanian AV, Bakris GL, Black HR *et al*. Seventh report of the Joint National Committee on Prevention, Detection, Evaluation, and Treatment of High Blood Pressure. *Hypertension* 2003; 42:1206–1252.
17. Scranton RE, Sesso HD, Glynn RJ *et al*. Characteristics associated with differences in reported versus measured total cholesterol among male physicians. *J Prim Prev* 2005; 26:51–61.
18. Taher T, Khan NA, Devereaux PJ, Fisher BW, Ghali WA, McAlister FA. Assessment and reporting of perioperative cardiac risk by Canadian general internists: art or science? *J Gen Intern Med* 2002; 17:933–936.
19. Haffner SM, Lehto S, Ronnemaa T, Pyorala K, Laakso M. Mortality from coronary heart disease in subjects with type 2 diabetes and in nondiabetic subjects with and without prior myocardial infarction. *N Engl J Med* 1998; 339:229–234.
20. Summary of revisions for the 2006 Clinical Practice Recommendations. *Diabetes Care* 2006; 29(suppl 1):S3.
21. Selvin E, Wattanakit K, Steffes MW, Coresh J, Sharrett AR. HbA1c and peripheral arterial disease in diabetes: the atherosclerosis risk in communities study. *Diabetes Care* 2006; 29:877–882.
22. Selvin E, Coresh J, Golden SH, Brancati FL, Folsom AR, Steffes MW. Glycemic control and coronary heart disease risk in persons with and without diabetes: the atherosclerosis risk in communities study. *Arch Intern Med* 2005; 165:1910–1916.
23. Sarnak MJ, Greene T, Wang X *et al*. The effect of a lower target blood pressure on the progression of kidney disease: long-term follow-up of the modification of diet in renal disease study. *Ann Intern Med* 2005; 142:342–351.
24. Gaede P, Vedel P, Larsen N, Jensen GV, Parving HH, Pedersen O. Multifactorial intervention and cardiovascular disease in patients with type 2 diabetes. *N Engl J Med* 2003; 348:383–393.
25. Casas JP, Chua W, Loukogeorgakis S *et al*. Effect of inhibitors of the renin-angiotensin system and other antihypertensive drugs on renal outcomes: systematic review and meta-analysis. *Lancet* 2005; 366:2026–2033.
26. Lea J, Greene T, Hebert L *et al*. The relationship between magnitude of proteinuria reduction and risk of end-stage renal disease: results of the African American study of kidney disease and hypertension. *Arch Intern Med* 2005; 165:947–953.
27. De Zeeuw D, Remuzzi G, Parving HH *et al*. Proteinuria, a target for renoprotection in patients with type 2 diabetic nephropathy: lessons from RENAAL. *Kidney Int* 2004; 65:2309–2320.
28. Atkins RC, Briganti EM, Lewis JB *et al*. Proteinuria reduction and progression to renal failure in patients with type 2 diabetes mellitus and overt nephropathy. *Am J Kidney Dis* 2005; 45:281–287.
29. Nakao N, Seno H, Kasuga H *et al*. Effects of combination treatment with losartan and trandolapril on office and ambulatory blood pressures in non-diabetic renal disease: a COOPERATE-ABP substudy. *Am J Nephrol* 2004; 24:543–548.
30. Morris S, Tiller R. Ezetimibe for hypercholesterolemia. *Am Fam Physician* 2003; 68:1595–1596.
31. Yatskar L, Fisher EA, Schwartzbard A. Ezetimibe: rationale and role in the management of hypercholesterolemia. *Clin Cardiol* 2006; 29:52–55.
32. McKenney JM, Farnier M, Lo KW *et al*. Safety and efficacy of long-term co-administration of fenofibrate and ezetimibe in patients with mixed hyperlipidemia. *J Am Coll Cardiol* 2006; 47:1584–1587.
33. Landray M, Baigent C, Leaper C *et al*. The second United Kingdom Heart and Renal Protection (UK-HARP-II) Study: a randomized controlled study of the biochemical safety and efficacy of adding ezetimibe to simvastatin as initial therapy among patients with CKD. *Am J Kidney Dis* 2006; 47:385–395.
34. Belcher G, Lambert C, Goh KL. Cardiovascular effects of treatment of type 2 diabetes with pioglitazone, metformin and gliclazide. *Int J Clin Pract* 2004; 58:833–837.
35. Chiquette E, Ramirez G, Defronzo R. A meta-analysis comparing the effect of thiazolidinediones on cardiovascular risk factors. *Arch Intern Med* 2004; 164:2097–2104.
36. Holleman F, Gerdes VE, de Vries JH, Hoekstra JB. Trial of pioglitazone for the secondary prevention of cardiovascular events in patients with diabetes mellitus type 2: insufficient evidence. *Ned Tijdschr Geneeskd* 2006; 150:358–360.
37. Gedulin BR, Nikoulina SE, Smith PA *et al*. Exenatide (exendin-4) improves insulin sensitivity and {beta}-cell mass in insulin-resistant obese fa/fa Zucker rats independent of glycemia and body weight. *Endocrinology* 2005; 146:2069–2076.
38. Park S, Dong X, Fisher TL *et al*. Exendin-4 uses Irs2 signaling to mediate pancreatic beta cell growth and function. *J Biol Chem* 2006; 281:1159–1168.

8

Should there be any reluctance to initiate combination antihypertensive therapy for patients with blood pressure of 160/100 mmHg or higher?

W. J. Elliott

INTRODUCTION

Hypertension is a powerful risk factor for cardiovascular and renal disease, and is expected to be even a more important public health problem worldwide by the year 2025 [1]. Despite more than three decades' work by government, academia, and the pharmaceutical industry, the proportion of people with controlled hypertension in the United States is lower (at 34% in the National Health and Nutrition Educational Survey, 1999–2002) than the 50% target set by Healthy People 2000 (which has not changed for Healthy People 2010) [2]. Hypertension control rates are lower in other countries than in the United States [3, 4]. Although some of the shortfall in hypertension control rates has been attributed to reluctance of patients to take their prescribed medications, many physicians appear to be reluctant to intensify treatment, by either increasing the dose of an already-prescribed medication or adding another medication, as required [5]. Recent clinical trials have shown that most hypertensive individuals require more than a single drug to achieve the blood pressure target. This is particularly true for those with diabetes or chronic kidney disease, for whom nearly all guideline committees recommend a lower-than-usual goal (<130/80 mmHg in the Seventh Report of the Joint National Committee on Prevention, Detection, Evaluation and Treatment of High Blood Pressure, JNC 7) [6]. The logical extension of these facts is the recommendation of JNC 7 [6], for individuals who start with blood pressures 20/10 mmHg higher than their blood pressure goal, 'Consideration should be given to initiating therapy with a two-drug combination.' This chapter reviews the possible risks and potential benefits of this approach, which is becoming ever more popular, given the wide array of antihypertensive drugs currently available as combination products (Table 8.1).

CLINICAL TRIALS INVOLVING MONOTHERAPY AND/OR COMBINATION THERAPY

ESTIMATES OF BLOOD PRESSURE-LOWERING EFFICACY IN MONOTHERAPY TRIALS

For ethical reasons, it is now unusual (if not impossible) to perform a clinical trial with morbidity and mortality endpoints using only a single drug in a randomized treatment

William J. Elliott, MD, PhD, Professor of Preventive Medicine, Internal Medicine and Pharmacology, Department of Preventive Medicine, Rush Medical College of RUSH University Medical Center, Chicago, Ilinois, USA

Table 8.1 Combination antihypertensive products available in the United States (as of October 1, 2005), listed within subtype in chronological order of regulatory approval

Combination	Brand name
*Diuretic/diuretic combinations****	
Triamterene/hydrochlorothiazide (37.5/25, 50/25, 75/50)	Dyazide**, Maxzide**
Spironolactone/hydrochlorothiazide (25/25, 50/50)	Aldactone**
Amiloride/hydrochlorothiazide (5/50)	Moduretic**
β-blocker/diuretic combinations	
Propranolol/hydrochlorothiazide (40/25, 80/25)	Inderide
Metoprolol/hydrochlorothiazide (50/25, 100/25)	Lopressor/HCT
Atenolol/chlorthalidone (50/25, 100/25)	Tenoretic
Nadolol/bendroflumethiazide (40/5, 80/5)	Corzide
Timolol/hydrochlorothiazide (10/25)	Timolide
Propranolol LA (long-acting)/hydrochlorothiazide (80/50, 120/50, 160/50)	Inderide LA
Bisoprolol/hydrochlorothiazide (2.5/6.25, 5/6.25, 10/6.25)	Ziac*
Centrally-acting drug/diuretic combinations	
Guanethidine/hydrochlorothiazide (10/25)	Esimil
Methyldopa/hydrochlorothiazide (250/15, 250/25, 500/30, 500/50)	Aldoril
Methyldopa/chlorothiazide (250/150, 250/250)	Aldochlor
Reserpine/chlorothiazide (0.125/250, 0.25/500)	Diupres
Reserpine/chlorthalidone (0.125/25, 0.25/50)	Demi-Regroton
Reserpine/hydrochlorothiazide (0.125/25, 0.125/50)	Hydropres
Clonidine/chlorthalidone (0.1/15, 0.2/15, 0.3/15)	Combipres
ACE inhibitor/diuretic combinations	
Captopril/hydrochlorothiazide (25/15, 25/25, 50/15, 50/25)	Capozide*
Enalapril/hydrochlorothiazide (5/12.5, 10/25)	Vaseretic
Lisinopril/hydrochlorothiazide (10/12.5, 20/12.5, 20/25)	Prinzide, zestoretic
Fosinopril/hydrochlorothiazide (10/12.5, 20/12.5)	Monopril/HCT
Quinapril/hydrochlorothiazide (10/12.5, 20/12.5, 20/25)	Accuretic
Benazepril/hydrochlorothiazide (5/6.25, 10/12.5, 20/12.5, 20/25)	Lotensin/HCT
Moexipril/hydrochlorothiazide (7.5/12.5, 15/25)	Uniretic
Angiotensin II receptor antagonist/diuretic combinations	
Losartan/hydrochlorothiazide (50/12.5, 100/25)	Hyzaar
Valsartan/hydrochlorothiazide (80/12.5, 160/12.5)	Diovan/HCT
Irbesartan/hydrochlorothiazide (75/12.5, 150/12.5, 300/12.5, 300/25)	Avalide
Candesartan/hydrochlorothiazide (16/12.5, 32/12.5)	Atacand/HCT
Telmisartan/hydrochlorothiazide (40/12.5, 80/12.5)	Micardis/HCT
Eprosartan/hydrochlorothiazide (600/12.5)	Teveten/HCT
Olmesartan medoxomil/hydrochlorothiazide (20/12.5, 40/12.5, 40/25)	Benicar/HCT
Calcium antagonist/ACE inhibitor combinations	
Amlodipine/benazepril (2.5/10, 5/10, 5/20, 10/20)	Lotrel
Diltiazem/enalapril (180/5)	Teczem
Verapamil (extended release)/trandolapril (180/2, 240/1, 240/2, 240/4)	Tarka
Felodipine (extended release)/enalapril (5/5)	Lexxel
Vasodilator/diuretic combinations	
Hydralazine/hydrochlorothiazide (25/25, 50/25, 100/25)	Apresazide
Prazosin/polythiazide (1/0.5, 2/0.5, 5/0.5)	Minizide

Table 8.1 (continued)

Triple-combination	
Reserpine/hydralazine/hydrochlorothiazide (0.10/25/15)	Ser-Ap-Es
Combination with other drug classes	
Amlodipine/atorvastatin (5/10, 5/20, 5/40, 5/80, 10/10, 10/20, 10/40, 10/80)	Caduet*

*Approved for initial therapy.
**Indicated for initial therapy only for individuals in whom the development of hypokalaemia cannot be risked.
***Numbers in parentheses indicate the strength (in mg) of each drug in a particular combination product.
Updated from JNC7 [6].

arm. Because blood pressure is seldom controlled with a single drug (as discussed in detail below), it would be inappropriate to execute a study that, by design, deprived hypertensive people of the drugs required to achieve their individual blood pressure targets. Some trials, e.g. the Treatment of Mild Hypertension Study (TOMHS) [7] and the Department of Veterans Affairs Monotherapy trial [8, 9], were intended as comparative studies of single-drug therapy, with the primary endpoint of blood pressure reduction (and not morbidity or mortality), but even these allowed a second antihypertensive drug to be added if the blood pressure was not adequately controlled. Some trials have published subgroup analyses of the blood pressure lowering obtained with the initial randomized monotherapy (e.g. Perindopril Protection Against Recurrent Stroke Study [PROGRESS] [10], and the Study on Cognition and Prognosis in the Elderly [SCOPE] [11, 12]). These estimates of antihypertensive efficacy may well be biased, as typically monotherapy is adequate only in those with lower baseline levels of blood pressure. Lastly, several studies have been designed to add a single antihypertensive drug to whatever other therapies (including antihypertensive drugs) that a person might need for their blood pressure or other conditions. Aside from The Diabetes Hypertension Cardiovascular events (DIABHYCAR) trial, these studies (e.g. PROGRESS, the Heart Outcomes Prevention Evaluation [HOPE] [13], EUropean Reduction of cardiac events with Perindopril in stable coronary Artery disease study [EUROPA] [14], Prevention of Events with Angiotensin Converting Enzyme inhibition [PEACE] trial [15], A Coronary disease Trial Investigating Outcome with Nifedipine gastrointestinal therapeutic system [ACTION] [16, 17] and Comparison of Amlodipine vs. Enalapril to Limit Occurrences of Thombosis [CAMELOT] [18]) have largely focused on secondary prevention in patients with a history of prior cardiovascular disease. Because not all patients in these trials have been hypertensive at randomization, and because many included patients who were not previously known to be hypertensive, the blood pressure-lowering efficacy of the antihypertensive drugs used in these trials tends to be biased toward the null (i.e. underestimated).

Despite these caveats, it is possible to compute the average reduction in blood pressure (and its standard deviation) in the nine trials that reported changes in blood pressure attributed to a single antihypertensive drug: TOHMS, HOPE, PROGRESS, EUROPA, SCOPE, DIABHYCAR, PEACE, ACTION and CAMELOT. On average, a single antihypertensive agent reduced blood pressure in these trials by $7.9 \pm 5.5/4.7 \pm 3.3$ mmHg. These data suggest that there is a 2.5% chance of lowering blood pressure more than 18.8/11.3 mmHg using a single antihypertensive drug.

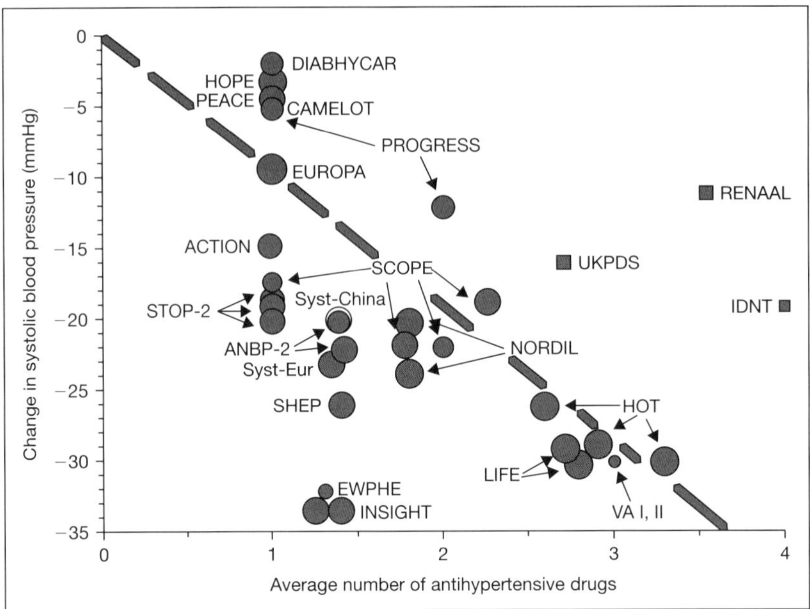

Figure 8.1 Correlation between the number of antihypertensive drugs used (on the *x*-axis) and the observed change (from baseline) in systolic blood pressure (on the *y*-axis) for 41 randomized arms of 27 different clinical trials. Trials in diabetics are denoted by squares. The area of each point is weighted by the square root of the number of patients receiving treatment. The lower bound of the 95% confidence limit of the multiple regression line at $x = 1$ (i.e. monotherapy) is 19.9 mmHg, suggesting that there is a 2.5% chance that a single antihypertensive drug will lower systolic blood pressure >19.9 mmHg. For expansions of abbreviations of clinical trials, see text or list of abbreviations (p. 169).

ESTIMATES OF BLOOD PRESSURE-LOWERING EFFICACY IN MULTIPLE-DRUG THERAPY TRIALS

Because of the limitations of clinical trials that reported the blood pressure-lowering efficacy of a single antihypertensive drug, it is appropriate to consider these results in the context of the many more trials that started with a suitable 'run-in' period (typically placebo), and then added antihypertensive agents to achieve the desired degree of blood pressure lowering. Unfortunately, many of the larger and more recent studies of antihypertensive agents simply 'switched' patients at randomization from their previous antihypertensive drug therapy to whatever drug was being studied. The Antihypertensive and Lipid-Lowering treatment to prevent Heart Attack Trial (ALLHAT) [19], Controlled-Onset Verapamil Investigation of Cardiovascular Endpoints (CONVINCE) trial [20], International Verapamil/trandolapril Study (INVEST) [21], Valsartan Antihypertensive Long-term Use Evaluation (VALUE) [22], and the Anglo-Scandinavian Cardiac Outcomes Trial (ASCOT) [23] did not have a 'run-in' period, so the degree of blood pressure lowering seen in each depends somewhat on the drug therapy that the patients were taking prior to randomization. These studies are therefore excluded from the following analyses, and are reviewed separately below.

Figure 8.1 shows the regression line for the number of antihypertensive drugs used and the observed change (from baseline) in systolic blood pressure for 41 randomized arms of 27 different clinical trials. As might be expected from pharmacological principles, the greater the number of antihypertensive agents used, the greater was the observed lowering of blood

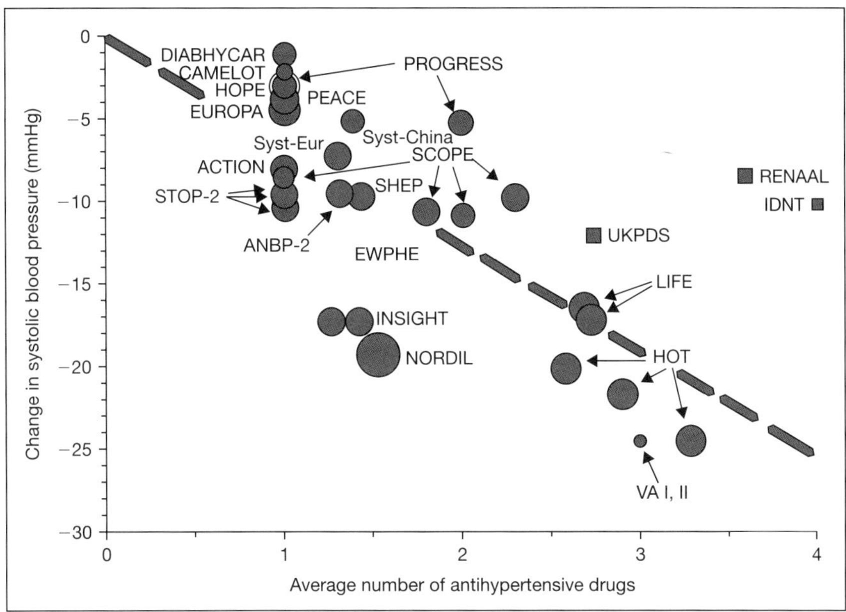

Figure 8.2 Correlation between the number of antihypertensive drugs used (on the *x*-axis) and the observed change (from baseline) in diastolic blood pressure (on the *y*-axis) for 41 randomized arms of 27 different clinical trials. Trials in diabetics are denoted by squares. The area of each point is weighted by the square root of the number of patients receiving treatment. The lower bound of the 95% confidence limit of the multiple regression line at $x = 1$ (i.e. monotherapy) is 10.1 mmHg, suggesting that there is a 2.5% chance that a single antihypertensive drug will lower diastolic blood pressure >10.1 mmHg. For expansions of abbreviations of clinical trials, see text or list of abbreviations (p. 169).

pressure. The correlation shown in the figure is highly significant ($r = 0.42$; $P < 0.001$ if an intercept is allowed, or $r = 0.89$; $P < 0.0001$, if the regression line is forced through zero), especially if one adds the initial systolic blood pressure as a covariate (multiple $r = 0.91$; $P < 0.0001$). This regression line can be used to predict the blood pressure lowering expected with a single antihypertensive drug, as well as its 95% confidence limits. According to these data from nearly 90 000 patients, a single antihypertensive drug has less than a 2.5% chance of lowering systolic blood pressure from 160 mmHg by more than 19.9 mmHg.

Figure 8.2 is identical to Figure 8.1, except that it shows the change in diastolic blood pressure as a function of the number of antihypertensive drugs used in the same 41 randomized arms in 27 trials. The regression line is again highly significant ($r = 0.59$; $P < 0.001$ if an intercept is allowed, or $r = 0.90$; $P < 0.0001$ if the line is forced through zero), especially if the baseline diastolic blood pressure is added as a covariate (multiple $r = 0.94$; $P < 0.0001$). From these data, a single antihypertensive drug has less than a 2.5% chance of lowering diastolic blood pressure from 100 mmHg by more than 10.1 mmHg.

NUMBER OF ANTIHYPERTENSIVE AGENTS USE IN RECENT OUTCOME-BASED CLINICAL TRIALS

The importance of multiple-drug therapy for hypertension in long-term clinical trials can be highlighted by the fact that, in nearly all recent trials, more than a single drug was required in a majority of the patients. Even in ALLHAT, which excluded patients with untreated blood pressure >180/110 mmHg (because it was designed as a trial comparing initial drug treatments), 2.0 drugs were needed, on average, per patient/day at the end of the trial (when the blood pressure target of <140/90 mmHg was achieved in more than 65% of patients) [24]. In CONVINCE, only 27% of patients were successfully treated with monotherapy; the average number of antihypertensive drugs required to get blood pressure <140/90 mmHg in 66% of the subjects was about 2.0 [20]. Hypertensive patients with coronary heart disease were treated initially with either verapamil or atenolol in the INVEST trial, but the average number of drugs required per patient was about 2.1 [21]. In VALUE, only 35% of those treated initially with valsartan and 35.3% of patients given amlodipine achieved the blood pressure target with monotherapy. On average, 2.1 medications were required to achieve a blood pressure <140/90 mmHg in 59% of patients [22]. In ASCOT, only 15% or 9% of the patients initially assigned to amlodipine or atenolol, respectively, were taking monotherapy, and 52% had achieved the blood pressure target of <140/90 mmHg [23]. The average number of antihypertensive drugs used, per patient per day, was 2.2 and 2.3, respectively [24].

In trials involving diabetic patients or patients with chronic kidney disease (in whom the blood pressure target now recommended by JNC 7 and nearly all other authoritative bodies is <130/80 mmHg), even more drugs have been required. The current record was set in the Irbesartan Diabetic Nephropathy Trial, in which 4.0, 4.0, and 4.0 drugs were required per patient/day in the placebo/control, irbesartan, or amlodipine arms, to achieve blood pressures of 144/80, 140/77, and 141/77 mmHg, respectively [25]. In the quite similar Reduction of Endpoints in Non-Insulin Dependent Diabetes Mellitus with the Angiotensin II Antagonist Losartan (RENAAL) study, 3.5 antihypertensive medications/day were required in the group randomized to losartan to lower the blood pressure, on average, to 140/74 mmHg [26]. In the African American Study of Kidney diseases and hypertension (AASK) study, patients required 2.66, 2.65, and 2.79 medications in the ramipril, amlodipine, or metoprolol succinate groups, to achieve blood pressures of 135/82, 133/81, and 135/81 mmHg, respectively [27]. In the earlier Ramipril Efficacy in Nephropathy (REIN) trial, about 1.8 drugs per patient/day were required to lower blood pressure from about 149/92 to 144/88 mmHg in the group randomized to ramipril [28, 29]. In the ACE-Inhibition for Progressive Renal Insufficiency (AIPRI) trial, it took 1.7 drugs per patient/day to lower blood pressure, on average, by 4.5–8.0/3.5–5.0 mmHg (from a baseline of 142/87 mmHg) [30, 31]. All of these studies were designed and essentially completed before the recommendation to achieve a lower blood pressure in patients with chronic kidney disease, so it is likely that even more drugs would have been required if the patients in these studies had the current blood pressure target of <130/80 mmHg. In fact, in the AASK study, 3.04 drugs were required, on average, to achieve the low blood pressure goal of <125/75 mmHg (vs. 128/78 mmHg actually achieved) [27]. A measure of how difficult it is to achieve the lower blood pressure target in chronic kidney disease patients can be discerned from the REIN study #2 (REIN-2), in which felodipine 5–10 mg/d or placebo was added to ramipril (2.5–5 mg/d), in an effort to see if the lower blood pressure prevented the progression of non-diabetic kidney disease [32]. The average blood pressures during follow-up in the two randomized groups differed in this study by only 4.1/2.8 mmHg, despite the addition of a fairly potent dihydropyridine calcium antagonist. Achieving the full 10/10 mmHg difference (between <140/90 mmHg, recommended for uncomplicated hypertensive patients, and <130/80 mmHg, recommended for diabetics and patients with chronic kidney disease) will therefore typically take multiple extra drugs.

POTENTIAL DRAWBACKS TO COMBINATION THERAPY

The major reason that a healthcare provider should be reluctant to prescribe an initial combination of antihypertensive drugs is the concern that blood pressure will be lowered excessively, and the patient may thereafter develop hypotension, shock, and irreversible tissue ischaemia. It is generally not possible to predict with certainty which individual will have a much larger-than-usual fall in blood pressure after being given a specific drug. Early recommendations from national authorities therefore recommended a 'start low, and go slow' approach to drug therapy for hypertension, particularly in older people (who were and are more likely to have hypertension and take drugs to control it).

During the 1960s–1990s, nearly all medical students were taught that a good physician should *never* prescribe a fixed-dose combination drug for hypertension. This precept was based on the collected experience and common practices of that era, when fixed-dose combination drugs had many disadvantages. Combination pills were available then for a small minority of the doses that might be required. Even for the best case, the combination of hydrochlorothiazide and metoprolol tartrate, only three of the eight possible dose combinations were marketed. The limited number of available combinations made it very difficult to titrate each component individually, particularly since only the lower doses were combined. As a result, many patients who ended up taking reasonable doses had to take two of the combination pills at each administration. This mitigated any possible decrease in pill burden or increase in adherence with the combination pills available at that time. Before about 1997, combination antihypertensive pills were typically priced at a premium over the cost for two separate prescriptions, especially when generic drugs were compared. For example, according to the August 1996 *Red Book* [33], the average wholesale price for generic propranolol (40 mg bid) + hydrochlorothiazide (25 mg bid) was 65% higher for the fixed-dose combination ($45.62) than two separate prescriptions for the components ($15.33 + $12.24). Propranolol 80 mg bid and hydrochlorothiazide 25 mg bid was 114% higher as the fixed-dose combination ($67.40) than two separate drugs ($19.20 + $12.24). The more commonly-used atenolol 50 mg + chlorthalidone 25 mg was 634% more expensive as a fixed-dose combination ($213.27), and the 100 mg dose of atenolol + 25 mg chlorthalidone cost 586% more as a single pill ($314.81), as opposed to prescribing two separate tablets ($17.92 + $11.35, and $34.50 + $11.35, respectively). The major objections to using combination pills as initial therapy were therefore [34]: (1) it was difficult (if not impossible) to predict which patients would respond sufficiently to initial monotherapy, thereby making combination therapy unnecessary; and (2) a more potent combination product might precipitate acute hypotension and/or other adverse effects in some patients.

POTENTIAL ADVANTAGES FOR COMBINATION THERAPY

The five major potential advantages of combination therapy for hypertension today are: (1) greater blood pressure-lowering effect; (2) reduced adverse effects, compared to high-dose monotherapy; (3) improved long-term adherence to pill-taking; (4) greater likelihood of achieving the goal blood pressure; (5) economic benefits (both in reduced cost to the pharmacist and healthcare system and reduced co-payment from the patient).

Probably the most important reason to consider combination therapy is the *greater likelihood of blood pressure lowering* resulting from co-prescribing two agents with different (or perhaps synergistic) mechanisms. Analyses of many recent clinical trials have had difficulty in teasing out specific benefits (if any) of antihypertensive agents that are independent of blood pressure lowering [35–37]. The cardiovascular protective effects of all antihypertensive drugs are clearly related to lowering of blood pressure; other effects (if any) are much more difficult to discern. In today's world, physicians, patients, and those paying for treatment are all interested in achieving the target blood pressure, to maximize benefit in reducing cardiovascular and renal morbidity and mortality. There are many clinical studies that prove that two agents, even in low doses, are much more effective in lowering blood pressure than either agent administered alone. Most initial two-drug combinations for hypertension that are approved or are often used as initial therapy contain very low doses, that typically do not result in statistically significant blood pressure reductions (compared to placebo) when administered alone. Thus, hydrochlorothiazide at a dose of 6.25 mg/d has been combined with small doses of bisoprolol, or with a small dose of benazepril, and these combinations do lower blood pressure significantly better than either drug given alone [38, 39]. Small doses of two agents with differing mechanisms of action also lower blood pressure significantly better than a higher dose of a single agent [40]. Physicians now recognize that multiple mechanisms are involved in the genesis and maintenance of hypertension, some of which are amenable to specific drug therapy. Diuretics were originally thought to be useful in volume-expanded hypertensive patients; ACE inhibitors have been alleged to be more effective in volume-contracted people with high circulating levels of angiotensin I. The combination of these two agents should therefore address whichever situation is operative in a particular individual. Thus there are several reasons why, when blood pressure control is not achieved with a single agent, combination therapy may be an attractive option.

Perhaps the next most important reason to consider combination therapy is that some combinations of two different drug classes have *fewer adverse effects* than higher doses of either drug class alone. Diuretics typically cause hypokalemia in a dose-dependent fashion, whereas both ACE inhibitors and angiotensin II receptor blockers cause dose-dependent hyperkalaemia. It is no surprise therefore that the combination of a diuretic and either an ACE inhibitor or an angiotensin II receptor blocker is more likely to lower blood pressure, and less likely to cause derangements in serum potassium than either drug given at a higher dose. One reason why the fixed-dose combination of hydrochlorothiazide (25 mg) + triamterene (37.5 mg) became so popular in the 1970s and 1980s was that hypokalaemia was less common with the combination, and therefore fewer blood tests and even fewer foul-tasting potassium supplements were required. More recently, the combination of a dihydropyridine calcium antagonist and an ACE inhibitor has been shown in several studies to be associated with a lower incidence and severity of pedal oedema (the most common complaint of women taking the former drug type) [41, 42].

It is very likely that combination therapy *enhances adherence* to pill-taking. Generally, the more pills that are required, the lower is the probability that the patient will take them correctly [43]. Many patients can easily cope with taking one or two pills a day, especially if there are no restrictions on the timing of medications (e.g. time of day, relationship to food intake or physical activity). Prescribing more medications increases the pill burden, reduces the chances that the patient will be able to execute the physician's orders correctly, and often leads to abandonment of the prescription [44, 45]. The negative psychological effects of adding more pills should not be ignored, as many patients feel that their condition has deteriorated when more medication is required to control it. This may be part of why, as more pills are added, the economic and adherence burden increases, and patients are more likely to become discouraged, and eventually give up treatment [46]. Recent research suggests that long-term adherence to prescribed antihypertensive drug therapy is more important than either the initial drug chosen for treatment or the initial blood pressure level in preventing cardiovascular events [47]. Thus, simple steps that will enhance the probability that a patient will take the prescribed therapy can be considered especially advantageous [48].

A fourth attraction for combination antihypertensive therapy is the *greater probability of achieving both short- and long-term goals of therapy*. The greater efficacy of combination pills in meeting or exceeding target blood pressures has been shown for many specific combinations, and is one of the requirements of the US Food and Drug Administration (FDA) for marketing a combination. Furthermore, in some demographic groups, certain agents appear to be somewhat less effective than others in lowering blood pressure; these differences typically disappear when a combination approach is adopted. Thus, low-dose ACE inhibitors reduce blood pressure somewhat less in African-American hypertensives than in whites, but addition of a low-dose diuretic wipes out these differences [49]. Perhaps more important, however, are the long-term reductions in morbidity and mortality observed in certain subgroups of the hypertensive population. Beta-blockers have been alleged to be ineffective (compared to placebo) in reducing cardiovascular events in older hypertensives [50], yet when they are used with (or after) a diuretic, they appear to be very effective indeed [51–53].

The most direct evidence-base for combination antihypertensive therapy in preventing cardiovascular events consists primarily of two randomized clinical trials. In the Fosinopril Amlodipine Cardiac Events Trial (FACET), 380 Italian hypertensive diabetics were randomized originally to either a calcium antagonist or an ACE inhibitor. Unlike what is done in most studies in the US, if the blood pressure did not achieve the target with the randomized drug, the other drug was added. Although originally designed to study metabolic effects of the two drugs, cardiovascular events were tallied during 4 years of follow-up [54]. Among the 191 diabetics originally randomized to amlodipine, 27 suffered a stroke, myocardial infarction, or cardiovascular death. This was significantly ($P < 0.008$) more than in those initially given fosinopril (14 of 189 patients). However, among those given *both* drugs, only 4 of 108 patients suffered an event ($P < 0.001$ vs. amlodipine). Similarly, and perhaps more clearly, the results of PROGRESS clearly showed the superiority of combination antihypertensive therapy (perindopril + diuretic, compared to their two corresponding placebos), over monotherapy (perindopril compared to its corresponding placebo) [10]. Not only was the blood pressure lowering much greater over 4 years (12/5 mmHg vs. two placebos, compared to 5/3 mmHg vs. a single placebo), but the prevention of both recurrent stroke (43% vs. 5%) and cardiovascular events (40% vs. 4%) was much better with combination antihypertensive therapy than with monotherapy. Some of these advantages of combination therapy in the PROGRESS study can probably be attributed to 'indication bias' (since the use of the diuretic was left to the investigator, rather than randomization), but both the data and the implications are persuasive in the argument that combination therapy was associated with better blood pressure lowering and long-term prevention of stroke and cardiovascular events.

In addition to post-stroke, there are several clinical situations in which combination therapy with antihypertensive drugs improves outcomes, but both drugs are not usually provided simultaneously from diagnosis. There are several reports of proteinuria being reduced more effectively with the combination of an ACE inhibitor and an angiotensin receptor blocker (ARB), in either diabetic nephropathy [55] or chronic kidney disease without diabetes [56]. Similarly, in heart failure, outcomes have been improved when an ARB was added to an ACE inhibitor [57, 58]. Many clinical trials attest to the benefits of adding a beta-blocker to an ACE inhibitor in patients with heart failure and reduced systolic function [59, 60].

Last, but certainly not least important in today's cost-conscious healthcare environment, are the *potential economic benefits of combination therapy*. Although most combination pills are currently more expensive (at least in average wholesale prices, if not at all pharmacies) than one of the components, some pharmaceutical companies are now marketing combination pills that include one medication (typically a low-dose diuretic) free of charge! Currently, bisoprolol, fosinopril, quinapril, benazepril, and the 100 mg dose of losartan are marketed at the same average wholesale price, whether alone or in combination with low-dose hydrochlorothiazide [61]. Most of the recently introduced combination pills for hypertension cost less than the price of two separate prescriptions. This is true not only for the average wholesale price paid by the pharmacy to acquire the pills for distribution to patients, but also for the out-of-pocket co-payment from patients that has become commonplace in managed care plans. Aside from these potential direct economic benefits of combination pills, there may also be indirect savings: reduced physician visits for dose-titration, less time off work, and fewer visits to pharmacies to pick up new pills. These economic benefits are likely when the combination pill is more likely to achieve goal blood pressure than individually-titrated doses of separately prescribed antihypertensive agents [46]. A recent economic analysis of heart failure patients who were given an ACE inhibitor and a dihydropyridine calcium antagonist either as a fixed-dose combination, or as two separate pills, showed better adherence (by about 28 days/year, on average), and about a 50% reduction in overall healthcare costs in those who took the fixed-dose combination. Whether the economic benefit is due to the greater likelihood of having taken the therapy in the long term, or from the reduction in Emergency Department visits, hospitalizations, and other sequelae of non-adherence, is uncertain [62].

ADVANTAGES AND DISADVANTAGES OF INITIAL COMBINATION ANTIHYPERTENSIVE DRUG THERAPY

As noted above, the major disadvantage to initial combination drug therapy for hypertension is the possibility of lowering blood pressure too far, too fast. A second concern is the possibility that if the two agents chosen have similar adverse effects, it would be challenging to attribute an observed side effect to one drug and not the other; thus, both drugs would likely be discontinued. In reality, most combination antihypertensive pills now marketed contain drugs with different mechanisms of action and very different adverse effect profiles, making this a minor concern.

There are many potential advantages to initial combination antihypertensive drug therapy, many of which are very similar to those discussed above (in the context of 'eventual' transformation of a multiple drug regimen into one that contains fixed-dose antihypertensive drugs). In nearly every clinical trial so far reported, achieving blood pressure goal more quickly has been associated with better prevention of cardiovascular events. Perhaps the three most recent illustrations of this are ALLHAT, VALUE, and ASCOT. In each of these studies, the regimen that achieved lower blood pressure initially was associated with fewer cardiovascular events. Stroke prevention appears to be particularly sensitive to the extent of blood pressure lowering in the preceding few months. During the first 3 months of follow-up in VALUE, systolic blood pressure was significantly worse (by 3.8 mmHg) in the group randomized to valsartan, and both stroke and the primary cardiac endpoint were significantly more common in this group (by about 2-fold) during this period [22]. As time of follow-up progressed, and more medications were added, the blood pressure difference between the two randomized groups shrank, and the hazard ratio for both the primary endpoint and stroke moved toward unity. At least one interpretation of the VALUE data concluded that early control of blood pressure is a strong determinant of cardiovascular outcomes [35].

Using initial combination therapy is likely to have other benefits, as well. Fewer physician visits for dose-titration are likely to be needed if combination antihypertensive therapy is prescribed at the outset, rather than waiting for it to be needed eventually during follow-up. This is particularly true among individuals who begin treatment at a blood pressure that is more than 20/10 mmHg higher than the target (<140/90 mmHg for uncomplicated hypertensives; <130/80 mmHg for diabetics and those with chronic kidney disease) [6]. The economic benefits of less expensive combination products, and the reduced out-of-pocket co-payment with a single prescription are as important for initial therapy as in the long term (as detailed above). Lastly, several recent reports have shown better adherence with a single pill prescribed at the outset, compared to adding a second pill [63, 64].

PRECEDENTS FOR INITIAL COMBINATION THERAPY

There are some historical precedents for allowing fixed-dose combination products to be used for initial treatment. For more than 25 years, the most commonly prescribed antihypertensive product in the USA was a fixed-dose combination of 25 mg of hydrochlorothiazide and 37.5 mg of triamterene; it was frequently used as initial therapy. The 'standard of care' initial therapy for dysuria and presumed urinary tract infection in females is still a

Table 8.2 Examples of 'synergy' between individual antihypertensive agents that could result in clinical benefits for combination therapy over monotherapy

- Fewer problems with abnormal potassium levels due to a thiazide-type diuretic in combination with either a potassium-sparing diuretic, an ACE-I [65], or an ARB [66]
- Reduced pedal oedema with DHP-CCB + ACE-I (compared to DHP-CCB alone) [42, 67, 68]
- Reduced proteinuria with NDHP-CCB + ACE-I (compared to half-doses of either) [69]
- Reduced proteinuria with ACE-I + ARB (compared to half-doses of either alone [55], or compared to either alone at full doses) [56]
- Better blood pressure control and (perhaps) reduced proteinuria with ACE-I + ARB [55]
- Better stroke prevention with diuretic + ACE-I (compared to ACE-I alone) [10]
- Potentiation of blood pressure-lowering effects beyond those of placebo using mini-dose (6.25 mg/d) diuretic + ACE-I [39] or beta-blocker [38]
- Make an intrinsically short-acting agent into a longer-acting combination (e.g. captopril + hydrochlorothiazide) [70]
- Potential drug–drug interaction that can increase serum levels of one or both antihypertensive agents (e.g. DHP-CCB + NDHP-CCB [71], or α-blocker + CCB [72])

ACE-I = angiotensin-converting enzyme inhibitor; ARB = angiotensin receptor blocker; CCB = calcium channel blocker; DHP-CCB = dihydropyridine calcium channel blocker; NDHP-CCB = non-dihydropyridine calcium channel blocker.

fixed-dose combination of 160 mg of trimethoprim and 800 mg of sulphamethoxazole. Many post-menopausal women were formerly given a fixed-dose combination of 0.625 mg of conjugated equine oestrogens and 2.5 or 5 mg of methoxyprogresterone acetate, rather than two individual pills containing the same drugs. The most commonly prescribed first-line antibiotic for otitis media, sinusitis, asthma, and/or other common infections in children is still a fixed-dose combination of amoxicillin and clavulanate. These data indicate that a combination drug has become 'standard of care' for many clinical situations faced by physicians in everyday practice.

REGULATORY REQUIREMENTS FOR COMBINATION THERAPY

The USFDA and other regulatory bodies have clear expectations about data that should lead to marketing approval for a combination product. These include: (1) better efficacy (e.g. lowering blood pressure) than the identical dose of the components given individually; and (2) a 'synergy', (e.g. an improvement in side effects) with the combination compared to the same doses of the components given individually (Table 8.2). In addition, it is unlikely that the combination product will be commercially successful without a better pharmacoeconomic profile than the individual components. As a result, most combination products are sold at a 'discount', compared to the combined prices of their components.

The first expectation of regulatory bodies is typically addressed by one or more 'factorial design studies' in which patients are randomized to one of several doses of the two components to be incorporated in the combination product [38, 66, 67, 73, 74]. The second expectation of regulatory bodies can sometimes be addressed in the same study. For example, in the irbesartan + hydrochlorothiazide trial with a factorial design, the dose-dependent hypokalaemic effect of the diuretic was nicely balanced by the dose-dependent hyperkalaemic effect of the ARB, resulting in no net change in serum potassium in those receiving the highest doses of each drug, compared to those taking two placebos [66].

ADDITIONAL REGULATORY REQUIREMENTS FOR INITIAL COMBINATION THERAPY

If a combination therapy is to be considered for approval as a 'first-line' treatment, an additional set of regulatory requirements must be met. After placebo run-in, randomization must be followed by simultaneous administration of *both* agents in the desired doses, and careful, deliberate, and specialized investigations directed at surveillance of all subjects for untoward adverse effects (especially hypotension). Because both *safety* and *efficacy* of the combination must be demonstrated, regulatory agencies expect to see, e.g. hourly blood pressure measurements in both the seated and upright positions, and careful assessments of all subjects for lightheadedness, dizziness, and/or fainting. Because the probability of any of these symptoms is finite in any acutely dosed antihypertensive agent, most companies marketing combination products in the last 15 years have not attempted this kind of study. Sponsors have instead consigned their combination drug to a 'second-step' niche, and the regulatory agencies have typically required a statement in the prescribing information that the product is 'not indicated for initial therapy'. There are six exceptions to this general rule (Table 8.1). One is a very-low dose diuretic (which has little hypotensive efficacy by itself) combined with various doses of bisoprolol. The others are anomalies of history, all of which were approved for initial therapy years before the current expectations of regulatory authorities were codified.

CHARACTERISTICS OF POTENTIAL CANDIDATES FOR INITIAL COMBINATION THERAPY

The most obvious candidates for initial combination drug therapy are those who need treatment for a very high blood pressure, or those who have a lower-than-usual target blood pressure. According to JNC 7 and nearly all guidelines committees and expert panels, a lower blood pressure is recommended for diabetics and patients with chronic kidney disease [6, 75, 76]. Table 8.3 summarizes some of the characteristics of patients who are good candidates for initial combination drug therapy for their hypertension.

ONGOING RESEARCH IN INITIAL COMBINATION THERAPY

The largest ongoing outcomes-based comparative trial of two initial combination therapies for hypertension is the Avoiding Cardiovascular events through Combination therapy in Patients Living with Systolic Hypertension (ACCOMPLISH) [78]. This multicentre study has enrolled more than 12 600 patients with systolic blood pressures ≥160 mmHg, but diastolic blood pressures <115 mmHg, and randomized them to begin treatment with either amlodipine/benazepril or benazepril/hydrochlorothiazide. The benazepril doses are equal across all steps of the titration scheme, so that the trial could be considered a test of whether a diuretic or a dihydropyridine calcium antagonist is the better drug to use with an initial ACE inhibitor. The primary outcome measure is cardiovascular morbidity and mortality, and 1642 primary events are expected so that it will be completed in late 2009 or 2010. Because there is no 'placebo run-in phase' and patients were immediately switched from their previous antihypertensive therapy to the randomized combination pills, some would not consider this a trial of *initial* combination therapy, as the incidence of acute hypotension after the first dose is likely to be underestimated.

The largest outcome-based study that includes a combination of antihypertensive pills in one randomized arm is the Ongoing Telmisartan alone and in combination with Ramipril Global Endpoint Trial (ON TARGET). This study has successfully enrolled 25 620 patients, aged 55 years and older, with a history of coronary disease, stroke, peripheral vascular

Table 8.3 Some potential candidates for initial combination drug therapy of hypertension*

- Individuals with uncomplicated Stage 2 hypertension (initial blood pressure ≥160/100 mmHg), in whom a single drug is unlikely to achieve a blood pressure <140/90 mmHg, as recommended by JNC7
- Individuals with diabetes mellitus with an initial blood pressure ≥150/90 mmHg, for whom a diuretic, ACE inhibitor, or angiotensin II receptor blocker is unlikely to reduce the blood pressure to <130/80 mmHg, as recommended by the ADA and NKF
- Individuals with chronic kidney disease (abnormal urinary protein excretion, serum creatinine, or estimated glomerular filtration rate) with an initial blood pressure ≥150/90 mmHg, for whom an ACE inhibitor or angiotensin II receptor blocker is unlikely to reduce the blood pressure to <130/80 mmHg, as recommended by JNC7
- Individuals with a 'compelling indication' that involves two drugs (e.g. secondary stroke prevention [10], and others, as discussed in the text)

*Updated from Materson [77]. ACE = angiotensin-converting enzyme; ADA = American Diabetes Association [76]; JNC7 = The Seventh Report of the Joint National Committee on Prevention, Detection, Evaluation, and Treatment of High Blood Pressure [6]; NKF = National Kidney Foundation [75].

disease, or diabetes with target-organ damage (similar to HOPE [13]). Randomized treatment options include ramipril 10 mg/d, telmisartan 80 mg/d, or their combination. The primary endpoint is the first occurrence of stroke, myocardial infarction, cardiovascular death, or hospitalization for heart failure [79]. The parallel Telmisartan Randomized Assessment Study in ACE intolerant subjects with cardiovascular Disease (TRANSCEND) enrolled 5926 patients who were otherwise eligible for ON TARGET, but who were unable to tolerate an ACE inhibitor; they were randomized to either telmisartan 80 mg/d or placebo. These studies are expected to complete their average 4.5 years of follow-up in 2007.

Guidelines committees, regulatory agencies, pharmaceutical companies, and many physicians now recognize that hypertension is seldom the only condition that needs drug treatment in most patients. Perhaps because insulin resistance, dyslipidaemia, obesity, and impaired glucose tolerance often accompany hypertension, combination drug therapies for more than one aspect of the 'metabolic syndrome' are being developed. The combination of amlodipine + atorvastatin has already been approved for marketing in the US, and the ASCOT results have been interpreted as showing a 44% reduction of fatal or non-fatal coronary heart disease and a 48% reduction in stroke for the group receiving the combination [23]. Because the registration trials for the combination included a placebo run-in phase, and patients were given both agents immediately after randomization, the combination is approved for *initial* therapy. Other examples of such combinations being considered for further development include ACE inhibitor + 3-hydroxy-3-methylglutaryl (HMG-CoA) reductase inhibitor [80], angiotensin II receptor antagonist + HMG-CoA reductase inhibitor [81], and insulin sensitizer and ACE inhibitor [82]. Research is currently underway to assess whether such combination therapies that include at least one antihypertensive drug may be more beneficial than either drug alone on such endpoints as endothelial dysfunction, LDL cholesterol levels, and peripheral glucose utilization rates. At least two large, long-term outcome-based studies are underway with such combinations: In the Diabetes Reduction with ramipril and rosiglitazone Medications (DREAM) trial, 5269 people with impaired fasting glucose (or glucose intolerance) have been randomized in a 2 × 2 factorial design to placebo, ramipril (15 mg/d), rosiglitazone (8 mg/d), or their combination. In 2006, 3 years of average follow-up should be accrued to address which therapy best prevents diabetes [83]. In the

Nateglinide and Valsartan in Impaired Glucose [A] Tolerance Outcomes Research (NAVIGATOR) trial, a similar 2 × 2 factorial design is being carried out in 9518 patients with impaired glucose tolerance. Randomization options include 60 mg/d of nateglinide, 160 mg/d of valsartan, both or placebo, but the endpoint is cardiovascular morbidity and mortality [84]. These interesting trials portend a bright future for combination therapies, either as initial or 'second-step' therapies, even apart from the more traditional marriage of two representatives from established antihypertensive drug classes. The major obstacle to more widespread acceptance of combination therapies is reluctance on the parts of some formulary committees to believe that the advantages outweigh the potential drawbacks. This may be amenable to lowering the price of combination products, relative to their components.

SUMMARY

In today's world, there are very few reasons for reluctance to prescribe combination antihypertensive drug therapy for most patients. Fear that the antihypertensive effect will be larger than the patient can tolerate is probably the only serious objection; the availability of low doses of nearly all combination pills makes this a weak argument. The fact is that most patients will eventually require more than a single drug to achieve current blood pressure targets. The US FDA has approved several combination antihypertensive pills for initial therapy of hypertension. Many of the rest have no such indication because the registration trials were done when, and in a way that, the FDA did not find the study designs acceptable for a drug as initial therapy. Since most antihypertensive combination pills are less expensive than their components prescribed separately, the patient saves one co-payment, adherence has been better with fewer pills, and clinical trial evidence for combination pills now exists, it is likely that these drugs will play an increasing role in antihypertensive therapy in the near future.

REFERENCES

1. Kearney PM, Whelton M, Reynolds K, Muntner P, Whelton PK, He J. Global burden of hypertension: analysis of worldwide data. *Lancet* 2005; 365:217–223.
2. Glover MJ, Greenlund KJ, Ayala C, Croft JB. Racial/ethnic disparities in prevalence, treatment and control of hypertension – United States, 1999–2002. *Morb Mortal Wkly Rep* 2005; 54:7–9.
3. Erdine S. How well is hypertension controlled in Europe? *J Hypertens* 2000; 18:1348–1349.
4. Wolf-Maier K, Cooper RS, Banegas JR *et al.* Hypertension prevalence and blood pressure levels in 6 European countries, Canada, and the United States. *JAMA* 2003; 289:2363–2369.
5. Berlowitz DR, Ash AS, Hickey EC *et al.* Inadequate management of blood pressure in a hypertensive population. *N Engl J Med* 1998; 339:1957–1963.
6. National High Blood Pressure Education Program Coordinating Committee. Seventh report of the Joint National Committee on Prevention, Detection, Evaluation and Treatment of High Blood Pressure. *Hypertension* 2003; 42:1206–1252.
7. Neaton JD, Grimm RH, Prineas RJ *et al.* Treatment of mild hypertension study: final results. *JAMA* 1993; 270:713–724.
8. Materson BJ, Reda DJ, Cushman WC. Department of Veterans Affairs Cooperative Study Group on Antihypertensive Agents. Single-drug therapy for hypertension in men. *N Engl J Med* 1993; 328:914–921.
9. Materson BJ, Reda DJ, Cushman WC. Department of Veterans Affairs Cooperative Study Group on Antihypertensive Agents. Single-drug therapy of hypertension study. Revised figures and new data. *Am J Hypertens* 1995; 8:189–192.
10. Progress Collaborative Group. Randomized trial of a perindopril-based blood-pressure-lowering regimen among 6105 individuals with previous stroke or transient ischaemic attack. *Lancet* 2001; 358:1033–1041.
11. Lithell H, Hansson L, Skoog I *et al.* The study on cognition and prognosis in the elderly (SCOPE): principal results of a randomized double-blind intervention trial. *J Hypertens* 2003; 21:875–886.

12. Lithell H, Hansson L, Skoog I *et al.* The SCOPE Study Group. The study on cognition and prognosis in the elderly (SCOPE): outcomes in patients not receiving add-on therapy after randomization. *J Hypertens* 2004; 22:1605–1612.
13. The Heart Outcomes Prevention Evaluation (HOPE) Study Investigators. Effects of an angiotensin-converting-enzyme inhibitor, ramipril, on death from cardiovascular causes, myocardial infarction, and stroke in high-risk patients. *N Engl J Med* 2000; 342:145–153.
14. Fox KM. EUROPA Investigators. Efficacy of perindopril in reduction of cardiovascular events among patients with stable coronary artery disease: randomized, double-blind, placebo-controlled, multicentre trial (The EUROPA study). *Lancet* 2003; 362:782–788.
15. Braunwald E, Domanski MJ, Fowler SE *et al.* The PEACE Trial Investigators. Angiotensin-converting-enzyme inhibition in stable coronary artery disease. *N Engl J Med* 2004; 351:2058–2068.
16. Poole-Wilson PA, Lubsen J, Kirwan BA *et al.* A Coronary Disease Trial Investigating Outcome with Nifedipine Gastrointestinal Therapeutic System Investigators. Effect of long-acting nifedipine on mortality and cardiovascular morbidity in patients with stable angina requiring treatment (ACTION trial): randomized controlled trial. *Lancet* 2004; 364:849–857.
17. Lubsen J, Wagener G, Kirwan B-A, de Brouwer S, Poole-Wilson PA. A Coronary Disease Trial Investigating Outcome with Nifedipine GITS Investigators. Effect of long-acting nifedipine on mortality and cardiovascular morbidity in patients with symptomatic stable angina and hypertension: the ACTION trial. *J Hypertens* 2005; 23:641–648.
18. Nissen SE, Tuzcu EM, Libby P *et al.* Effect of antihypertensive agents on cardiovascular events in patients with coronary disease and normal blood pressure: the CAMELOT Study: a randomized controlled trial. *JAMA* 2004; 292:2217–2225.
19. The ALLHAT Officers and Coordinators for the ALLHAT Collaborative Research Group. Major outcomes in high-risk hypertensive patients randomized to angiotensin-converting enzyme inhibitor or calcium channel blocker vs. diuretic: the antihypertensive and lipid lowering treatment to prevent heart attack trial (ALLHAT). *JAMA* 2002; 288:2981–2997.
20. Black HR, Elliott WJ, Grandits G *et al.* The CONVINCE Research Group. Principal results of the controlled onset Verapamil investigation of cardiovascular endpoints (CONVINCE) trial. *JAMA* 2003; 289:2073–2082.
21. Pepine CJ, Handberg EM, Cooper-DeHoff RM *et al.* The INVEST Investigators. A calcium antagonist vs. a non-calcium antagonist hypertension treatment strategy for patients with coronary artery disease: A randomized controlled trial. *JAMA* 2003; 290:2805–2816.
22. Julius S, Kjeldsen S, Weber M *et al.* Outcomes in hypertensive patients at high cardiovascular risk treated with regimens based on valsartan or amlodipine: the VALUE randomized trial. *Lancet* 2004; 363:2022–2031.
23. Dahlöf B, Sever PS, Poulter NR *et al.* Prevention of cardiovascular events with an antihypertensive regimen of amlodipine adding perindopril as required versus atenolol adding bendroflumethiazide as required, in the Anglo-Scandinavian cardiac outcomes trial-blood pressure lowering arm (ASCOT-BPLA): a multicentre randomized controlled trial. *Lancet* 2005; 366:895–906.
24. Cushman WC, Ford CE, Cutler JA *et al.* Success and predictors of blood pressure control in diverse North American settings: the antihypertensive and lipid-lowering treatment to prevent heart attack trial (ALLHAT). *J Clin Hypertens (Greenwich)* 2002; 4:393–404.
25. Lewis EJ, Hunsicker LG, Clarke WR *et al.* Collaborative Study Group. Renoprotective effect of the angiotensin-receptor antagonist irbesartan in patients with nephropathy due to Type 2 diabetes. *N Engl J Med* 2001; 345:841–860.
26. Brenner BM, Cooper ME, de Zeeuw D *et al.* Reduction of Endpoints in Non-Insulin Dependent Diabetes Mellitus with the Angiotensin II Antagonist Losartan (RENAAL) Study Group. Effects of losartan on renal and cardiovascular outcomes in patients with Type 2 diabetes and nephropathy. *N Engl J Med* 2001; 345:861–869.
27. Wright JT Jr, Bakris GL, Greene T *et al.* Effect of blood pressure lowering and antihypertensive drug class on progression of hypertensive kidney disease: results from the AASK trial. *JAMA* 2002; 288:2421–2431.
28. The GISEN Group (Gruppo Italiano di Studi Epidemiologici in Nefrologia). Randomized placebo-controlled trial of effect of ramipril on decline in glomerular filtration rate and risk of terminal renal failure in proteinuric, non-diabetic nephropathy. *Lancet* 1997; 349:1857–1863.
29. Ruggenenti P, Perna A, Zoccali C *et al.* Gruppo Italiano di Studi Epidemologici in Nefrologia (GISEN). Chronic proteinuric nephropathies. II. Outcomes and response to treatment in a prospective cohort of

352 patients: differences between women and men in relation to the ACE gene polymorphism. *J Am Soc Nephrol* 2000; 11:88–96.

30. Maschio G, Alberti D, Janin G *et al.* Angiotensin-Converting Enzyme Inhibition in Progressive Renal Insufficiency Study Group. Effect of the angiotensin-converting enzyme inhibitor benazepril on the progression of chronic renal insufficiency. *N Engl J Med* 1996; 323:939–945.
31. Locatelli F, Carbarns IR, Maschio G *et al.* The Angiotensin-Converting-Enzyme Inhibition in Progressive Renal Insufficiency Study Group. Long-term progression of chronic renal insufficiency in the AIPRI Extension Study. *Kidney Int* 1997; 63:S63–S67.
32. Ruggenenti P, Perna A, Loriga G *et al.* Blood-pressure control for renoprotection in patients with non-diabetic chronic renal disease (REIN-2): multicentre, randomized controlled trial. *Lancet* 2005; 365:939–946.
33. Drug Topics Red Book, August Update: Medical Economics Data, Montvale, NJ, 1996.
34. Drugs for hypertension. *Med Lett Drugs Ther* 2001; 43:41–45.
35. Weber MA, Julius S, Kjeldsen SE *et al.* Blood pressure dependent and independent effects of antihypertensive treatment on clinical events in the VALUE trial. *Lancet* 2004; 363:2049–2051.
36. Verdecchia P, Reboldi G, Angeli F *et al.* Angiotensin-converting enzyme inhibitors and calcium channel blockers for coronary heart disease and stroke prevention. *Hypertension* 2005; 46:386–392.
37. Elliott WJ, Jonsson MC, Black HR. It's Not Beyond the Blood Pressure, It IS the Blood Pressure! *Circulation* 2006; (in press).
38. Frishman WH, Bryzinski BS, Coulson LR *et al.* A multifactorial trial design to assess combination therapy in hypertension: treatment with bisoprolol and hydrochlorothiazide. *Arch Intern Med* 1994; 154:1461–1468.
39. Chrysant SG, Fagan T, Glazer R, Kriegman A. Effects of benazepril, given alone or in low- and high-dose combinations, on blood pressure in patients with hypertension. *Arch Family Med* 1996; 5:17–24.
40. Elliott WJ, Montoro R, Smith D, Liebowitz M, Schleman M, Klibaner M. Enalapril-Felodipine ER vs. Enalapril (LEVEL) Study Group. Comparison of two strategies for intensifying antihypertensive treatment: low-dose combination (enalapril + felodipine ER) vs. increased dose of monotherapy (enalapril). *Am J Hypertens* 1999; 14:691–696.
41. Morgan TO, Anderson A, Jones E. Comparison and interaction of low-dose felodipine and enalapril in the treatment of essential hypertension in elderly subjects. *Am J Hypertens* 1992; 5:238–243.
42. Messerli FH, Weir MR, Neutel JM. Combination therapy of amlodipine/benazepril versus monotherapy of amlodipine in a practice-based setting. *Am J Hypertens* 2002; 15:550–556.
43. Iskedjian M, Einarson TR, MacKeigan LD *et al.* Relationship between daily dose frequency and adherence to antihypertensive pharmacotherapy: Evidence from a meta-analysis. *Clin Ther* 2002; 24:302–316.
44. Jones JK, Gorkin L, Lian JF, Staffa JA, Fletcher AP. Discontinuation of and changes in treatment after start of new courses of antihypertensive drugs: a study of a United Kingdom population. *BMJ* 1995; 311:293–296.
45. Caro JJ, Salas M, Speckman JL, Raggio G, Jackson JD. Persistence with treatment for hypertension in actual practice. *CMAJ* 1999; 160:31–37.
46. Caro JJ, Speckman JL, Salas M, Raggio G, Jackson JD. Effect of initial drug choice on persistence with antihypertensive therapy: the importance of actual practice data. *CMAJ* 1999; 160:41–60.
47. Mar J, Rodriguez-Artalejo F. Which is more important for the efficiency of hypertension treatment: hypertension stage, type of drug, or therapeutic compliance? *J Hypertens* 2001; 19:149–155.
48. Haynes RB, McDonald HP, Garg AX. Helping patients follow prescribed treatment: Clinical applications. *JAMA* 2002; 288:2880–2883.
49. Sehgal AR. Overlap between whites and blacks in response to antihypertensive drugs. *Hypertension* 2004; 43:566–572.
50. Messerli FH, Grossman E, Goldboourt U. Are beta-blockers efficacious as first-line therapy for hypertension in the elderly: a systematic review. *JAMA* 1998; 279:1903–1907.
51. Systolic Hypertension in the Elderly Program Research Group. Prevention of stroke by antihypertensive drug treatment in older persons with isolated systolic hypertension. *JAMA* 1991; 265:3255–3264.
52. Psaty BM, Lumley T, Furberg CD *et al.* Health outcomes associated with various antihypertensive therapies used as first-line agents: a network meta-analysis. *JAMA* 2003; 289:2534–2544.
53. Wassertheil-Smoller S, Psaty B, Greenland P *et al.* Association between cardiovascular outcomes and antihypertensive drug treatment in older women. *JAMA* 2004; 292:2849–2859.
54. Tatti P, Pahor M, Byington RP *et al.* Outcome results of the fosinopril amlodipine cardiovascular events randomized trial (FACET) in patients with hypertension and NIDDM. *Diabetes Care* 1998; 21:1779–1780.

55. Mogensen CE, Neldam S, Tikkanen I *et al.* Randomized controlled trial of dual blockade of renin-angiotensin system in patients with hypertension, microalbuminuria, and non-insulin dependent diabetes: the candesartan and lisinopril microalbuminuria (CALM) study. *BMJ* 2000; 321:1440–1444.
56. Nakao N, Yoshimura A, Morita H, Takeda M, Kayano T, Ideura T. Combination treatment of angiotensin-II receptor blocker and angiotensin-converting-enzyme inhibitor in non-diabetic renal disease (COOPERATE): a randomized controlled trial. *Lancet* 2003; 361:117–124.
57. Cohn JN, Tognoni G. The Val-HeFT Investigators. A randomized trial of the angiotensin-receptor blocker valsartan in chronic heart failure. *N Engl J Med* 2001; 345:1667–1675.
58. McMurray JJV, Östergren J, Swedberg K *et al.* CHARM Investigators and Committees. Effects of candesartan in patients with chronic heart failure and reduced left-ventricular systolic function taking angiotensin-converting-enzyme inhibitors: the CHARM-added trial. *Lancet* 2003; 362:767–771.
59. Brophy JM, Joseph L, Rouleau JL. Beta-blockers in congestive heart failure: a Bayesian meta-analysis. *Ann Intern Med* 2001; 134:550–560.
60. Foody JM, Farrel MH, Krumholz HM. Beta-blocker therapy in heart failure: scientific review. *JAMA* 2002; 287:883–889.
61. Drugs for hypertension. *Treat Guidel Med Lett* 2003; 1:31–42.
62. Taylor AA, Shoheiber O. Adherence to antihypertensive therapy with fixed-dose amlodipine besylate/benazepril HCl vs. comparable component-based therapy. *Congest Heart Fail* 2003; 9:324–332.
63. Chapman RH, Benner JS, Petrilla AA *et al.* Predictors of adherence with antihypertensive and lipid-lowering therapy. *Arch Intern Med* 2005; 165:1147–1152.
64. Sturkenboom MCJM, Picelli G, Dieleman JP, Mozaffari E, Pompen M, van der Lei J. Patient adherence and persistence with antihypertensive therapy: one- versus two-pill combinations [abstract]. *J Hypertens* 2005; 23(suppl 2):S269.
65. Weinberger MH. Influence of an angiotensin converting-enzyme inhibitor on diuretic-induced metabolic effects in hypertension. *Hypertension* 1983; 5:132–138.
66. Kochar M, Guthrie R, Triscari J, Kassler-Taub K, Reeves RA. Matrix study of irbesartan with hydrochlorothiazide in mild-to-moderate hypertension. *Am J Hypertens* 1999; 12:797–805.
67. Gradman AH, Cutler NR, Davis PJ *et al.* Enalapril-Felodipine ER Factorial Study Group. Combined enalapril and felodipine extended release (ER) for systemic hypertension. *Am J Cardiol* 1997; 79:431–435.
68. Jamerson KA, Nwose O, Jean-Louis L *et al.* Initial angiotensin-converting enzyme inhibitor/calcium channel blocker combination therapy achieves superior blood pressure control compared with calcium channel blocker monotherapy in patients with Stage 2 hypertension. *Am J Hypertens* 2004; 17:495–501.
69. Bakris GL, Weir MR, DeQuattro V, McMahon FG. Effects of an ACE inhibitor/calcium antagonist combination on proteinuria in diabetic nephropathy. *Kidney Int* 1998; 54:1283–1289.
70. Schoenberger JA, Wilson DJ. One-daily treatment of essential hypertension with captopril. *J Clin Hypertension* 1986; 2:379–387.
71. Saseen JJ, Carter BL, Brown TER, Elliott WJ, Black HR. Comparison of nifedipine alone and in combination with diltiazem or verapamil in hypertension. *Hypertension* 1996; 28:109–114.
72. Brown MJ, Dickerson JE. Alpha-blockade and calcium antagonism: An effective and well-tolerated combination for the treatment of resistant hypertension. *J Hypertens* 1995; 13:701–707.
73. Burris J, Weir M, Oparil S *et al.* An assessment of diltiazem and hydrochlorothiazide in hypertension. *JAMA* 1990; 263:1507–1512.
74. DeQuattro V, Lee D, Messerli FH. Trandolapril Study Group. Efficacy of combination therapy with trandolapril and verapamil SR in primary hypertension: a 4×4 trial design. *Clin Exp Hypertension* 1997; 19:373–387.
75. K/DOQI clinical practice guidelines on hypertension and antihypertensive agents in chronic kidney disease. *Am J Kidney Dis* 2004; 43(suppl 2):1–290.
76. American Diabetes Association. Hypertension Management in Adults with Diabetes. *Diabetes Care* 2004; 27(suppl 1):S65–S67.
77. Materson BJ. Combination therapy as the initial drug treatment for hypertension: When is it appropriate? *Am J Hypertens* 2001; 14:293–295.
78. Jamerson KA, Bakris GL, Wun CC *et al.* Rationale and design of the avoiding cardiovascular events through combination therapy in patients living with systolic hypertension (ACCOMPLISH) trial: the first randomized controlled trial to compare the clinical outcome effects of first-line combination therapies in hypertension. *Am J Hypertens* 2004; 17:793–801.
79. Teo K, Yusuf S, Anderson C *et al.* Rationale, design, and baseline characteristics of 2 large, simple, randomized trials evaluating telmisartan, ramipril, and their combination in high-risk patients: the

ongoing telmisartan alone and in combination with ramipril global endpoint trial/telmisartan randomized assessment study in ACE intolerant subjects with cardiovascular disease (ONTARGET/TRANSCEND) trials. *Am Heart J* 2004; 148:52–61.

80. Teo KK, Burton JR, Buller CE *et al.* Long-term effects of cholesterol lowering and angiotensin-converting enzyme inhibition on coronary atherosclerosis. the simvastatin/enalapril coronary atherosclerosis trial (SCAT). *Circulation* 2000; 102:1748–1754.
81. Nickenig G, Baumer AT, Temur Y, Keben D, Jockenhovel F, Bohm M. Statin-sensitive dysregulated AT1 receptor function and density in hypercholesterolemic men. *Circulation* 1999; 100:2131–2134.
82. Yoshida K, Kohzuki M, Xu HL, Wu SM, Kamimoto M, Sato T. Effects of troglitazone and temocapril in spontaneously hypertensive rats with chronic renal failure. *J Hypertens* 2001; 19:503–510.
83. Gerstein HC, Yusuf S, Holman R, Bosch J, Pogue J. Rationale, design and recruitment characteristics of a large, simple international trial of diabetes prevention: the DREAM trial. DREAM Trial Investigators. *Diabetologia* 2004; 47:1519–1527.
84. Leiter LA, Lewanczuk RZ. Of the renin-angiotensin system and reactive oxygen species: type 2 diabetes and angiotensin II inhibition. *Am J Hypertens* 2005; 18:121–128.

9

Is pulse pressure a predictor of therapeutic outcome?

G. M. London, M. E. Safar

For many years systolic blood pressure (SBP) and diastolic blood pressure (DBP) were the exclusive mechanical factors used to predict cardiovascular (CV) risk in populations of normotensive and hypertensive individuals. However, the weight of evidence suggests that if hypertension is considered as a mechanical factor acting on the arterial wall with possible deleterious consequences, the totality of the blood pressure (BP) curve should give more information than SBP or DBP alone. The purpose of this review is to show that, in addition to SBP and DBP, other haemodynamic indexes with particular relevance for CV complications and that originate from pulsatile pressure should have to be taken into account, namely brachial pulse pressure (PP).

The main findings of this review based on the study of normotensive and hypertensive populations are: (i) increased PP is an independent predictor of CV risk, mainly myocardial infarction, but also congestive heart failure and CV death; (ii) increased PP is a major predictor of death in high risk populations such as subjects with diabetes mellitus, ischaemic heart disease and, in particular, patients with end-stage renal disease (ESRD). Furthermore, in recent years, therapeutic trials reducing CV risk have demonstrated the predictive value of PP regarding myocardial infarctus in subjects with end-stage renal failure and, to a lesser extent, in old subjects with systolic hypertension.

PATHOPHYSIOLOGICAL BACKGROUND

Many epidemiological studies have emphasized the close correlation observed between the elevation of BP and the incidence of CV events [1]. Within this context, in the past, clinical hypertension was classified almost exclusively on the basis of DBP level [2]. The hypertensive haemodynamic changes were attributed exclusively to a reduction in the calibre and/or number of small arteries, with a resulting increase in systemic vascular resistance and consistent alterations in the structure and function of the arterioles and the heart. More recently, prospective studies [3–5] have directed attention to SBP as a better guide than DBP to evaluate CV and all mortality. Furthermore, it has been shown that drug treatment of hypertension frequently results in adequate control of DBP (≤90 mmHg in 80% cases), whereas the ability to control SBP (≤140 mmHg in 60% cases) is achieved to a much smaller extent [6–8]. Such studies have finally focused attention on the haemodynamic factors that determine the level of SBP and PP and CV risk in hypertensive individuals, and therefore on the role of increased arterial stiffness and wave reflections in the mechanism of CV morbidity and mortality.

Gérard M. London, MD, Chief, Department of Nephrology, Manhes Hospital Fleury-Mérogis, France
Michel E. Safar, PhD, PU-PH Consultant, Diagnosis Center, Hôtel-Dieu Hospital, Paris, France

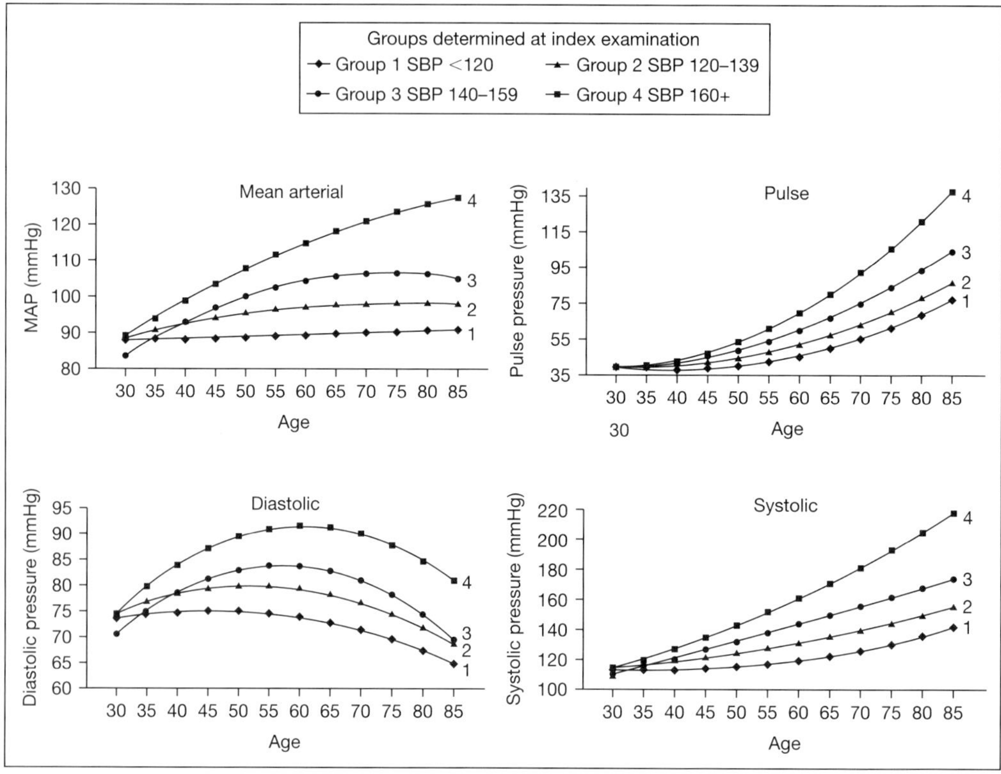

Figure 9.1 Relationship between BP (divided into four subgroups according to SBP level) and age in the Framingham population [12].

A characteristic function of large arteries is to instantaneously accommodate the volume of blood ejected from the heart, storing part of the stroke volume during systolic ejection and draining this volume during diastole, thereby ensuring a continuous perfusion of organs and tissues. This 'Windkessel' effect is usually described in terms of compliance, distensibility or stiffness of the aorta of an individual artery [9, 10] (see appendix). The most direct method to evaluate arterial stiffness is based on the study of pulse wave velocity (PWV) along a given large artery such as the aorta [10]. Nevertheless, in patients over 50 years of age, a quite common but indirect method consists of determining brachial PP. For a given cardiac function, increased arterial stiffness is the major determinant of PP in large populations of normotensive and hypertensive subjects [9, 10].

HISTORICAL BACKGROUND

Cross-sectional and longitudinal studies have extensively shown that BP increases markedly with age [11, 12]. However, this aspect is mainly observed for SBP. In individuals over 50–60 years of age [12], DBP becomes stable and even tends to fall spontaneously (Figure 9.1). From this classic description, it appears that PP increases more markedly with age than does mean arterial pressure (MAP). As a result, in terms of pathophysiological mechanisms, the role played by large arteries overrides that of small arteries after 50 years of age. The increase in aortic PP with age is expected to have important consequences in the complications of hypertensive disease. The increase in SBP enhances the metabolic needs of the myocardium through an increase in end-systolic stress, and thus development of cardiac hypertrophy, whereas the decrease in DBP compromises coronary perfusion and then favours myocardial ischaemia [9, 10]. However, such possibilities require confirmation from clinical findings issued from CV epidemiology.

In clinical research, from a methodological viewpoint, the concept that PP *per se* plays a role in CV morbidity and mortality in addition to (or independently of) SBP, DBP and MAP is difficult to demonstrate. Indeed, PP is the mathematical difference between SBP and DBP, and therefore raises the problem of artefactual interpretations [11, 12]. Some reports [13, 14] have suggested that PP was no better than SBP alone in predicting coronary heart disease in either sex. However, in such studies, the description of the BP curve was based mainly on one or two points (SBP and/or DBP) and did not take into account that the BP curve involved two different components, a steady and a pulsatile one, and that the statistical analysis requires each component to be investigated independently.

In 1988 and later [15, 16], we observed that in patients treated for hypertension, whose DBP was adequately controlled (≤90 mmHg), approximately one-third of the population exhibited an elevated SBP (≥140 mmHg) and PP for the same MAP as the remaining individuals. This group was characterized both by a higher aortic PWV and a higher degree of cardiac hypertrophy. Later, the Systolic hypertension in the Elderly Program (SHEP) study [17] noted similar findings. Because the drug treatment in patients with isolated systolic hypertension reduced SBP more than DBP, it resulted in a sustained increase in PP. The same findings were observed in several other large populations of therapeutic trials [6–8, 18], including mainly old subjects with isolated systolic or with systolic–diastolic hypertension. Thus, the drug treatment of hypertension caused a very peculiar haemodynamic pattern associating a low DBP and an elevated SBP. Taken together, these observations pointed to the importance of normalizing SBP in individuals with hypertension and focused attention on PP as a possible significant factor playing a role in CV risk (Figure 9.2).

PULSE PRESSURE AS AN INDEPENDENT PREDICTOR OF CARDIOVASCULAR RISK

In 1989, in a French study including a large population of normotensive and untreated hypertensive adults [19], a pulsatile component index, clearly defined as a strong correlate of PP, was derived by principal-components analysis from brachial SBP and DBP measurements. An association was found between this index and electrocardiographic evidence of left ventricular hypertrophy. During a 10-year follow-up, the index was independently associated with an increased risk of death from coronary artery disease, but not from stroke. The relationship was found to be significant mainly in women over 55 years of age. In another prospective study evaluating hypertensive subjects [20], those in the highest tertile of PP before the initiation of therapy (≥63 mmHg) had an increased risk of myocardial infarction and, to a lesser extent, of stroke. This result was obtained during an average follow-up of 5 years. In a later study [21], multivariate analysis revealed that PP as a categorical variable (but not as a continuous variable) was an independent predictor of myocardial infarction. Finally, the results were observed whether PP was measured by sphygmomanometry or ambulatory measurements [22].

In a few years, Franklin and colleagues [23] from the Framingham Heart Study, Millar and co-workers [24] from the Medical Research Council trial, and Blacher and colleagues [25] from the EWPHE, Syst-China and Syst-Eur trials, clearly showed that brachial PP was a stronger CV risk factor than SBP alone for myocardial infarction in populations of individuals with hypertension. The best predictor function of all possible linear combinations of SBP and DBP was shown to be similar to that of PP, indicating that their association was not merely a statistical artefact caused by the correlation between SBP and PP [23, 24, 26].

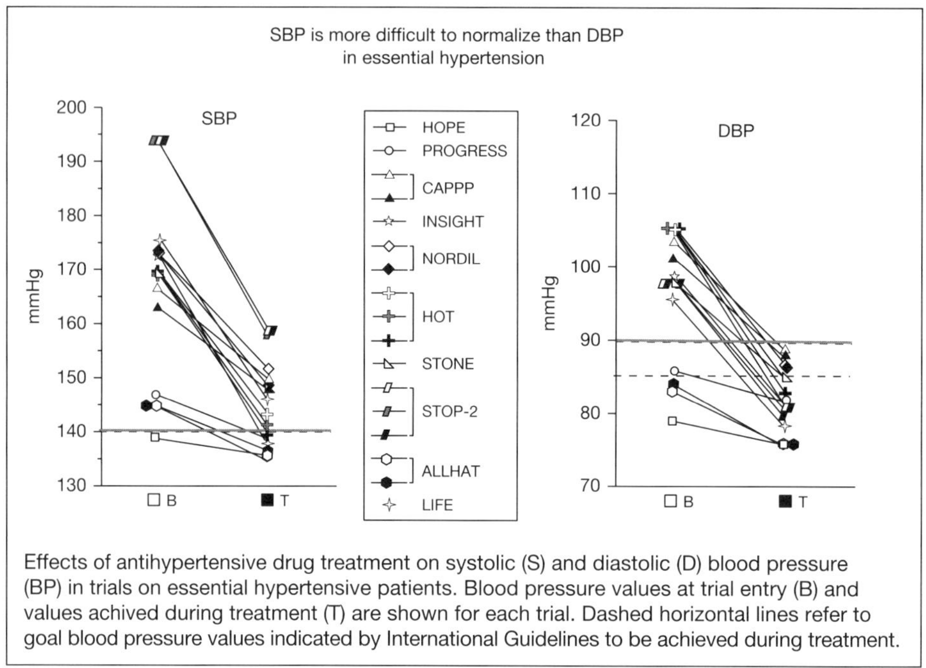

Figure 9.2 Therapeutic trials in hypertension: whereas DBP is constantly controlled, SBP remains elevated in the majority of subjects [8].

Furthermore, studies clearly indicated that CV risk was related not only to an increase in SBP but also to a decrease in DBP [25]. As shown in Figure 9.3, CV risk increases markedly with SBP level. However, at any given value of SBP, CV risk was higher when DBP was lower [25]. This important finding was confirmed by a longitudinal study [27] indicating that, during a 20-year follow-up, subjects with the higher CV mortality rates were those who developed in parallel an increase in SBP and a decrease in DBP. CV mortality was significantly higher in such individuals than in individuals developing both an increase in SBP and DBP [27]. Furthermore, it was shown that, above 59 years of age, neither SBP nor DBP were superior to PP in predicting coronary risk [23]. Finally, PP was demonstrated to be an independent predictor of CV mortality, even in individuals with recurrent myocardial infarction, congestive heart failure and myocardial dysfunction [28–32]. In addition, in selected populations of patients with coronary ischaemic disease but preserved ejection fraction, intra-aortic PP was shown to be superior to brachial PP in predicting CV risk [32].

PULSE PRESSURE AS AN INDEPENDENT CARDIOVASCULAR RISK FACTOR IN NORMOTENSIVE AND TREATED HYPERTENSIVE INDIVIDUALS

In a large population of 19083 normo- and hypertensive men followed for 20 years, Benetos and colleagues [33] not only confirmed that increased PP was a strong predictor of myocardial infarction but also that this predictive value was observed in the normotensive population, particularly in men over 55 years of age.

From the studies of Benetos and co-workers [33, 34], it appeared that the evaluation of PP is of major interest, even in individuals with a mean blood pressure (MBP) of 107 mmHg or less, i.e. with BP within the normal range. According to these results, normotensive men who are in the higher PP group (mean values of SBP 131 mmHg; DBP 73 mmHg; MBP

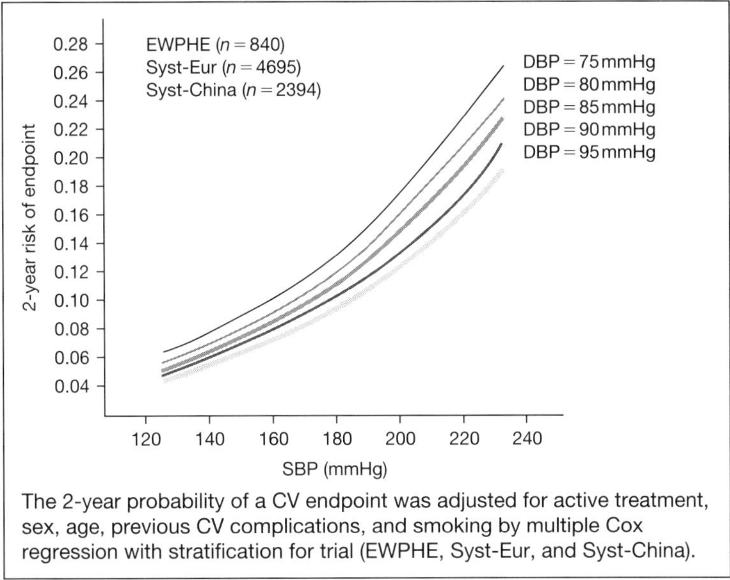

The 2-year probability of a CV endpoint was adjusted for active treatment, sex, age, previous CV complications, and smoking by multiple Cox regression with stratification for trial (EWPHE, Syst-Eur, and Syst-China).

Figure 9.3 Relationship between CV risk and SBP. Risk estimates for all CV endpoints based on three large therapeutic trials (n = 7929) [25] as a function of SBP. Note that the risk increases with the level of SBP. However, at any given value of SBP, the risk is higher when DBP is lower.

92 mmHg; PP 58 mmHg) have: (i) an increased relative risk of 40% compared with normotensive individuals who belong in the lower PP group (SBP 120 mmHg; DBP 78 mmHg; MBP 92 mmHg; PP 42 mmHg), and (ii) a similar CV risk to hypertensive individuals who belong in the lower PP group (SBP 145 mmHg; DBP 105 mmHg; MBP 118 mmHg; PP 40 mmHg). This analysis could be applied even to treated hypertensive individuals [35]. As a result, even within normotensive BP ranges (SBP ≤140 mmHg; DBP ≤90 mmHg) after successful drug therapy, increased PP predicts a reduced CV mortality, a finding mainly observed in diabetic patients [35]. Finally, such findings showed clear interactions between drug treatment and the strength of PP as a CV risk factor [35, 36].

The more recent therapeutic trials of the literature have confirmed such an overview. In the SHEP study [17], which involved elderly subjects with isolated systolic hypertension, and in which increased SBP was the exclusive criterion of inclusion, the reduction in CV risk was associated with a decrease in SBP, whereas, in contrast, a decrease in DBP was rather associated with an increase in CV risk [36]. Furthermore, in therapeutic trials performed in the elderly, CV mortality was indeed substantially reduced but, at the end of such trials, the population was still characterized by a low DBP contrasting with an elevated SBP. Taken together, these findings indicate that, in elderly subjects treated for hypertension, the classic haemodynamic pattern of isolated systolic hypertension with increased PP is still present despite an 'adequate' but not 'optimal' drug treatment [6, 18]. These observations suggested that not only should more attention be paid to the level of SBP and PP in relation to CV risk, but also that it is worth evaluating the CV risk induced by the haemodynamic factors influencing SBP and PP: namely ventricular ejection, aortic stiffness, and wave reflections. Finally, in recent years, the validity of PP as a significant CV risk factor over 59 years of age, has been confirmed by the demonstration of the role of aortic PWV in the development of CV risk [37, 38].

PP AS A CV RISK FACTOR IN SELECTED POPULATIONS

Numerous clinical reports have shown that arterial stiffening in subjects with diabetes mellitus and in ESRD patients is typically associated with changes in BP profile, characterized by isolated increase in SBP and/or increased PP [39–41]. Epidemiological studies have shown that increased PP is associated with a risk of death in subjects with diabetes mellitus and in ESRD patients undergoing haemodialysis [40]. In the latter, cardiac hypertrophy is closely related to SBP or PP. The arterial stiffness and early wave reflections are the principal determinants of SBP and PP in such ESRD patients and are characterized by increased cardiac mass and its progression over time. The arterial stiffness is responsible for earlier return of wave reflections that affect the central arteries during systole rather than diastole, thus amplifying aortic and left ventricular pressures during systole and reducing aortic BP during diastole. By favouring early wave reflections, arterial stiffening increases peak- and end-systolic pressures in the ascending aorta, increasing pressure load and myocardial oxygen consumption and decreasing the DBP as a determinant of coronary perfusion and blood-flow distribution. Furthermore, increased SBP induces myocardial hypertrophy, and impairs diastolic myocardial function and left ventricular ejection [40]. An example of the consequences of such alterations on CV mortality is presented in Figure 9.4.

TARGET TRIALS SHOWING SELECTIVE PP REDUCTION IN HYPERTENSIVE SUBJECTS

Pharmacological studies indicate that any antihypertensive drug reducing arteriolar tone, and therefore MAP, may decrease SBP through a passive reduction of arterial stiffness and change in the timing of wave reflections. However, in the case of subjects with a disproportionate increase of SBP over DBP, the target mechanisms are rather a decrease of ventricular ejection and/or an active increase of arterial stiffness or change in wave reflections. The former, observed with ventricular pacing and treatment of atrioventricular blocks, is not within the scope of this review [41]. The latter is one of the main objectives of this report, where it will be shown that: (i) some drugs, such as nitrates or converting enzyme inhibitors, may act predominantly on large artery structures and function independently of MAP and vascular resistance changes, particularly in the elderly, and (ii) prolongation of survival in hypertensive subjects requires reduction not only of BP but also of arterial stiffness and/or wave reflections.

Nitrates are known to dilate larger rather than smaller arteries, whether or not the endothelium is intact [41–43]. Early studies showed that nitrates cause an acute and selective decrease of SBP over DBP in healthy volunteers, as well as in subjects with borderline or sustained essential hypertension [43]. Since the baroreflex response following nitrates is known to be attenuated with age, an acute and selective reduction of SBP is thus constantly observed in older subjects with systolic hypertension [44]. Low-dose nitrates weakly modify stroke volume, venous tone and aortic PWV while aortic wave reflections, as a consequence of a significant increase in the diameter of peripheral (but not central) muscular arteries, play a major role in the mechanism of this SBP reduction [41–43]. Taylor [45] previously reported that an increase of the arterial cross-sectional area at peripheral bifurcations theoretically causes a delay of wave reflections with subsequent selective decreases of SBP and PP through changes of peripheral reflection patterns. In clinical situations, such changes of SBP and PP have been widely observed in acute randomized studies [41–43, 46]. However, in many cases, they are difficult to detect clinically. Indeed, under nitrates, the PP amplification is modified from the central aorta to the brachial artery, making the SBP changes more pronounced at the thoracic aorta level than at the site of brachial artery [41]. Finally, for a therapeutic approach, the major point to consider regarding nitrates is that a selective and chronic decrease of aortic SBP may be constantly obtained as a consequence of changes of muscular artery geometry and subsequent modifications in reflection coefficients [41–48]. Results on nitrates were the first to show that a

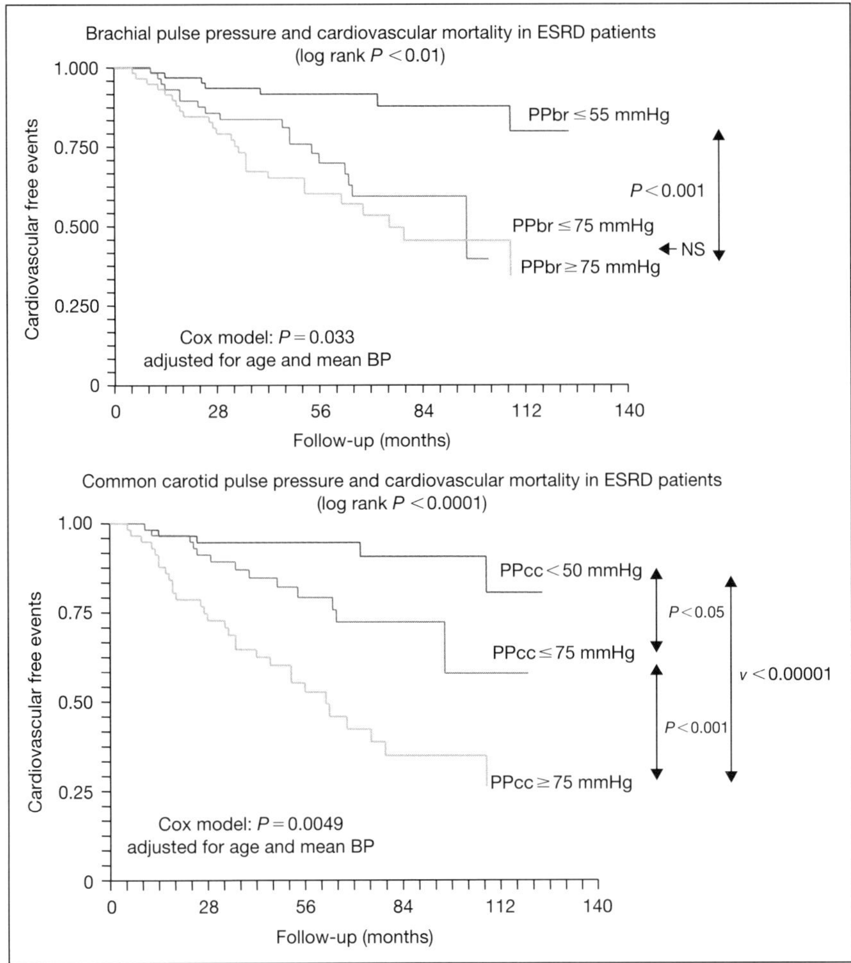

Figure 9.4 Relationship brachial and carotid PP vs. CV mortality in ESRD patients (personal data). Receiver operating characteristic (ROC) curves show that PP is superior as a predictor than SBP, DBP or MAP (data not shown).

pharmacological approach based on arterial stiffness and wave reflections should be sufficient to obtain a selective SBP reduction in hypertensive subjects [47, 48]. In recent years, a more complete demonstration of this possibility has been shown using the angiotensin-converting enzyme inhibitor (ACE-I) perindopril in subjects with hypertension treated for one year, by comparison with the beta-blocking agent atenolol. For the same DBP reduction, SBP was more reduced with ACE-I than with atenolol, as a consequence of reduction in arterial stiffness, and in particular, normalization of carotid wave reflections (Figure 9.5) [49].

The main therapeutic trial demonstrating the role of PP, arterial stiffness and wave reflections in the control of SBP and PP in hypertensive subjects was performed in patients with ESRD undergoing haemodialysis [50]. Many studies have shown that the clinical and haemodynamic profile of ESRD patients is very close to that described in systolic hypertension in the elderly [47, 50] and even constitutes a caricature of the old hypertensive population. The primary objective of the trial in ESRD patients was to reduce CV mortality through a therapeutic regimen involving successively: salt and water depletion by haemodialysis;

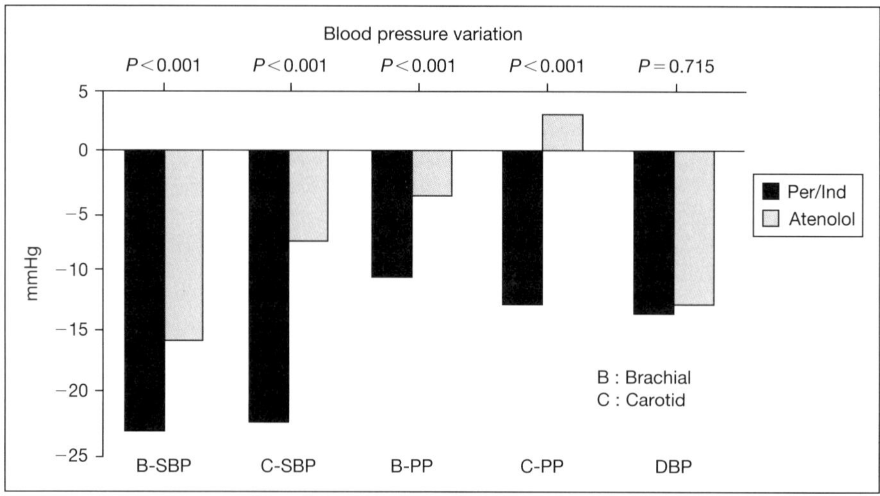

Figure 9.5 The Reason study: double-blind study comparing ACE-I (in association with small doses of diuretic) to atenolol. For the same reduction of DBP, brachial and mostly central SBP was more reduced under ACE-I than under atenolol, resulting in a significant reduction of brachial and central PP under ACE-I and practically no change under atenolol [49].

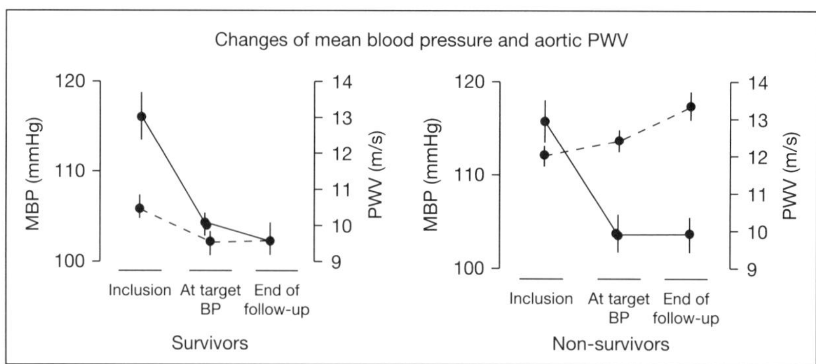

Figure 9.6 Therapeutic trial in subjects with chronic renal failure undergoing haemodialysis [50]: MBP reduction is observed both in survivor and non-survivor subjects. The main difference is that non-survivors have no reduction of PWV. Here MBP is mean arterial pressure (MAP) and the changes in PP have the same profile [50].

then, after randomization, ACE-I or calcium-entry blockade; finally the combination of the two agents and/or their association with a beta-blocker. Using this procedure, it was possible to evaluate over a long-term follow-up (51 months) whether the drug-induced MAP reduction was associated (or not) with a parallel decrease of PP and aortic PWV and resulting consequences on CV risk [50]. During the follow-up, it was clearly shown that MAP, brachial PP and aortic PWV were reduced in parallel in the surviving population. In contrast, in subjects who died from CV events, MAP was lowered to the same extent as in survivors, but neither brachial PP nor PWV were significantly modified by drug treatment (Figure 9.6). From the results of this trial, it seemed likely that a lack of aortic PWV attenuation despite a significant drug-induced MAP reduction can be considered a significant predictor of CV death in subjects with ESRD.

In old subjects with systolic hypertension the Syst-Eur trial enabled similar observations as those observed in ESRD subjects. The predictive value of conventional and ambulatory PP for CV morbidity and mortality was studied after adjustment for all significant confounding covariables, along the overall follow-up [51]. In the placebo group, conventional and mostly ambulatory PP – but not MAP – predicted total and CV mortality, all CV events, stroke and cardiac events. In the active treatment group compared with the placebo group, the relation between clinical outcomes and ambulatory (and conventional) PP was consistently attenuated and even reached non-significant levels. Furthermore, at any given level of 24-h SBP, a lower 24-h DBP was achieved and was shown to be significantly associated with a worsening of CV risk. Finally, the results of the Syst-Eur trial clearly confirmed that PP in the elderly is a significant predictor of CV risk and that its lowering is a necessary goal in old hypertensive subjects to improve CV morbidity and mortality.

Taken together, all these therapeutic studies have shown the need in hypertensive subjects, particularly in the elderly, to develop drugs acting specifically on the large artery wall, i.e. either on arterial stiffness or on wave reflections or on a combination of both, with resulting improvements in CV risk [52]. The recent finding of aortic PWV as an independent predictor of CV risk has largely confirmed this conceptual approach in recent years.

APPENDIX: ARTERIAL HAEMODYNAMIC INDICES

Compliance (C)	Measure of the volume/pressure relationship, generally an absolute volume change (ΔV) for a given pressure step (ΔP): $$C = \Delta V/\Delta P \ (\text{cm}^3/\text{mmHg})$$ In the arteries, compliance is expressed as arterial diameter (or cross-sectional area) change (ΔD) for a given pressure step (ΔP): $$C = \Delta D/\Delta P \ (\text{cm/mmHg; cm}^2/\text{mmHg})$$ The inverse of compliance is elastance.
Distensibility (Di)	Measure of relative volume (or diameter) change for a given pressure step: $$Di = \Delta V/\Delta P \ (\text{mmHg}^{-1})$$ where ΔV is absolute volume change, V is the initial volume, and ΔP is pressure change. Distensibility reflects the capacitive properties of the arteries as a hollow structure.
Elastic modulus	Elastic incremental modulus (E_{inc}). The stretching force per unit areas required for 100% stretch from resting values: $$E_{inc} = \Delta P \cdot V/\Delta V \cdot h \ (\text{mmHg/cm})$$ where ΔP is pressure step, V is initial volume (or diameter), ΔV is absolute volume (or diameter) change, and h is wall thickness. E_{inc} reflects the intrinsic elastic properties of wall material.
Pulse wave velocity	Speed of travel of the pressure wave along an arterial segment (cm/s). According to the Moens–Korteweg equation: $$(PW)^2 = E_{inc} \cdot h/pD$$ where E_{inc} is elastic modulus, h is wall thickness, p is density, and D is arterial diameter.

ACKNOWLEDGMENTS

This study was performed with the help of GEPIR (Group d'Etude de la Pathophysiologie de l'Insuffisance Rénale) and GPH-CV (Groupe de Pharmacologie et d'Hémodynamique Cardiovasculaire), Paris. We thank Mrs. Deboute for her helpful assistance.

REFERENCES

1. Kannel WB. Blood pressure as a cardiovascular risk factor: prevention and treatment. *JAMA* 1996; 24:1571–1576.
2. Collins R, Peto R, MacMahon S *et al.* Blood pressure, stroke, and coronary heart disease: Part 2. Short-term reductions in blood pressure: overview of randomized drug trials in their epidemiological context. *Lancet* 1990; 335:827–838.
3. National Heart, Lung, and Blood Institute. Morbidity and Mortality 1996. *Chartbook on Cardiovascular, Lung, and Blood Diseases*. National Institute of Health, Bethesda, MD, 1996.
4. Sagie A, Larson MG, Levy D. The natural history of borderline isolated systolic hypertension. *N Engl J Med* 1993; 329:1912–1917.
5. Actuarial Society of America. *Blood Pressure Study*. Actuarial Society of America and Association of Life Insurance Medical Directors, New York, 1939, 1940.
6. Black HR. The paradigm has shifted to systolic blood pressure. *Hypertension* 1999; 34:386–387.
7. Staessen JA, Wang JG, Thijs L. Cardiovascular prevention and blood pressure reduction: a quantitative overview updated until 1 March 2003. *J Hypertens* 2003; 21:1055–1076.
8. Mancia G, Grassi G. Systolic and diastolic blood pressure control in antihypertensive drug trials. *J Hypertens* 2002; 20:1461–1464.
9. Safar ME, Levy BI, Struijker-Boudier H. Current perspectives on arterial stiffness and pulse pressure in hypertension and cardiovascular diseases. *Circulation* 2003; 107:2864–2869.
10. Nichols WW, O'Rourke M. *McDonald's Blood Flow in Arteries. Theoretical, Experimental and Clinical Principles*, 4th edition. E. Arnold, London, Sydney, Auckland, 1998, pp 54–401.
11. Kannel WB, Stokes JLL. hypertension as a cardiovascular risk factor. In: Bulpitt CJ (ed.). *Handbook of Hypertension. Epidemiology of Hypertension*. Elsevier Science, Amsterdam, 1985, pp 15–34.
12. Franklin SS, Gustin W IV, Wong ND *et al.* Hemodynamic patterns of age-related changes in blood pressure. The Framingham Heart Study. *Circulation* 1997; 96:308–315.
13. Prospective Studies Collaboration, Age specific relevance of usual blood pressure to vascular mortality: one million adults in 61 prospective studies. *Lancet* 2002; 360:1903–1913.
14. Miura K, Dyer AR, Greenland P *et al.* Pulse pressure compared with other blood pressure indexes in the prediction of 25-year cardiovascular and all-cause mortality rates. The Chicago Heart Association Detection Project in Industry Study. *Hypertension* 2001; 38:232–237.
15. Safar ME. Therapeutic trials and large arteries in hypertension. *Am Heart J* 1988; 115:702–710.
16. Asmar R, Benetos A, London G *et al.* Aortic distensibility in normotensive untreated and treated hypertensive patients. *Blood Press* 1995; 4:48–54.
17. Systolic Hypertension in the Elderly Program Cooperative Research Group. Prevention of stroke by antihypertensive drug treatment in older persons with isolated systolic hypertension: final results of the Systolic Hypertension in the Elderly Program (SHEP). *JAMA* 1991; 265:3255–3264.
18. Safar ME, Blacher J, Mourad JJ *et al.* What does STOP-2 tell us about management of hypertension? *Lancet* 2000; 19:651–652; discussion 653.
19. Darne B, Girerd X, Safar M *et al.* Pulsatile versus steady component of blood pressure: a cross-sectional analysis and a prospective analysis on cardiovascular mortality. *Hypertension* 1989; 13:392–400.
20. Madhavan S, Ooi WL, Cohen H *et al.* Relation of pulse pressure and blood pressure reduction to the incidence of myocardial infarction. *Hypertension* 1994; 23:395–401.
21. Fang J, Madhavan S, Cohen H *et al.* Measures of blood pressure and myocardial infarction in treated hypertensive patients. *J Hypertens* 1995; 13:413–419.
22. Verdecchia P, Schillaci G, Borgioni C *et al.* Ambulatory pulse pressure. A potent predictor of total cardiovascular risk in hypertension. *Hypertension* 1998; 32:983–988.
23. Franklin SS, Khan SA, Wong ND *et al.* Is pulse pressure useful in predicting risk for coronary heart disease? The Framingham Heart Study. *Circulation* 1999; 100:354–360.

24. Millar JA, Lever AF, Burke V. Pulse pressure as a risk factor for cardiovascular events in the MRC mild hypertension trial. *J Hypertens* 1999; 17:1065–1072.
25. Blacher J, Gasowski J, Staessen JA *et al.* Pulse pressure – not mean pressure – determines cardiovascular risk in older hypertensive patients. *Arch Med* 2000; 160:1085–1089.
26. Domanski MJ, Davis BR, Pfeffer MA *et al.* Isolated systolic hypertension, prognostic information provided by pulse pressure. *Hypertension* 1999; 34:375–380.
27. Benetos A, Zureik M, Morcet J *et al.* A decrease in diastolic blood pressure combined with an increase in systolic blood pressure is associated with high cardiovascular mortality. *J Am Coll Cardiol* 2000; 35:673–680.
28. Mitchell GF, Moye LM, Braunwald E *et al.* Sphygmomanometrically determined pulse pressure is a powerful independent predictor of recurrent events after myocardial infarction in patients with impaired left ventricular function. *Circulation* 1997; 96:4254–4260.
29. Chae CU, Pfeffer MA, Glynn RJ *et al.* Increased pulse pressure and risk of heart failure in the elderly. *JAMA* 1999; 281:634–639.
30. Domanski ML, Mitchell GF, Norman JE *et al.* Independent prognostic information provided by sphygmomanometrically determined pulse pressure and mean arterial pressure in patients with left ventricular dysfunction. *J Am Coll Cardiol* 1999; 33:951–958.
31. Haider AW, Larson MG, Franklin SS *et al.* Pulse pressure predicts the new onset of overt heart failure in the community: The Framingham Heart Study. *Circulation* 1998; 98:1–324.
32. Nakayama Y, Tsumura K, Yamashita N, Yoshimaru K, Hayashi T. Pulsatility of ascending aortic pressure waveform is a powerful predictor of restenosis after percutaneaous transluminal coronary angioplasty. *Circulation* 2000; 101:470–472.
33. Benetos A, Safar M, Rudnichi A *et al.* Pulse pressure: a predictor of long-term cardiovascular mortality in a French male population. *Hypertension* 1997; 30:1410–1415.
34. Benetos A, Rudnichi A, Safar M *et al.* Pulse pressure and cardiovascular mortality in normotensive and hypertensive subjects. *Hypertension* 1998; 35:560–564.
35. Alderman MH, Cohen H, Madhavan S. Distribution and determinants of cardiovascular events during 20 years of successful antihypertensive treatment. *J Hypertens* 1998; 16:761–769.
36. Somes GW, Pahor M, Shorr RI *et al.* The role of diastolic blood pressure when treating isolated systolic hypertension. *Arch Intern Med* 1999; 159:2004–2009.
37. Laurent S, Boutouyrie P, Asmar R *et al.* Aortic stiffness is an independent predictor of all-cause and cardiovascular mortality in hypertensive patients. *Hypertension* 2001; 37:1236–1241.
38. Meaume S, Benetos A, Henry OF, Rudnichi A, Safar ME. Aortic pulse wave velocity predicts cardiovascular mortality in subjects >70 years of age. *Arterioscler Thromb Vasc Biol* 2001; 21:2046–2050.
39. Schram MT, Kostense PJ, van Dijk RA *et al.* Diabetes, pulse pressure and cardiovascular mortality: The Hoorn Study. *J Hypertens* 2002; 20:1743–1751.
40. Klassen PS, Lowrie EG, Reddan DN *et al.* Association between pulse pressure and mortality in patients undergoing hemodialysis. *JAMA* 2002; 287:1548–1555.
41. London GM, Guerin AP, Pannier B, Marchais SJ, Benetos A, Safar ME. Increased systolic pressure in chronic uremia: role of arterial wave reflections. *Hypertension* 1992; 20:10–19.
42. Milnor WR. *Hemodynamics*, 2nd edition. W. Wilkins, Baltimore, 1989, pp 211–241.
43. Safar ME. Antihypertensive effects of nitrates in chronic human hypertension. *J Appl Cardiol* 1990; 5:69–81.
44. Simon AC, Safar ME, Levenson JA, Kheder AM, Levy BI. Systolic hypertension: hemodynamic mechanism and choice of antihypertensive treatment. *Am J Cardiol* 1979; 44:505–511.
45. Taylor MG. Wave travel in arteries and the design of the cardiovascular system. In: Attinger EO (ed.). *Pulsatile Blood Flow*. McGraw Hill, New York, 1964, pp 343–347.
46. Stokes GS, Ryan M, Brnabic A, Nyberg G. A controlled study of the effects of isosorbide mononitrate on arterial blood pressure and pulse wave form in systolic hypertension. *J Hypertens* 1999; 17:1767–1773.
47. Safar ME, Blacher J, Mourad JJ, London GM. Stiffness of carotid artery wall matrial and blood pressure in humans. *Stroke* 2000; 31:782–790.
48. Duchier J, Iannascoli F, Safar M. Antihypertensive effect of sustained-release isosorbide dinitrate for isolated systolic hypertension in the elderly. *Am J Cardiol* 1987; 60:99–102.
49. London GM, Asmar RG, O'Rourke MF, Safar ME, on behalf of the REASON Project Investigators. Mechanism(s) of selective systolic blood pressure reduction after a low-dose combination of perindopril/indapamide in hypertensive subjects: comparison with atenolol. *J Am Coll Cardiol* 2004; 43:92–99.

50. Guerin AP, Blacher J, Pannier B, Marchais SJ, Safar ME, London GM. Impact of aortic stiffness attenuation on survival of patient in end-stage renal failure. *Circulation* 2001; 103:987–992.
51. Safar ME. Systolic hypertension in the elderly: arterial wall mechanical properties and the renin-angiotensin-aldosterone system. *J Hypertens* 2005; 23:673–681.
52. Staessen JA, Thijs L, O'Brien ET *et al.*, for the Syst-Eur Trial Investigators. Ambulatory pulse pressure as predictor of outcome in older patients with systolic hypertension. *Am J Hypertens* 2002; 15:835–843.

10

Should selection of antihypertensive therapy be focused on other markers for cardiovascular risk besides blood pressure?

J. M. Flack, S. A. Nasser, S. M. O'Connor

INTRODUCTION

The idea that the pharmacological targeting of non-blood pressure (BP) physiological parameters in hypertensive patients might result in clinical benefit is not new or unreasonable. However, this therapeutic approach has not been widely embraced in clinical practice despite evidence that it probably causes measurable benefits, at least on intermediate outcomes such as albuminuria, left ventricular hypertrophy (LVH), endothelial function and vascular stiffness. It is probably an incorrect premise that non-BP therapeutic targets are wholly independent of BP because they are not. Accordingly, non-BP physiological targets are linked to BP in several important ways.

This chapter will explore various aspects of BP such as ambulatory and cuff BP, the interrelationships of BP with albuminuria, LVH, endothelial function and vascular stiffness, and both the physiological rationale as well as the evidence for targeting the so-called non-BP physiological targets. Considered briefly will be commonly used non-BP cardiovascular drugs taken by hypertensive patients that have been shown to lower BP. Why? Because these agents likely manifest their BP-lowering effects through improving endothelial function and vascular stiffness, two of the non-BP therapeutic targets under review.

Despite the existence of evidence in support of this therapeutic approach, a more robust database is needed. Such supporting investigations will include prospective clinical endpoint-driven trials, clinical databases, basic science investigations, and physiological as well as genetic studies. Strengthening the database in support of targeting non-BP physiological parameters in hypertensive patients will be critical to gain endorsement from guideline-issuing organizations that propound evidence-based therapeutic algorithms for the diagnosis, risk stratification, and treatment of hypertensive patients. It should, however, become very clear that purposeful targeting of non-BP physiological parameters vs. the approach of simply targeting BP, though not identical, overlap to a greater degree than has been recognized. It should be further noted that attributing cardiovascular disease (CVD) risk reduction in a

John M. Flack, MD, MPH, Professor and Interim Chairman of Internal Medicine, Division of Clinical Epidemiology and Translational Research and Endocrinology, Metabolism and Hypertension, Department of Internal Medicine, Wayne State University School of Medicine and the Detroit Medical Center, Detroit, Michigan, USA

Samar A. Nasser, PA-C, MPH, Physician Assistant, Division of Clinical Epidemiology and Translational Research, Department of Internal Medicine, Wayne State University and the Detroit Medical Center, Detroit, Michigan, USA

Shannon M. O'Connor, BS, Research Assistant, Division of Clinical Epidemiology and Translational Research, Department of Internal Medicine, Wayne State University and the Detroit Medical Center, Detroit, Michigan, USA

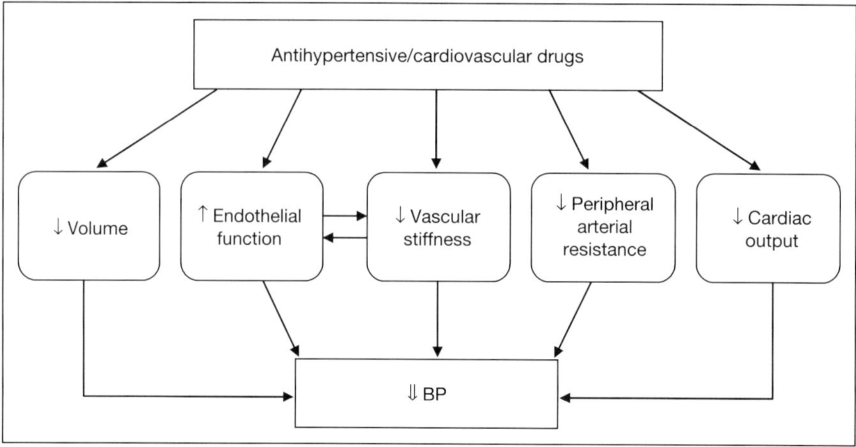

Figure 10.1 This simplified schematic depicts an overview of the likely mechanisms through which antihypertensive and cardiovascular drugs lower BP. The fall in BP is the sum of these physiological changes net the counter regulatory responses induced by the fall in BP that attenuate the maximal possible BP reduction. Until recently the therapeutic focus was almost entirely on BP, though these more proximal mechanisms were targeted albeit in a non-purposeful fashion. However, the clinician now has access to validated devices in their offices that quantify these mechanisms for individual patients.

multivariate statistical model to BP by no means proves that BP is the actual mediator of the risk reduction. Instead, some non-BP physiological variable that moves in parallel with BP may be involved. Such physiological variables (e.g. vascular stiffness) might also be determinants of the fall in BP (Figure 10.1).

BLOOD PRESSURE

Though the focus of this chapter is on non-BP targets, it is imperative that BP must be understood both as a physiological entity and a pharmacological target. It is also important to examine what cardiac and haemodynamic factors actually determine BP levels.

BP represents the confluence of vascular properties such as arterial stiffness, endothelial dysfunction, cardiac output, peripheral vascular resistance and extracelluar/intravascular volume. Accordingly, successful antihypertensive therapy often favourably affects these determinants of BP without actually targeting them in a conscious and purposeful manner [1].

Any physiological measure meriting serious consideration during the management of hypertensive patients in ambulatory office settings must also be routinely available and measured ideally and accurately. Cuff BP readings are certainly convenient and form the basis for most ambulatory clinical practice decisions in hypertension treatment. However, these readings may be grossly inaccurate because of the pervasiveness of both random and systematic errors in BP measurement. These errors occur because rigorous measurement protocols that can minimize or even prevent their occurrence are infrequently utilized. Such errors include utilization of the incorrect BP cuff size and highly variable measurement conditions. Despite the compelling rationale that can be put forward for BP measurement protocols, the chief reason why they have been infrequently utilized outside of research settings is because of the perceived interruption in the smooth flow of patients.

Cuff BP readings are often obtained at random rather than specific time points (e.g. just before the morning medication doses). These readings may certainly be similar yet represent distinctly different ambulatory BP patterns and therefore differing 24-h BP loads as well as patterns of diurnal BP variation [2]. Even in hypertension clinical trials where standardized

BP measurement is the norm, the number of BP measurements to be included in multivariate analyses has often been insufficient to ensure that observed CVD risk reductions were truly independent of BP changes (residual confounding). Accordingly, several studies have suggested BP independent effects of antihypertensive agents on cardiovascular outcomes [3, 4]. However, no study could reliably eliminate residual confounding in the magnitude of BP changes as an explanation for CVD risk reductions. Even large hypertension studies such as the Antihypertensive and Lipid Lowering Treatment to Prevent Heart Attack (ALLHAT) study [5] may have too few BP readings of sufficient precision to rule this out as the explanation for risk reductions that cannot be statistically linked solely to the magnitude of BP lowering.

In traditional antihypertensive pharmacotherapeutics, lowering BP is the major therapeutic goal. Nevertheless, BP changes and attained BP levels serve as proxies for underlying vascular abnormalities that are often unmeasured in usual clinical settings. Many antihypertensive agents have well-documented effects on endothelial dysfunction, vascular stiffness, peripheral vascular resistance, and extracelluar/intravascular fluid volume [6–9]. Up until recently, these physiological measures were unavailable in clinical settings. Consideration of these measures has been shown to improve BP control rates and, in turn, those who attained better BP control more often had normalization of selected vascular parameters [1].

Ambulatory BP levels are more closely linked to cardiovascular events than cuff BP levels [10]. Intuitively this makes sense because BP readings are obtained throughout the 24-h sleep–wake cycle providing a relatively accurate determination of BP level as well as insight into the pattern and magnitude of diurnal BP variation. However, ambulatory BP determinations are simply not practical for most large-scale clinical trials.

Finally, brachial artery BP levels do not appear fully to explain the relationship of BP to cardiovascular events. Recent data have shown that estimated central aortic BP levels can diverge from brachial artery BP levels and that lower central aortic pressures are associated with lower rates of composite cardiovascular–renal endpoints [11]. Antihypertensive drugs appear to differentially impact central aortic pressures despite similar effects on brachial artery BP [11, 12]. Accordingly, atenolol-based therapy does not appear to lower central aortic BP as effectively as either amlodipine or eprosartan, two mechanistically dissimilar vasodilators. It appears that the β-blocker, for example, does not reduce the reflected waves from the peripheral arteries as effectively. These pharmacological differences on central aortic and peripheral brachial artery pressures have been suggested as plausible explanations for the differences in CVD risk reduction. This has been observed in two recent active controlled hypertension endpoint trials where cuff BP readings were virtually identical between the two treatment arms [11, 13]. Central aortic pressure can now be derived non-invasively in office settings *via* radial artery applanation tonometry and pulse wave analysis.

What does all of this mean? First, there should be a high degree of suspicion that residual confounding, even in large studies, may explain at least some of the cardiovascular–renal risk reduction that has been described as 'beyond BP'. This explanation is particularly likely in the absence of a rigorous BP measurement protocol as well as when BP measurements during follow-up are less than plentiful. Large-scale clinical trials, particularly those adequately powered statistically for the collection of hard clinical endpoints, rarely ascertain ambulatory BP measurements, unless in a sub-sample of randomized participants, for reasons of practicality [14]. Finally, changes in BP levels are determined by the use of various combinations of antihypertensive agents that reverse abnormalities in cardiac and vascular function, structure, as well as in intravascular volume. There is a likely correlation between changes in BP and changes in these non-BP physiological parameters. Even if BP and non-BP physiological parameters were measured simultaneously and it was statistically determined that BP lowering accounted for all of the risk reduction, this does not mean that the non-BP physiological parameters did not contribute to risk reduction. Simply put, a statistical model cannot determine the physiological determinants of CVD risk reduction or even

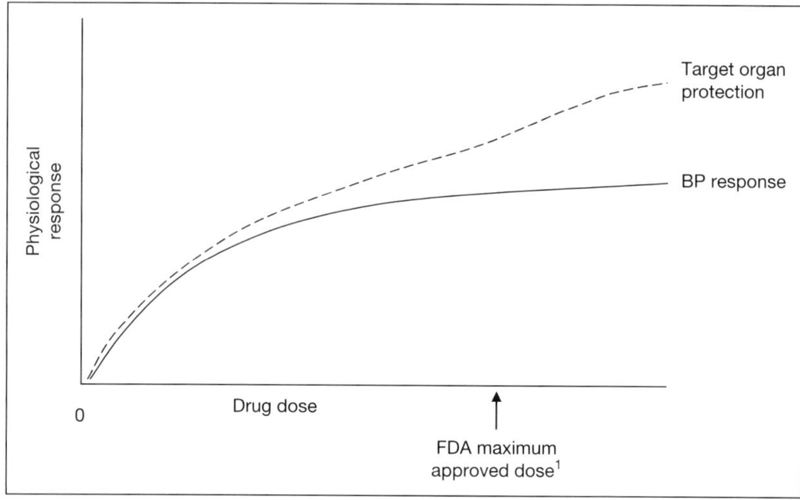

Figure 10.2 Putative dose–response relationship of antihypertensive drugs with BP and target organ function. Depicted is the typical curvilinear dose–response curve for antihypertensive agents and BP response. The fall in BP begins to flatten with most antihypertensive drugs once the mid-point of the FDA approved hypertension dose range is exceeded. However, some antihypertensive agents, particularly the RAS antagonists, have beneficial effects on target organ function at incrementally higher doses that do not lower BP, at least as ascertained from the peripheral brachial artery. [1]For the indication of essential hypertension.

BP changes. However, these models can identify factors that are correlated with changes in both. Multivariate statistical models may be unable to disentangle the correlations of BP change to changes in non-BP physiological parameters (thus assigning all of the risk reduction to changes in BP), especially if BP is measured more precisely (with less random error) than the non-BP parameters. Even the most accurate traditional peripheral BP measurements may be misleading in regards to absolute or relative estimates of CVD–renal risk reduction unless derivations of central aortic pressure are considered.

A plausible case can be made that non-BP physiological parameters should guide therapeutic selections as well as to function as specific targets of therapy when attempting to control BP. It is also reasonable to posit that these non-BP targets should be pharmacologically targeted for normalization even if BP has come under control. There is no legitimate reason to believe that the BP lowering dose–response curve of antihypertensive agents or other vasculoactive drugs is identical to the dose–response curve for target-organ protection (Figure 10.2). There is evidence that higher doses, than approved for hypertension treatment, of selected antihypertensive agents confer measurable improvements in target-organ function [15]. It is also reasonable to pose the question as to whether persons with BP levels below current diagnostic thresholds for the diagnosis of hypertension, who have abnormalities in non-BP physiological parameters, should be treated with vasculoactive agents to normalize these parameters. At present, there is simply insufficient evidence to answer this important question. Nevertheless, this issue will likely serve as the basis for important future clinical trials.

VASCULAR STIFFNESS

Vascular stiffness or reduced arterial compliance occurs with ageing of the vascular tree and also manifests prematurely in persons with diabetes mellitus [16, 17]. Other factors contributing to vascular stiffness include dietary sodium intake [18], obesity [19, 20], and sedentary lifestyle [21]. The non-enzymatic glycation of collagen and elastin produces advanced glycation endproducts that cross-link these arterial wall components, thereby increasing vascular stiffness. Increased vascular stiffness also occurs as a consequence of endothelial dysfunction which contributes to increased smooth muscle tone [22]. It is thus reasonable to propose that vascular stiffness is a physiological plausible therapeutic target.

Vascular stiffness contributes to the typically observed BP phenotype of higher systolic BP (SBP) and lower diastolic BP (DBP), the so-called wide pulse pressure hypertension. Vascular stiffness also contributes to endothelial dysfunction as stretching of the vessel wall in response to pulsatile flow appears to be an important vascular property resulting in the stimulation of endothelial nitric oxide synthase and thus the release of nitric oxide by vascular endothelial cells [23]. Vascular stiffness also increases cardiac work as higher end-systolic pressures are required to generate the same stroke volume compared to when the heart ejects blood into a more compliant arterial tree [24]. The reduced vascular compliance coupled with the increased arterial tone that accompanies vascular stiffness, changes cardiac loading conditions resulting in increased cardiac work.

Vascular stiffness also results in structural changes and remodelling as well as in ventricular function and mechanics (e.g. increased ventricular stiffness) that augments the risk for sudden cardiac death and heart failure and also contributes to changes in coronary blood flow. Accordingly, aortic stiffness prolongs systole, shifts some of the coronary blood flow that is typically confined to the diastolic phase of the cardiac cycle into the systolic phase, and also reduces both resting and hyperaemic coronary flow velocity reserve [25]. These changes in coronary blood flow increase myocardial susceptibility to ischaemia.

ALBUMINURIA

Albuminuria is the result of increased glomerular permeability and/or increased glomerular hydrostatic pressure and can be easily measured in clinical office settings by the collection of a random spot for ascertainment of the ratio of albumin to creatinine (mg/g). Albuminuria has been linked to more rapid decline in glomerular filtration rate [26], increased prevalence of pressure-related target-organ injury [27], and higher cardiovascular event rates [28]. Furthermore, there are physiologically plausible explanations as to why albuminuria predicts increased cardiovascular risk. Accordingly, albuminuria has been linked to endothelial dysfunction and also to a plethora of local renal inflammatory responses that, if unchecked, would cause progressive tissue injury/scarring and loss of kidney function. On the other hand, albuminuria has several important links to BP.

Persons with albuminuria have higher levels of BP compared to those with no albuminuria [29]. Also, persons with essential hypertension and albuminuria have an attenuated nocturnal decline in BP compared to essential hypertensives without albuminuria [30]. We have shown that albuminuria is linked to a lesser longitudinal fall in both SBP and DBP in complex drug-treated hypertensive patients within an academic referral practice (personal observations). Thus, it is very reasonable to postulate that at least part of the higher cardiovascular–renal risk attributable to albuminuria is mediated through persistently higher levels of BP.

Despite the inadequate appreciation of the link between albuminuria and BP, albuminuria remains a logical physiologic target for normalization independent of BP. At least one study showed that escalation of angiotensin receptor blocker therapy to dose levels that produced little change in cuff BP readings resulted in significant incremental reductions in albuminuria [15]. This confirms the thesis that the BP and target-organ protection dose–response curves are probably not identical.

How might albuminuria be pharmacologically targeted? Aggressive BP lowering with just about any antihypertensive drug regimen may lower urinary albumin excretion. Clearly, inclusion of at least one of the renin–angiotensin system (RAS) antagonists – an angiotensin-converting enzyme inhibitor or angiotensin receptor blocker – in the antihypertensive drug regimen will augment reductions in albuminuria over and above that observed in drug regimens that do not include a RAS blocker. Prescription of RAS blocker doses higher than the Food and Drug Administration (FDA) approved doses for hypertension, or combining an ACE with an ARB even within the FDA approved dosing range for both drugs, has also been shown to incrementally lower urinary albumin excretion. Aldosterone antagonists lower albuminuria to a degree similar to traditional RAS antagonists [31]. It also appears that statin drugs lower urinary albumin excretion [32]. Finally, at least three lifestyle modifications can significantly lower urinary albumin excretion – smoking cessation, dietary salt restriction [33], as well as weight loss.

Albuminuria is readily available in most clinical settings and, in fact, should be obtained from virtually all hypertensive patients in order to risk stratify them and to determine the appropriate target BP according to JNC7 guidelines. However, single albuminuria readings can be highly variable. Confirming albuminuria with determinations separated in time should be routine. There are multiple non-pharmacological and pharmacological approaches to lowering urinary albumin excretion. An interesting paradox exists in hypertensive patients. Patients with albuminuria are less likely to attain their goal BP and, when they do, the time to attainment is longer as they do not respond as well to antihypertensive drug therapy. This is evidenced by their higher medication requirements and longer time to attainment of goal BP levels (personal observations).

What do clinical outcome studies tell us in regard to the potential clinical benefits of albuminuria/proteinuria reductions? The most relevant studies are randomized, active comparator drug trials that have tracked not only renal but non-renal cardiovascular endpoints [34]. It has been very clear that antihypertensive regimens containing RAS blocker drugs slow renal disease progression more than those without RAS blocker drugs [34, 35]. Interestingly, there is some evidence that at least part of the lesser risk of renal disease progression is related to the attainment of lower BP levels with RAS antagonists [36]. The superiority of RAS blocker treatment regimens does, however, appear to depend significantly on the magnitude of proteinuria [34–36]. Even when RAS blocking agents slow the progressive loss of renal disease, non-RAS agents (calcium antagonists), appear to offer greater protection against non-renal CVD events such as stroke and myocardial infarction (though not congestive heart failure [CHF]) despite the fact that these agents do not reduce proteinuria as much [37]. There is an interesting paradox in the interpretation of data from studies focused on renoprotection. That is, RAS blockers do not appear to provide equal protection (relative to calcium antagonists) against non-renal CVD endpoints, save CHF, yet they provide greater protection against the progressive loss of kidney function. In the real world of caring for hypertensive patients with chronic kidney disease this is much less of an issue because the vast majority of these patients will need more than two drugs for control of BP. Thus, there is ample opportunity to combine RAS and non-RAS drugs in a manner that provides optimal risk reduction from renal and non-renal clinical events.

LEFT VENTRICULAR HYPERTROPHY

LVH represents a maladaptive cardiac response to persistently elevated BP. Though BP is an important determinant of left ventricular (LV) mass, other patient characteristics such as body size, height, age, physical activity and even dietary sodium intake all are correlated positively with LV mass [38, 39]. We have previously shown that echocardiographic LV mass is more closely associated with SBP than DBP even in young, mostly healthy young adults [38].

LVH is not reliably detected *via* the surface electrocardiogram. M-mode echocardiograpy has been the gold standard for measurement of LV mass; however, a major problem with this modality of measurement, despite its widespread availability, is the relatively high measurement error. For example, mean intra-reader and inter-reader variability, respectively, approximates 10% and 17% [40]. Newer computed tomography (CT) and magnetic resonance imaging (MRI) determinations of LV mass have much promise, particularly since LV mass measurements can be made with these modalities with significantly greater precision.

The majority of antihypertensive drug classes reduce LV mass over time when they are used in a manner that also lowers BP [13]. Differences in LV mass regression between antihypertensive drug classes are beyond the scope of this review. It has been shown that over 10 years in drug-treated hypertensive patients regression of LVH is associated with a lower risk of non-fatal CVD events [41]. Thus, should LV mass be measured and followed in all hypertensive patients?

At the present time, the answer to this question is probably no, though the definitive answer in unknown. Undoubtedly, M-mode echocardiography LV mass measurements are too variable to allow for changes in serial measurements within a person over time to be the basis of therapeutic decisions – even when obtained using rigorous research measurement and reading protocols. The newer CT and MRI LV mass measurements can be obtained with much greater precision and thus less variation within a person over time. Accordingly, these modalities are better suited than echocardiography for obtaining accurate serial measurements and detecting changes in LV mass during therapy. Nevertheless, the following are true. The frequency of persistent LVH even after BP normalization is not known. Without doubt, most antihypertensive drug regimens that effectively lower BP will also regress LV mass. If LV mass truly remains elevated after attainment of goal BP, it is an important question as to whether further therapy to regress LV mass should be undertaken by driving BP even lower. It is also not known whether LV mass should be used to select individuals for either antihypertensive drug therapy and/or non-drug interventions that have been shown to regress LVH. Weight loss and sodium restriction have both been shown to regress LVH [42, 43]. Interestingly, both of these interventions have also been shown to lower BP, improve endothelial function, and reduce urinary albumin excretion.

So how should the practitioner utilize LV mass measurements? More data are needed before definitive recommendations can be made with confidence. Until such data are available, these authors believe the following recommendations are prudent. Ascertainment of LV mass is not routinely warranted in the management of hypertension. However, the use of echocardiography can be invaluable in determining the level of ventricular function which is often necessary when middle-aged and older patients present with symptoms suggestive of either heart failure or LV dysfunction. In the majority of cases LV systolic function will be preserved and LVH will be incidentally documented. In most situations, LVH will not significantly impact antihypertensive drug selection as most patients with LVH will require multiple drugs for BP normalization and most drugs regress LVH. We occasionally utilize the presence or absence of LVH to determine whether to initiate therapy in patients with borderline BP elevations in the absence of micro- or macro-albuminuria. Finally, the International Society on Hypertension in Blacks (ISHIB) recommended a lower BP target (<130/80 mmHg) in hypertensive patients with LVH [44]. Though this recommendation is an extrapolation from the available clinical trial database, it is very logical. LVH is clearly a pressure-related manifestation of target-organ injury. Once target injury occurs, it is also logical to postulate that lower levels of BP for longer periods of time will be required to lower CVD risk back toward normal levels. At the present time there is virtually no evidence to suggest that either lowering BP to low levels – albeit without proven benefit – nor regressing LVH by any available means confers excessive risk or harms ventricular function.

BLOOD PRESSURE EFFECTS OF NON-BLOOD PRESSURE CARDIOVASCULAR DRUGS

Statin drugs have been shown to lower the risk of stroke in several hypertension trials [45, 46] despite the fact that cholesterol, *per se*, is not an epidemiological risk factor for stroke. It is also clear that statins not only lower cholesterol and triglyceride levels, but also have pleiotropic effects and improve endothelial function [47, 48]. Statins have also been shown to lower BP in several studies [49, 50]. One ambulatory BP study demonstrated that statins did not affect the nocturnal fall in BP but did impressively lower daytime BP [51]. Thus, one potential benefit of statin drugs may be augmentation of BP lowering. There are also data suggesting that statins lower urinary albumin excretion [52].

Thiazolidinediones are oral antidiabetic agents that improve insulin sensitivity. These agents have similar ancillary cardiovascular effects to the statins given their ability to lower BP as well as to reduce urinary albumin excretion [53–55]. These agents also improve endothelial function.

SUMMARY

There are multiple, physiologically attractive non-BP targets that, for the most part, are inadvertently rather than specifically targeted during antihypertensive drug therapy that is prescribed according to the JNC7 treatment algorithm. Now that at least some of these targets can be readily measured in clinical settings, they can be purposefully targeted. Interestingly, these non-BP targets are not totally distinct from BP because they likely represent the mechanisms through which many vasculoactive drugs actually lower BP. It does not appear that the dose–response curve for BP and target-organ protection are the same with the latter actually manifesting a steeper dose–response curve. At the very least, a convincing argument can be made to target the so-called non-BP physiological targets that can be measured in the office because this strategy leads to better BP control. Further data will, however, be needed. Nevertheless, non-BP physiological targets such as arterial stiffness, albuminuria, LVH, peripheral vascular resistance, and intravascular volume may ultimately prove to be viable targets independent of their impact on BP. There are also proven benefits on vascular function and BP even when treating dyslipidaemia and diabetes with statins and/or thiazolidinediones.

REFERENCES

1. Smith RD, Levy P, Ferrario CM. Value of noninvasive hemodynamics to achieve blood pressure control in hypertensive subjects. *Hypertension* 2006; 47:771–777.
2. Pickering TG. Principles and techniques of blood pressure measurement. *Cardiol Clin* 2002; 20:207–223.
3. Effects of ramipril on cardiovascular and microvascular outcomes in people with diabetes mellitus: results of the HOPE study and MICRO-HOPE substudy. Heart Outcomes Prevention Evaluation Study Investigators. *Lancet* 2000; 355:253–259.
4. Nissen SE, Tuzcu EM, Libby P *et al*. Effect of antihypertensive agents on cardiovascular events in patients with coronary disease and normal blood pressure: the CAMELOT study: a randomized controlled trial. *JAMA* 2004; 292:2217–2225.
5. Major outcomes in high-risk hypertensive patients randomized to angiotensin-converting enzyme inhibitor or calcium channel blocker vs diuretic. The Antihypertensive and Lipid-Lowering Treatment to Prevent Heart Attack Trial (ALLHAT). *JAMA* 2002; 288:2981–2997.
6. Courtney CH, McCance DR, Atkinson AB *et al*. Effect of the alpha-andergenic blocker, doxazosin, on endothelial function and insulin action. *Metabolism* 2003; 52:1147–1152.
7. Shargorodsky M, Leibovitz E, Lubimov L *et al*. Prolonged treatment with the AT1 receptor blocker, valsartan, increases small and large artery compliance in uncomplicated essential hypertension. *Am J Hypertens* 2002; 15:1087–1091.
8. Rocha R, Williams GH. Rationale for the use of aldosterone antagonists in congestive heart failure. *Drugs* 2002; 62:723–731.
9. Agabiti-Rosei E. Structural and functional changes of the microcirculation in hypertension: influence of pharmacological therapy. *Drugs* 2003; 63:19–29.
10. Verdecchia P, Reboldi G, Porcellati C *et al*. Risk of cardiovascular disease in relation to achieved office and ambulatory blood pressure control in treated hypertensive subjects. *J Am Coll Cardiol* 2002; 39:878–885.

11. Williams B, Lacy PS, Thom SM *et al.* Differential impact of blood pressure-lowering drugs on central aortic pressure and clinical outcomes. Principal Results of the Conduit Artery Function Evaluation (CAFÉ) Study. *Circulation* 2006; 113:1213–1225.
12. Dhakam Z, McEniery CM, Yasmin *et al.* Atenolol and eprosartan: differential effects on central blood pressure and aortic pulse wave velocity. *Am J Hypertens* 2006; 19:214–219.
13. Devereux RB, Dahlof B, Gerdts E *et al.* Regression of hypertensive left ventricular hypertrophy by losartan compared with atenolol: the Losartan Intervention for Endpoint Reduction in Hypertension (LIFE) trial. *Circulation* 2004; 110:1456–1462.
14. Messerli FH, White WB, Staessen JA. If only cardiologists did properly measure blood pressure. Blood pressure recordings in daily practice and clinical trials. *J Am Coll Cardiol* 2002; 40:2201–2203.
15. Rossing K, Schjoedt KJ, Jensen BR *et al.* Enhanced renoprotective effects of ultrahigh doses of irbesartan in patients with type 2 diabetes and microalbuminuria. *Kidney Int* 2005; 68:1190–1198.
16. Redfield MM, Jacobsen SJ, Borlaug BA *et al.* Age- and gender-related ventricular-vascular stiffening: a community-based study. *Circulation* 2005; 112:2254–2262.
17. Westerbacka J, Leinonen E, Salonen JT *et al.* Increased augmentation of central blood pressure is associated with increases in carotid intima-media thickness in type 2 diabetic patients. *Diabetologia* 2005; 48:1654–1662.
18. Safar ME, Thuilliez C, Richard V, Benetos A. Pressure-independent contribution of sodium to a large artery structure and function in hypertension. *Cardiovasc Res* 2000; 46:269–276.
19. Zebekakis PE, Nawrot T, Thijs L *et al.* Obesity is associated with increased arterial stiffness from adolescence until old age. *J Hypertens* 2005; 23:1839–1846.
20. Grassi G, Giannattasio C. Obesity and vascular stiffness: when body fat has an adverse impact on arterial dynamics. *J Hypertens* 2005; 23:1789–1791.
21. Tanaka H, DeSouza CA, Seals DR. Absence of age-related increase in central arterial stiffness in physically active women. *Arterioscler Thromb Vasc Biol* 1998; 18:127–132.
22. Kass DA. Ventricular arterial stiffening: integrating the pathophysiology. *Hypertension* 2005; 46:185–193.
23. Thuillez C, Richard V. Targeting endothelial dysfunction in hypertensive subjects. *J Hum Hypertens* 2005; 19:S21–S25.
24. McEniery CM, Yasmin, Wallace S *et al.* Increased stroke volume and aortic stiffness contribute to isolated systolic hypertension in young adults. *Hypertension* 2005; 46:221–226.
25. Nemes A, Forster T, Csanady M. Relationship between coronary flow velocity reserve and aortic stiffness. *Am J Physiol Heart Circ Physiol* 2006; 290:H1311.
26. Kong AP, So WY, Szeto CC *et al.* Assessment of glomerular filtration rate in addition to albuminuria is important in managing type II diabetes. *Kidney Int* 2006; 69:383–387.
27. Reboldi G, Gentile G, Angeli F, Verdecchia P. Microalbuminuria and hypertension. *Minerva Med* 2005; 96:261–275.
28. Nathan DM, Cleary PA, Backlund JY *et al.* Intensive diabetes treatment and cardiovascular disease in patients with type 1 diabetes. *N Engl J Med* 2005; 353:2643–2653.
29. Cirillo M, Lombardi C, Bilancio G *et al.* Urinary albumin and cardiovascular profile in the middle-aged population. *Semin Nephrol* 2005; 25:367–371.
30. Bianchi S, Bigazzi R, Baldari G *et al.* Diurnal variations of blood pressure and microalbuminuria in essential hypertension. *Am J Hypertens* 1994; 7:23–29.
31. Flack JM, Oparil S, Pratt JH *et al.* Efficacy and tolerability of eplerenone and losartan in hypertensive black and white patients. *J Am Coll Cardiol* 2003; 41:1148–1155.
32. Nakamura T, Ushiyama C, Hirokawa K *et al.* Effect of cerivastatin on urinary albumin excretion and plasma endothelin-1 concentrations on type 2 diabetes patients with microalbuminuria and dyslipidemia. *Am J Nephrol* 2001; 21:449–454.
33. Redon J. Treatment of patients with essential hypertension and microalbuminuria. *Drugs* 1997; 54:857–866.
34. Weekers L, Krzesinski JM, Clinical study of the month. Nephroprotective role of angiotensin II receptor antagonists in type 2 diabetes: results of the IDNT and RENAAL trials. *Rev Med Liege* 2001; 56:723–726.
35. Wright JT Jr, Bakris G, Greene T *et al.* Effect of blood pressure lowering and antihypertensive drug class on progression of hypertensive kidney disease: results from the AASK trial. *JAMA* 2002; 288:2421–2431.

36. Jafar TH, Stark PC, Schmid CH. Proteinuria as a modifiable risk factor for the progression of non-diabetic renal disease. *Kidney Int* 2001; 60:1131–1140.
37. Berl T, Hunsicker LG, Lewis JB *et al.* Cardiovascular outcomes in the Irbesartan Diabetic Nephropathy Trial of patients with type 2 diabetes and overt nephropathy. *Ann Intern Med* 2003; 138:542–549.
38. Flack JM, Gardin JM, Yunis C, Liu K. Static and pulsatile blood pressure correlates of left ventricular structure and function in black and white young adults: the CARDIA study. *Am Heart J* 1999; 138:856–864.
39. Liebson PR, Grandits G, Prineas R *et al.* Echocardiographic correlates of left ventricular structure among 844 mildly hypertensive men and women in the Treatment of Mild Hypertension Study (TOMHS). *Circulation* 1993; 87:476–486.
40. Gardin JM, Dabestani A, Matin K *et al.* Reproducibility of Doppler aortic blood flow measurements: studies on intraobserver, interobserver, and day-to-day variability in normal subjects. *Am J Cardiol* 1984; 54:1092–1098.
41. Okin PM, Devereux RB, Jern S *et al.* Regression of electrocardiographic left ventricular hypertrophy during antihypertensive treatment and the prediction of major cardiovascular events. *JAMA* 2004; 292:2343–2349.
42. Jennings G, Dart A, Meredith I *et al.* Effects of exercise and other nonpharmacological measures on blood pressure and cardiac hypertrophy. *J Cardiovasc Pharmacol* 1991; 17:S70–S74.
43. Hinderliter A, Sherwood A, Gullette EC *et al.* Reduction in left ventricular hypertrophy after exercise and weight loss in overweight patients with mild hypertension. *Arch Intern Med* 2002; 162:1333–1339.
44. Douglas JG, Bakris GL, Epstein M *et al.* Management of high blood pressure in African Americans: consensus statement of the Hypertension in African Americans Working Group of the International Society on Hypertension in Blacks. *Arch Intern Med* 2003; 163:525–541.
45. Sever PS, Dahlof B, Poulter NR *et al.* Prevention of coronary and stroke events with atorvastatin in hypertensive patients who have average or lower-than-average cholesterol concentrations, in the Anglo-Scandinavian Cardiac Outcomes Trial – Lipid Lowering Arm (ASCOT-LLA): a multicentre randomized controlled trial. *Drugs* 2004; 64:43–60.
46. Rouleau J. Improved outcome after acute coronary syndromes with an intensive versus standard lipid-lowering regimen: results from the Pravastatin or Atorvastatin Evaluation and Infection Therapy-Thrombolysis in Myocardial Infarction 22 (PROVEIT-TIMI 22) trial. *Am J Med* 2005; 118:28–35.
47. Dogra GK, Watts GF, Chan DC, Stanton K. Statin therapy improves brachial artery vasodilator function in patients with Type 1 diabetes and microalbuminuria. *Diabet Med* 2005; 22:239–242.
48. Mullen MJ, Wright D, Donald AE *et al.* Atorvastatin but not 1-arginine improves endothelial function in type I diabetes mellitus: a double-blind study. *J Am Coll Cardiol* 2000; 36:410–416.
49. Pelat M, Balligrand JL. Statins and hypertension. *Semin Vasc Med* 2004; 4:367–375.
50. Magen E, Viskoper R, Mishal J *et al.* Resistant arterial hypertension and hyperlipidemia: atorvastatin, not vitamin C, for blood pressure control. *Isr Med Assoc J* 2004; 6:742–746.
51. Terzoli L, Mircoli L, Raco R, Ferrari AU. Lowering of elevated ambulatory blood pressure by HMG-CoA reductase inhibitors. *J Cardiovasc Pharmacol* 2005; 46:310–315.
52. Sinzinger H, Kritz H, Furberg CD. Atorvastatin reduces microalbuminuria in patients with familial hypercholesterolemia and normal glucose tolerance. *Med Sci Monit* 2003; 9:PI88–PI92.
53. Sarafidis PA, Lasaridis AN, Nilsson PM *et al.* The effect of rosiglitazone on urine albumin excretion in patients with type 2 diabetes mellitus and hypertension. *Am J Hypertens* 2005; 18:227–234.
54. Pistrosch F, Herbrig K, Kindel B *et al.* Rosiglitazone improves Glomerular Hyperfiltration, Renal Endothelial Dysfunction, and Microalbuminuria of Incipient Diabetic Nephropathy in Patients. *Diabetes* 2005; 54:2206–2211.
55. Chana RS, Brunskill NJ. Thiazolidinediones inhibit albumin uptake by proximal tubular cells through a mechanism independent of peroxisome proliferator activated receptor gamma. *Am J Nephrol* 2006; 26:67–74.

11

Can aggressive control of blood pressure prevent progression of kidney disease?

A. E. Briglia, M. R. Weir

INTRODUCTION

The socioeconomic impact of hypertension is profound when one considers that approximately 50 million people have this disease in the United States and that only 25% of those individuals are adequately treated, according to the Third National Health and Nutrition Examination Survey (NHANES-III) [1]. Even more alarming, at least 8 million people have chronic kidney disease (CKD) [2], and renal disease substantially increases the risk for cardiovascular mortality [3]. The influence of hypertension on cause and progression of renal failure has been studied extensively, and optimal blood pressure (BP) control is one of several measures that can be employed to delay progression of CKD. Commonly accepted strategies to promote renoprotection have been summarized [4]. This chapter will discuss pertinent studies to support the notion that aggressive BP control can, in fact, delay progression of kidney disease and will provide focus on populations who are at high risk for renal failure, namely diabetics and patients with proteinuric nephropathy.

OVERVIEW

The topic of whether hypertension by itself contributes to progression of CKD in the absence of baseline renal dysfunction has led to several studies. Work by Klag and colleagues [5] and Perry and co-workers [6] indicated a relationship between higher BP at baseline and risk of developing end-stage renal disease (ESRD). However, these studies were unable to ascertain whether hypertension led to ESRD by creating renal disease or by worsening pre-existing renal disease [7]. Recently, Hsu *et al.* [8] evaluated 316 675 individuals with estimated glomerular filtration rate (eGFR) >60 ml/min/1.73 m^2 and absence of proteinuria at baseline. For those with BP <120/80 mmHg, the age-adjusted risk of ESRD over 100 000 person-years was 2.8 in white patients and 14 for black patients, and 3.8 in those without diabetes vs. 12.7 among individuals with diabetes. There was a 1.6-fold increase in risk for BP range 120–129/80–84, which rose to a 4.2-fold increase in risk for BP >210/120. Not only does this study demonstrate that hypertension predates the development of renal disease, but it also shows an increasing risk for development of ESRD in BP strata that were formerly considered

Andrew E. Briglia, DO, Assistant Professor of Medicine, Division of Nephrology, Department of Medicine, University of Maryland School of Medicine, Baltimore, Maryland, USA

Matthew R. Weir, MD, Professor of Medicine, Director, Division of Nephrology, Department of Medicine, University of Maryland School of Medicine, Baltimore, Maryland, USA

to be normotensive [7, 8]. Moreover, these risk ratios may be underestimated in light of elevated cardiovascular mortality incurred by the presence of CKD, even before the development of ESRD [7, 9, 10]. A prospective evaluation of the Framingham Heart Study cohort found that for individuals 65 years of age and older, the 10-year cumulative incidence of cardiovascular disease (CVD) (death due to CVD, recognized myocardial infarction [MI], stroke, or congestive heart failure) over a 12-year follow-up was 18% for women and 25% for men with high-normal BP (systolic pressure of 130–139 mmHg, diastolic pressure of 85–89 mmHg, or both) [11]. Compared with optimal BP, defined as systolic pressure <120 mmHg and diastolic pressure <80 mmHg, the hazard ratio was 2.5 among women and 1.6 among men. The reason for the graded increase in risk of cardiovascular events with increasing BP has not been firmly established. However, vascular endothelial dysfunction, which includes reduced levels of vasodilatory substances such as nitric oxide and increased expression of vasoconstrictive substances such as endothelin-1, has been implicated [12].

WHAT CONSTITUTES AGGRESSIVE BLOOD PRESSURE CONTROL?

There is abundant literature to substantiate the rationale for BP control in patients with kidney disease and in those who are at risk for target organ damage [13–17]. Of importance is the observation that patients with cardiovascular risk factors, including kidney disease, may require BP reduction to <140/90, a level that in the past has been considered to be optimal [15]. When discussing the topic of appropriate BP control at the nephrologic level, glomerular haemodynamics must be considered (Figure 11.1) [18]. Autoregulation is a physiologic property that allows for minute changes in preglomerular afferent arteriolar tone over a systolic blood pressure (SBP) range of 90–150 mmHg. Subsequently, intraglomerular and peritubular capillary pressure can be maintained at a constant mean arterial pressure (MAP) range of 60–80 mmHg. The ability to maintain glomerular perfusion pressure and GFR within normal limits in the face of wide changes in arterial BP is impaired in patients with insulin-dependent diabetes mellitus (IDDM) and nephropathy as well as hypertensive non-insulin-dependent diabetic patients [19]. As a result, the afferent arteriolar myogenic reflex is lost in certain populations. Consequently, glomeruli are exposed to elevated systemic pressures, and glomerular capillary permeability to macromolecules is increased. The ensuing vascular dysfunction results in microalbuminuria (MAU) (defined as 20–200 μg/min, or 30–300 mg/day) and later macro- or overt albuminuria (defined as >200 μg/min, or >300 mg/day), which are believed to trigger formation of vasoactive and inflammatory substances in renal tubular epithelial cells that induce renal parenchymal fibrogenesis (Figure 11.2) [20]. Therefore, patients with impaired prerenal autoregulation may benefit more substantially from lower levels of systemic BP than those with normal vasculature. In addition, increased sodium concentration in the distal tubular fluid produces stimulation of the renin–angiotensin–aldosterone system (RAAS), which has increasingly become a therapeutic target. Angiotensin II, in addition to its vasoconstrictive properties, also possesses mitogenic and fibrogenic capabilities, which further contribute to progressive renal damage. However, angiotensin II also causes vasoconstriction of the efferent glomerular arteriole, which can raise glomerular capillary pressure. This is particularly important when autoregulation is impaired.

Control of albuminuria, the 'barometer' of endothelial dysfunction, is essential. Not only has urinary albumin excretion been linked to cardiovascular events [21], but also a significant association between clinical proteinuria (>300 mg/day) and stroke has been identified in both non-diabetic and type 2 diabetic patients [22]. Therefore, the presence of proteinuria has become accepted as a marker of vascular endothelial dysfunction and microinflammation, and is viewed as the main prognostic factor for progression of renal disease. Some have argued that the Antihypertensive and Lipid-lowering Treatment to Prevent Heart Attack Trial (ALLHAT) [23] demonstrated no statistical difference between thiazide-based,

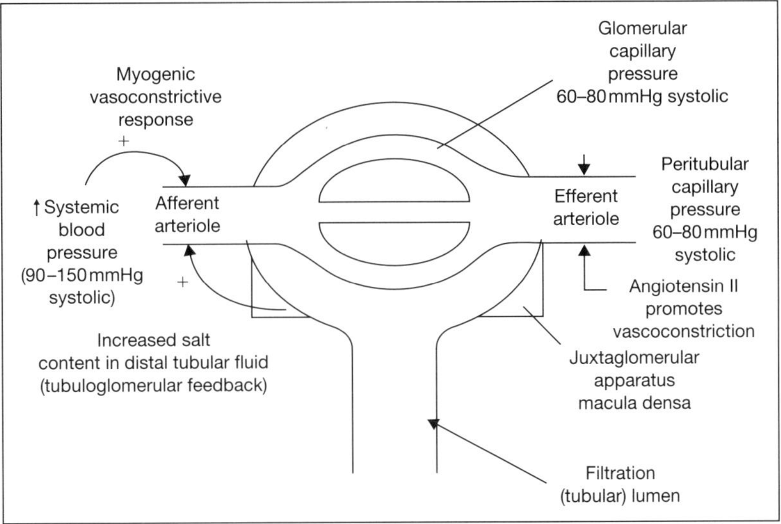

Figure 11.1 Relationships among systemic, glomerular capillary, and peritubular capillary pressures. Reproduced with permission from [14].

angiotensin-converting enzyme inhibitor (ACE-I)-based, or calcium channel blocker (CCB)-based antihypertensive regimens in reducing the incidence of ESRD despite varying degrees of renal insufficiency among study participants. However, there was no measurement of proteinuria in the study. Consequently, it is not possible to evaluate the influence of proteinuria on CVD outcomes based on different antihypertensive medications over the 5-year duration of this study [24]. Clinical trial data indicate that patients with less than 1 gram of proteinuria per day may need to be studied for more than 5 years to demonstrate possible differences between BP goals and therapies on the rate of progression of kidney disease [25, 26].

The subsequent sections deal with BP goals and treatment recommendations for patients with diabetes mellitus (DM) and varying strata of proteinuria: normoalbuminuria to MAU, MAU to overt proteinuria, and overt proteinuria to ESRD and CVD. The rationale for this format lies in the abundant clinical trial data that profile the therapeutic goals and treatment strategies for each subset. Following this is a discussion of therapeutic goals for non-diabetic kidney disease. Hypertension in renal transplantation will also be briefly discussed.

PROGRESSION OF NORMOALBUMINURIA TO MICROALBUMINURIA

The combination of hypertension and either types 1 or 2 DM increases the risk for progression of both renal and CVD. Recent reviews on management of hypertension in diabetic patients have been published [13, 27]. Several aetiologic factors have been postulated to explain the mechanisms of renal injury in DM (Table 11.1) [27]. The United Kingdom Prospective Diabetes Study Group demonstrated a 44% reduction in stroke, a 21% reduction in MI, a 37% reduction in microvascular disease, and a 32% reduction in risk of mortality for a 10/5 mmHg reduction in BP in 1148 hypertensive individuals with type 2 DM assigned to either tight BP control (<150/85 mmHg) or less tight BP control (BP goal <180/105) [28]. With regard to renal outcome, serum creatinine concentration was not significantly different between the tight vs. less tight BP control groups after 9 years, nor was there a significant reduction in risk for proteinuria and urinary albumin concentration >5 mg/dl. This may not be surprising given the considerably higher BP treatment goals targeted in this study. These goals are considerably higher than would be currently considered acceptable. While

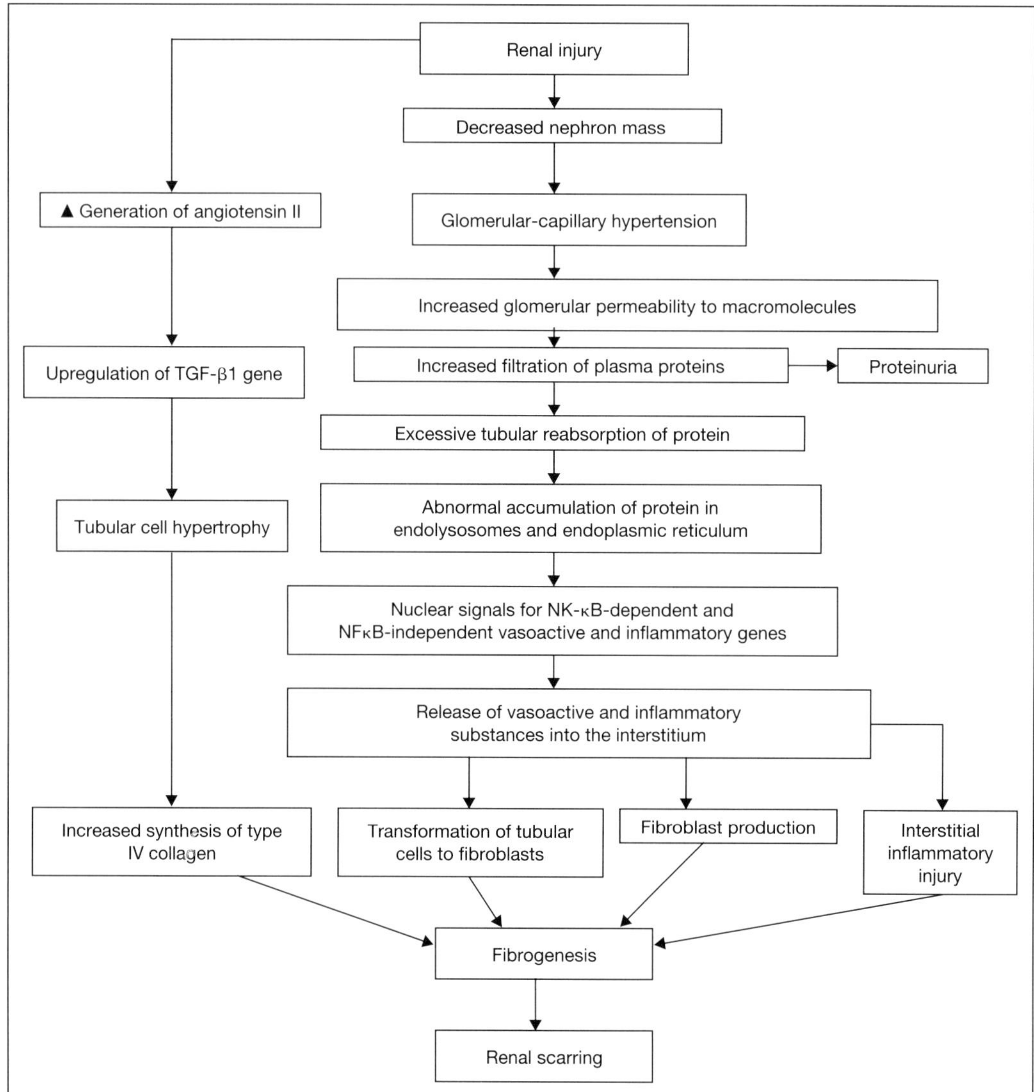

Figure 11.2 Mechanisms of disease. Effects of glomerular permeability to proteins on progressive renal injury. Reproduced with permission from [20].

most patients had normoalbuminuria at baseline, MAU (defined as >50 mg/l) was found in 18% of the patients randomized to tight control and in 16% of those randomized to less tight control. A smaller portion of patients (3% in the tight and 4% in the less tight control group) had overt proteinuria (defined as >300 mg/l). During study follow-up, progression to MAU and overt proteinuria was observed in both groups; however, the difference was significant only in patients who developed MAU after 6 years (20.3% in tight control group vs. 28.5% in less tight control group; $P = 0.0085$).

Interruption of the RAAS with an ACE-I or angiotensin II receptor blocking agent (ARB) has had favourable outcomes in delaying the progression of diabetic nephropathy. The beneficial effects of RAS inhibition in the diabetic population have been known for years.

Table 11.1 Theoretical mechanisms of progressive renal injury in DM

Haemodynamics
Systemic hypertension
Glomerular capillary hypertension
Hyperfiltration/transglomerular passage of albumin
Biochemical
Glomerular basement membrane charge defects
Glycation phenomena
Aldose reductase enzymatic changes
Endothelial dysfunction
Tubular reabsorption of albumin
Reproduced with permission from [27].

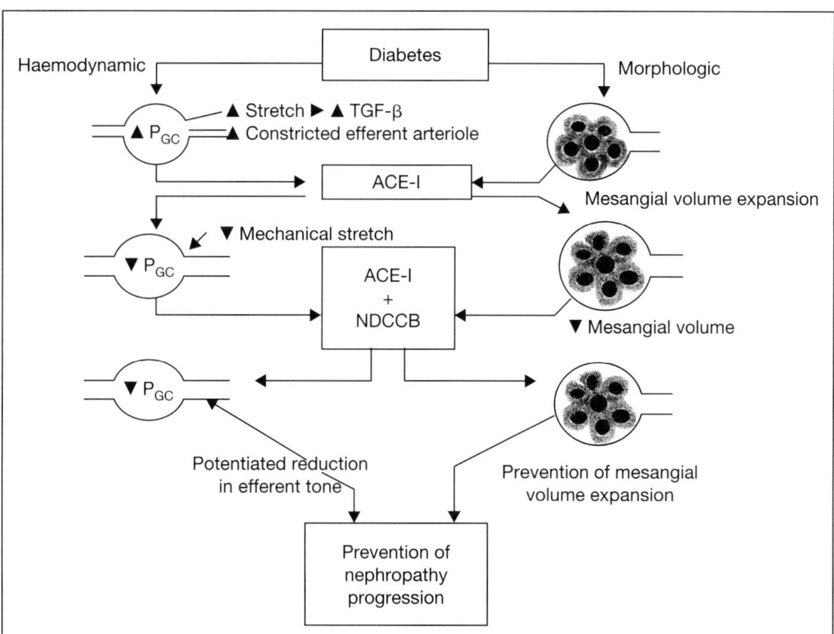

Figure 11.3 Effects of ACE-I and non-dihydropyridine calcium antagonists alone and in combination on intrarenal haemodynamics and glomerular morphology. Reproduced with permission from [30].

In fact, a meta-analysis of 16 trials containing 4925 patients with DM and normoalbuminuria (urinary albumin excretion <30 mg/day) demonstrated that only ACE-I therapy resulted in a significant reduction in the risk for developing MAU [29]. This effect is illustrated in Figure 11.3 [30].

PROGRESSION FROM MICROALBUMINURIA TO OVERT PROTEINURIA

Viberti and colleagues [31] randomized 92 patients with IDDM to receive either captopril 50 mg or placebo twice per day. All had persistent MAU (defined as <200 μg/min). Mean urinary albumin excretion increased with placebo (from 52 to 76 μg/min) but decreased with captopril (from 52 to 41 μg/min) ($P < 0.01$). Similarly, patients in the captopril group experienced a significant decrease in BP by 4/2 mmHg. Twelve patients in the placebo group and four in the captopril group progressed to clinical proteinuria over 24 months of follow-up, and BP rose independently of treatment for these individuals. Glomerular filtration rate did not change significantly between groups during the study interval. Ravid and co-workers [32] studied 94 normotensive patients with non-insulin dependent diabetes mellitus (NIDDM) whose serum creatinine was <1.4 mg/dl (123.76 μmol/l) and who had MAU (30–300 mg/24 h). Patients were randomized to receive either enalapril 10 mg or placebo daily for 5 years. Urinary albumin excretion and serum creatinine remained stable in the enalapril-treated group, and remained stable when the study was extended for another 2 years. Enalapril decreased the relative risk for development of nephropathy by 42% over 7 years. Patients who were initially treated with placebo for 5 years and then treated with enalapril over 2 years of study extension demonstrated stabilization in urinary albumin excretion and serum creatinine. The MAU, Cardiovascular, and Renal Outcomes substudy of the Heart Outcomes Prevention Evaluation (MICRO-HOPE) [33] demonstrated a significant reduction in progression from MAU to overt nephropathy with ACE-I therapy (117 [7%] on ramipril and 149 [8%] on placebo; $P = 0.027$), and treatment with ramipril resulted in a lower albumin-to-creatinine ratio at 1 and 4.5 years of follow-up compared with placebo.

The antiproteinuric effects of ARB have been demonstrated by the Irbesartan in Patients with Type 2 Diabetes and Microalbuminuria (IRMA2) Study Group [34]. This trial documented a significant reduction in the rate of progression from MAU to overt nephropathy in a cohort of 590 patients with similar hypertensive control. Greater benefit was achieved using a 300 mg daily dose of irbesartan as opposed to 150 mg over the 2-year follow-up period. Data published from the same institution several years later found that urinary albumin excretion was decreased further by 15% in type 2 diabetic patients treated with 'ultrahigh doses' of irbesartan (900 mg daily) instead of 300 mg/day [35]. Lastly, in the MAU Reduction With Valsartan in Patients With Type 2 Diabetes Mellitus (MARVAL) trial, patients experienced a 44% reduction in proteinuria with valsartan over 24 weeks vs. 8% reduction with amlodipine ($P < 0.001$ between groups) [36]. These results were achieved despite similar BP control in both groups.

PROGRESSION FROM OVERT PROTEINURIA TO END-STAGE KIDNEY DISEASE AND CARDIOVASCULAR DISEASE

Lewis and colleagues [37] studied patients with IDDM for at least 7 years duration and diabetic nephropathy, defined as urinary protein excretion ≥500 mg/24 h and serum creatinine concentration ≤2.5 mg/dl (221 μmol/l). Patients were randomized to captropril 25 mg vs. placebo three times per day, and BP was controlled to <140/90 mmHg. Of 409 patients originally randomized, 68 reached the primary endpoint of doubling of serum creatinine concentration (25 in captropril group; 43 in placebo group; $P = 0.007$), and 65 had died or required dialysis or transplantation (23 in captopril group; 42 placebo group; $P = 0.006$). In addition, the mean rate of increase in serum creatinine over 2.7 years follow-up was 0.2 ± 0.8 mg/dl (22 ± 67 μmol/l) per year in the captopril group vs. 0.5 ± 0.8 mg/dl (42 ± 67 μmol/l) per year in the placebo group ($P = 0.004$). Increases in serum creatinine and decrements in 24-h creatinine clearance were more substantive in patients whose baseline serum creatinine was ≥1.5 mg/dl.

The Irbesartan Diabetic Nephropathy Trial (IDNT) randomized 1715 patients with hypertension and type 2 DM to receive irbesartan 300 mg daily, amlodipine 10 mg daily, or placebo for a mean follow-up of 2.6 years. Treatment with irbesartan was associated with relative risk of doubling of serum creatinine that was 33% lower than for those treated with placebo ($P = 0.003$) and 37% lower than for those treated with amlodipine ($P < 0.001$), and

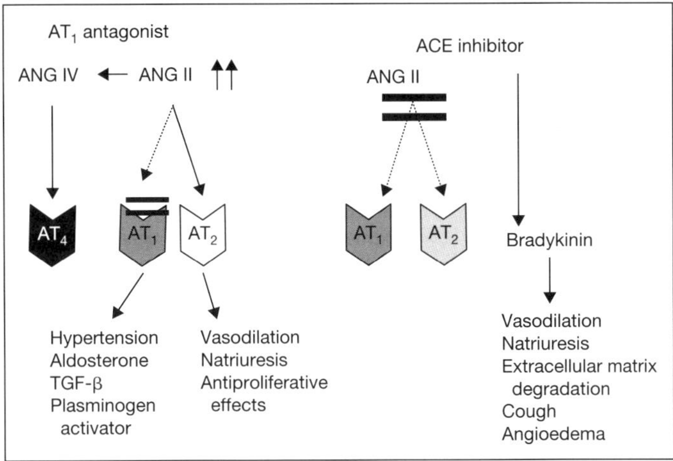

Figure 11.4 Differences between AT_1 receptor antagonists and ACE-I. Modified with permission from [41].

the unadjusted relative risk of developing ESRD was 23% lower in the irbesartan group than for either the placebo or amlodipine arm ($P = 0.07$). There was no significant difference in relative risk of death between the three groups [38]. Similarly, the Reduction of Endpoints in NIDDM with the Angiotensin II Antagonist Losartan (RENAAL) investigators [39] randomized 1513 patients with hypertension and type 2 DM to receive either losartan 50–100 mg daily or placebo with additional antihypertensive medication (not including ACE-I or ARBs) to reach target BP <140/90 mmHg. The mean follow-up was 3.4 years. Losartan reduced the incidence of doubling of serum creatinine 25% compared with placebo ($P = 0.006$) and ESRD (28% compared with placebo; $P = 0.002$) but yielded no difference in the rate of death.

Considerable attention has been paid to dual blockade of RAAS using both ACE-I and ARB [40, 41], particularly in individuals who have not achieved target BP control <125/75 in the setting of 24-h urinary protein excretion >1 g/day. The effects of ACE-I and ARB, including differences in mechanism of action, are characterized in Figure 11.4 [40, 41]. Investigators from the Candesartan and Lisinopril Microalbuminuria Study randomized participants with type 2 DM and hypertension to receive 4 weeks placebo run-in followed by 12 weeks of either candesartan 16 mg daily or lisinopril 20 mg daily followed by 12 more weeks of either monotherapy or combination therapy. Combination therapy was more effective at reducing urinary albumin:creatinine ratio (50% vs. 24% for candesartan and 39% for lisinopril; $P < 0.001$). Mean SBP was reduced by 25.3 mmHg in the combination group vs. 14.1 mmHg in the candesartan arm and 16.7 mmHg in the lisinopril group. Slight increases in serum creatinine, potassium, and urate were noted. Creatinine clearance, calculated by the Cockroft-Gault formula, at 24 weeks decreased by 0.0835 ml/s ($P = 0.04$) in the lisinopril group and by 0.0735 ml/s ($P = 0.05$) in the combination therapy group, but was not changed in the candesartan group. Response to combination therapy was not related to angiotensin converting enzyme genotype [42]. Other studies are available that have researched combination ARB and ACE-I therapy [43–46].

LEVEL OF BLOOD PRESSURE CONTROL: RENAL AND CARDIOVASCULAR OUTCOMES

The degree of BP control needed to prevent renal disease progression has also been a matter of controversy. A recent analysis of the IDNT cohort evaluated patients with type 2 diabetic nephropathy and overt proteinuria (>900 mg/24 h), mild to moderate renal insufficiency (serum creatinine up to 3.0 mg/dl or 266 μmol/l), and hypertension (seated office SBP >135 mmHg and diastolic blood pressure (DBP) >85 mmHg). Renal endpoints were defined as doubling of baseline serum creatinine or ESRD (serum creatinine >6 mg/dl or need for renal replacement therapy). Of note, these researchers found that the achieved follow-up SBP is an independent predictor of renal outcome regardless of baseline SBP. In addition, the best renal outcomes were observed for participants who achieved a follow-up SBP <134 mmHg, and there was no advantage to achieving a SBP <120 mmHg. In fact, patients with follow-up SBP <120 mmHg experienced the highest mortality, in a J-curve fashion. Therefore, a target SBP range of 120–130 mmHg was recommended in these patients [47]. Similarly, an analysis of the same cohort evaluated cardiovascular events and found an increased risk of cardiovascular death and hospitalization for congestive heart failure (CHF) at a SBP ≤120 mmHg. In addition, a DBP <85 mmHg was associated with increased risk of MI while simultaneously protecting against stroke. Lastly, increased pulse pressure >90 mmHg increased the risk of mortality, MI, and CHF, but did not increase risk of stroke [48].

These data are corroborated by a *post hoc* analysis of the RENAAL study cohort, which demonstrated that both baseline SBP and pulse pressure are equally predictive of progression of diabetic nephropathy and were stronger than DBP in predicting renal outcomes. Patients with baseline SBP range of 140–159 mmHg carried an increased risk for ESRD or death that was 38% greater than those with SBP <130 mmHg ($P = 0.05$). Losartan-treated patients with pulse pressure >90 mmHg experienced a 53.5% risk reduction for ESRD ($P = 0.003$) and a 35.5% risk reduction for ESRD or death ($P = 0.02$) compared with placebo-treated individuals [49]. Therefore, in patients with DM, lower BP and RAAS blockade have been shown to reduce MAU, as well as decrease the rate of progression of MAU to overt proteinuria and, subsequently, ESRD and CVD.

NON-DIABETIC KIDNEY DISEASE

The progression of kidney disease in non-diabetic patients with proteinuria has been addressed recently. Jafar and co-workers [58, 59] from the ACE Inhibition in Progressive Renal Disease (AIPRD) study group conducted a meta-analysis of eleven studies and 1860 patients. These investigators found that 16.8% of patients experienced kidney disease progression, defined as doubling of serum creatinine or kidney failure. Of these 124 (13.2%) were from the ACE-I treated group, and 187 (20.5%) were from the control group ($P = 0.001$). Of 176 (9.5%) of patients who developed kidney failure, 70 (7.4%) came from the treatment group and 106 (11.6%) came from the control group ($P = 0.002$). The relative risks observed for SBP control were for the range 110–119 mmHg and were higher for SBP <110 (RR 2.48), SBP 130–139 (RR 1.83), and >160 mmHg (RR 3.14) [58]. Figure 11.5 illustrates the increasing risk for kidney disease progression that is associated with each increasing decile of SBP for individuals with current urinary protein excretion >1 g/day. The observation that patients from the Modification of Diet in Renal Disease Study cohort in non-diabetic patients with baseline proteinuria >3 g/day demonstrated greater decrement in GFR at MAP >98 mmHg established proteinuria as an independent risk factor for progression of renal disease. This study led to the recommendation that patients with proteinuria in excess of 1 g/day be treated to a MAP <92 mmHg (or 125/75 mmHg). Because the rate of decline in GFR was unrelated to BP control in patients whose baseline urinary protein excretion was <0.25 g/day, recommendations to control BP to less than 98 mmHg mean or <130/80 mmHg systemic were made for those whose proteinuria was within the range of 0.25–1.0 g/day [26]. Of note, reduction of proteinuria in response to ACE-I therapy is more pronounced in patients with greater degrees of urinary protein excretion at baseline, and the degree of proteinuria after treatment with these agents is a better predictor of progression than the level of proteinuria at baseline. In addition, the timing of response to low vs. usual BP control can be seen as early as 8 months in patients with ≥3 g of proteinuria

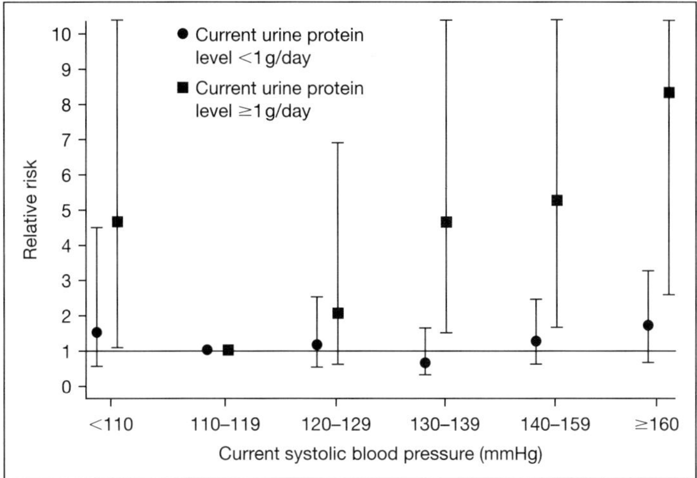

Figure 11.5 Relative risk for kidney disease progression based on current level of SBP and current urine excretion. Reproduced with permission from [58].

per day and at 24 months in patients with 1–3 g of proteinuria per day. In those with <1 g proteinuria per day, no difference between BP goals was observed (Figure 11.6) [26]. When adjusting for the antihypertensive and antiproteinuric effects of ACE-I on renal disease progression, the benefit of ACE inhibition on progression remained significant in the meta-analysis by Jafar and coworkers, which underscores the presence of another property of ACE-I that mediates their beneficial effect beyond control of hypertension and proteinuria [59].

The Ramipril Efficacy in Nephropathy study evaluated 352 patients with chronic, non-diabetic nephropathies who were stratified according to baseline proteinuria (stratum 1: 1–3 g/24 h vs. stratum 2: ≥3 g/24 h) and randomized to receive ramipril or placebo with further antihypertensive therapy as needed to achieve target DBP <90 mmHg [60]. Because GFR decline was significantly greater in the patients whose baseline proteinuria was >3 g/day (0.53 vs. 0.88 ml/min/month; $P = 0.03$), the Adjudicating Panel decided to open stratum 2 and allow the most effective therapy to be provided. At the time of the second interim analysis, 177 of 352 patients had three consecutive GFR measurements. The mean rate of GFR decline was 0.67 ml/min in the 87 patients with baseline urinary protein excretion rates >3 g/24 h and 0.25 ml/min in 90 patients with urinary protein excretion <3 g/24 h. Fifty-eight patients reached the endpoint of doubling of baseline serum creatinine concentration or end-stage renal failure (18 in ramipril group and 42 in placebo group; $P = 0.02$). A higher baseline urinary protein excretion rate was associated with a higher risk of reaching the combined endpoint in the placebo group, and this risk persisted after adjustments were made for changes in SBP and DBP. Therefore, ramipril was protective over placebo in slowing decline in renal function and halved the risk of doubling of baseline serum creatinine or reaching ESRD, and this effect was not fully explained by ramipril's ability to control systemic BP [60].

The African-American Study of Kidney Disease and Hypertension Study Group randomized 1094 African-Americans with GFR of 20–65 ml/min/1.73 m^2 to receive either the sustained release beta-blocker metoprolol 50–200 mg/day, the ACE-I ramipril 2.5–10 mg/day or the dihydropyridine calcium channel blocking agent (DHP-CCB) amlodipine 5–10 mg/day. Other agents were added to reach one of two BP goals: a usual MAP goal of 102–107 mmHg or a low MAP goal of ≤92 mmHg. Urinary protein excretion, measured as the protein:creatinine (UP/Cr) ratio, was also observed. The endpoints of the study were

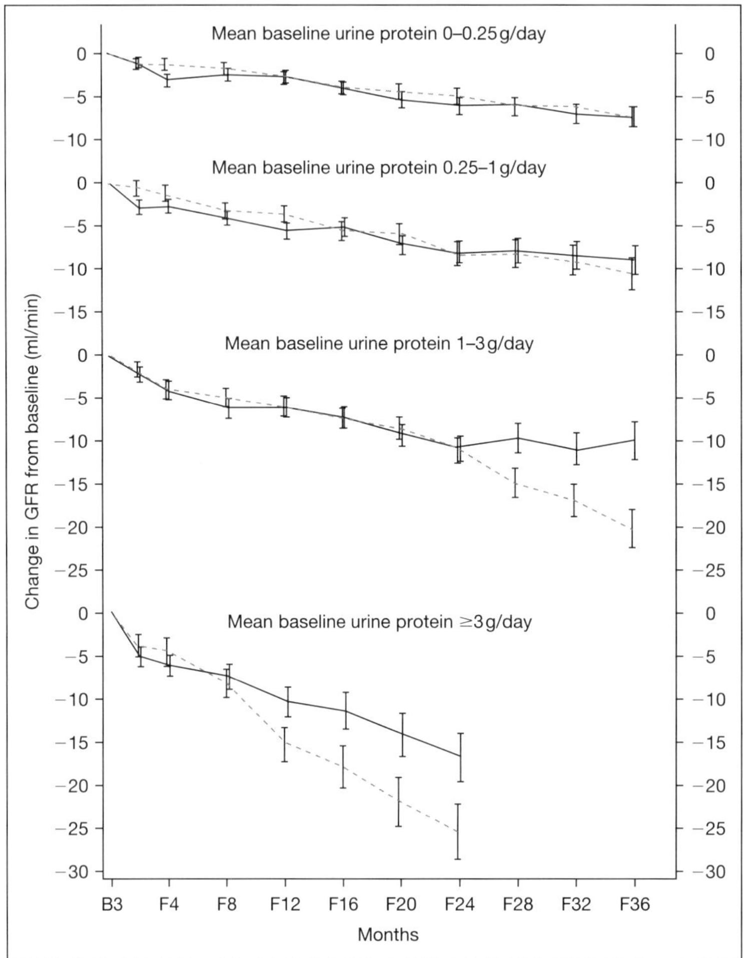

Figure 11.6 Changes in glomerular filtration rate based on graded levels of urinary protein excretion. Reproduced with permission from [26].

reduction in GFR by 50% or by 25 ml/min, onset of ESRD (need for renal replacement therapy), or death. The amlodipine arm was subsequently terminated in 2000. Overall, the mean decline in GFR was 1.15 ml/min/1.73 m^2/year, or 36%, slower in the ramipril group ($P = 0.002$). Of note, the GFR increased during the initial 3-month acute phase in participants treated with amlodipine; however, this change was only observed in those whose baseline UP/Cr was ≤0.22 (~300 mg/day). Although the decline in GFR to 3 years was 1.22 ± 0.44 ml/min per 1.73 m^2/year faster ($P = 0.006$) in the ramipril-treated patients whose UP/Cr was <0.22, ramipril delayed progression in those whose UP/Cr was >0.22 (rate of GFR decline 2.02 ± 0.74 ml/min/1.73 m^2/year, or 36%; $P = 0.006$). Among those with UP/Cr <0.22 at baseline, the rate of development of UP/Cr >0.22 was 56% lower for the ramipril arm than for the amlodipine arm ($P < 0.001$). Therefore, the investigators concluded that ACE-I have a renoprotective effect over DHP-CCB in patients with established kidney disease despite substantial reductions in BP conferred by those agents [25]. However, because of the extended duration of time needed to measure benefit in these patients, longer follow-up is indicated. Results from an additional 5-year investigation are forthcoming.

In summary, for patients with non-diabetic CKD, lower BP goals and RAAS blockade have been shown to provide benefit. However, no data on preventing progression of MAU to proteinuria exist in this population. Moreover, response to BP reduction and RAAS blockade depends on the level of proteinuria, such that for greater levels of urinary protein excretion, less time is required for therapeutic benefit to be observed.

WHAT IS GOOD FOR THE KIDNEY IS GOOD FOR THE HEART

The cardiovascular benefits of RAAS inhibition in addition to BP reduction also deserve mention. Three studies, including the Heart Outcomes Prevention Evaluation (HOPE) trial [50] the Appropriate Blood Pressure Control in Diabetes (ABCD) study [51], and the LIFE cohort [52] are landmarks in this regard. The HOPE study investigators reported on 9297 patients ≥55 years old with preserved left ventricular function and evidence of vascular disease or diabetes plus one other cardiovascular risk factor such as hypertension, MAU, cigarette smoking, high total cholesterol, or low levels of high density lipoprotein concentration. Patients were randomized to receive ramipril 10 mg or placebo daily for a mean follow-up of 5 years. Of 651 patients assigned to ramipril, 14% reached the primary composite endpoint of MI, stroke, or death from cardiovascular causes (vs. 17.8% of patients assigned to the placebo arm). Ramipril treatment was associated with a 6.1% death rate from cardiovascular causes (compared with 8.1% in the placebo group; relative risk [RR] 0.74; $P < 0.001$); a 9.9% MI rate (vs. 12.3% with placebo; RR 0.8; $P < 0.001$); and 3.4% risk of stroke (vs. 4.9% with placebo; RR 0.68; $P < 0.001$). Similarly, ramipril treatment was associated with significant risk reduction with regard to death from any cause, cardiac arrest, heart failure, revascularization procedures, complications related to DM, and new diagnosis of diabetes. These effects of ramipril were evident within one year of randomization.

Estacio and colleagues [51] from the ABCD trial studied 950 patients with NIDDM, with hypertension (DBP >90 mmHg) or without (DBP 80–90 mmHg). Patients were randomized to receive nisoldipine, enalapril, or placebo (for those in the normotensive arm only) and were followed for 5 years. The primary endpoint was the effect of intensive (target DBP 75 mmHg) vs. moderate (DBP 80–89 mmHg) BP control on 24-h creatinine clearance. However, the main finding of the study was based on a secondary endpoint, namely that fewer MI were observed in the enalapril group (fatal and non-fatal MI: 5 enalapril group vs. 25 nisoldipine group; $P = 0.001$). Other secondary endpoints included the effect of intensive vs. moderate BP control on left ventricular hypertrophy (LVH), urinary albumin excretion, neuropathy, and retinopathy. This study further supports the notion that a RAAS inhibitor should be considered a preferred first-line agent for prevention of cardiovascular complications, particularly MI, in patients with NIDDM [51]. Other studies have found favourable results of using ACE-I following MI [53–55] and CHF [56, 57].

Investigators for the Losartan Intervention for Endpoint in hypertension study (LIFE) randomized 9193 patients with hypertension (defined as sitting BP 160–200/95–115 mmHg) and LVH to losartan or atenolol once daily and followed them for 4 years. The primary composite endpoint (death, MI, or stroke) occurred in 508 losartan- and 588 atenolol-treated patients ($P = 0.021$) despite substantial BP reductions with both drugs. Losartan-based treatment was also protective against stroke (25% further reduction over and above BP control) and was associated with fewer cases of new-onset DM. MI occurred in more losartan-treated patients; however, the difference did not achieve statistical significance [52].

RENAL TRANSPLANTATION

Hypertension is commonly observed following renal transplantation and is often the result of parenchymal or atherosclerotic disease. Other aetiologies attributed to the 80–90% rate of post-transplant hypertension include immunosuppressive medications, particularly calcineurin inhibitors such as cyclosporine and tacrolimus as well as glucocorticoids, and lifestyle factors. In addition, properties of the transplanted allograft such as transplant renal artery stenosis or reduced nephron mass caused by parenchymal disease in the donor kidney have also been implicated. Several studies exist to support aggressive BP control in order to increase allograft survival [61–64]. These studies suggest that worsened renal transplant function occurs with graded increases in systolic, diastolic, and mean arterial pressures. This relationship applies particularly to African-American allograft recipients. In addition, the ideal degree of BP control and the preferred antihypertensive regimen, if any, remain to be settled in renal transplantation. Traditionally, RAAS inhibitors have been avoided due to the risk of elevated serum creatinine and hyperkalaemia, leading clinicians to rely more upon calcium channel antagonists, vasodilators, diuretics, and other agents. However, RAAS inhibitors may be used with greater frequency for their antifibrotic effects in an interest to delay chronic allograft nephropathy (CAN). Because the role of hypertension in progressive CAN has not been fully elucidated, the results of clinical trials are eagerly anticipated [65]. It is likely that lower BP coupled with RAAS blockade will result in better preservation of kidney transplant function, much as it does for native kidney function.

SUMMARY

There is abundant evidence from numerous clinical studies to substantiate the claim that aggressive BP control can delay progression of kidney disease. The most favourable results have been observed in patients with proteinuric nephropathy, for whom interruption of the RAAS system in conjunction with aggressive BP control provides the best first-line defence against progressive loss of kidney function. However, a number of questions remain to be answered, including the optimal doses of ACE-I and ARB in progressive kidney disease as well as the best method to assess optimal dose. In addition, the role of nocturnal BP control in proteinuric renal disease remains to be determined [66]. As of this writing, patients who are treated to goal BP reduction have not only been shown to benefit from fewer renal comorbid events, but also stand to experience better cardiovascular and cerebrovascular outcomes.

ACKNOWLEDGEMENT

The authors wish to acknowledge their gratitude to Ms. Geetha Stachowiak for her outstanding assistance in the preparation of the figures in this text and for her editorial contributions to this manuscript.

REFERENCES

1. Burt VL, Whelton P, Roccella EJ *et al.* Prevalence of hypertension in the US adult population. Results from the Third National Health and Nutrition Examination Survey, 1988–1991. *Hypertension* 1995; 25:305–313.
2. Coresh J, Astor BC, Greene T, Eknoyan G, Levey AS. Prevalence of chronic kidney disease and decreased kidney function in the adult US population: Third National Health and Nutrition Examination Survey. *Am J Kidney Dis* 2003; 41:1–12.
3. Foley RN, Parfrey PS, Sarnak MJ. Clinical epidemiology of CVD in CKD. *J Am Osteopath Assoc* 2005; 105:207–215.
4. Hebert LA, Wilmer WA, Falkenhain ME, Ladson-Wofford SE, Nahman NS Jr, Rovin BH. Renoprotection: one or many therapies? *Kidney Int* 2001; 59:1211–1226.
5. Klag MJ, Whelton PK, Randall BL *et al.* Blood pressure and end-stage renal disease in men. *N Engl J Med* 1996; 334:13–18.
6. Perry HM Jr, Miller JP, Fornoff JR *et al.* Early predictors of 15-year end-stage renal disease in hypertensive patients. *Hypertension* 1995; 25:587–594.

7. Ritz E. Which comes first–renal dysfunction or high BP? *J Am Soc Nephrol* 2005; 16:2817–2826.
8. Hsu CY, McCulloch CE, Darbinian J, Go AS, Iribarren C. Elevated blood pressure and risk of end-stage renal disease in subjects without baseline kidney disease. *Arch Intern Med* 2005; 165:923–928.
9. Go AS, Chertow GM, Fan D, McCulloch CE, Hsu CY. Chronic kidney disease and the risks of death, cardiovascular events, and hospitalization. *N Engl J Med* 2004; 351:1296–1305.
10. Ritz E, McClellan WM. Overview: increased cardiovascular risk in patients with minor renal dysfunction: an emerging issue with far-reaching consequences. *J Am Soc Nephrol* 2004; 15:513–516.
11. Vasan RS, Larson MG, Leip EP *et al*. Impact of high-normal blood pressure on the risk of cardiovascular disease. *N Engl J Med* 2001; 345:1291–1297.
12. Panza JA. High-normal blood pressure – more 'high' than 'normal'. *N Engl J Med* 2001; 345:1337–1340.
13. Bakris GL, Williams M, Dworkin L *et al*. National Kidney Foundation Hypertension and Diabetes Executive Committees Working Group. Preserving renal function in adults with hypertension and diabetes: a consensus approach. *Am J Kidney Dis* 2000; 36:646–661.
14. Weir MR. The role of combination antihypertensive therapy in the prevention and treatment of chronic kidney disease. *Am J Hypertens* 2005; 18:100S–105S.
15. Weir MR. How low should we treat blood pressure and why? *J Clin Hypertens* (Greenwich) 1999; 1:199–208.
16. Weir MR. Preventing renal disease progression: is it the drug or the blood pressure reduction, or both? *Curr Hypertens Rep* 2000; 2:497–499.
17. Weir M, Dworkin L. Antihypertensive drugs, dietary salt, and renal protection: how low should you go and with which therapy? *Am J Kidney Dis* 1998; 32:1–22.
18. Weir MR. Progressive renal and cardiovascular disease: optimal treatment strategies. *Kidney Int* 2002; 62:1482–1492.
19. Christensen PK, Hansen HP, Parving HH. Impaired autoregulation of GFR in hypertensive non-insulin dependent diabetic patients. *Kidney Int* 1997; 52:1369–1374.
20. Remuzzi G, Bertani T. Pathophysiology of progressive nephropathies. *N Engl J Med* 1998; 339:1448–1456.
21. Ibsen H, Olsen MH, Wachtell K *et al*. Reduction in albuminuria translates to reduction in cardiovascular events in hypertensive patients: losartan intervention for endpoint reduction in hypertension study. *Hypertension* 2005; 45:198–202.
22. Miettinen H, Haffner SM, Lehto S, Ronnemaa T, Pyorala K, Laakso M. Proteinuria predicts stroke and other atherosclerotic vascular disease events in nondiabetic and non-insulin-dependent diabetic subjects. *Stroke* 1996; 27:2033–2039.
23. Major outcomes in high-risk hypertensive patients randomized to angiotensin-converting enzyme inhibitor or calcium channel blocker vs diuretic: The Antihypertensive and Lipid-Lowering Treatment to Prevent Heart Attack Trial (ALLHAT). *JAMA* 2002; 288:2981–2997.
24. Weir MR. Clinical trials report. Chronic kidney disease: blood pressure, treatment goals, and cardiovascular outcomes. *Curr Hypertens Rep* 2003; 5:405–407.
25. Agodoa LY, Appel L, Bakris GL *et al*. Effect of ramipril vs amlodipine on renal outcomes in hypertensive nephrosclerosis: a randomized controlled trial. *JAMA* 2001; 285:2719–2728.
26. Peterson JC, Adler S, Burkart JM *et al*. Blood pressure control, proteinuria, and the progression of renal disease. The Modification of Diet in Renal Disease Study. *Ann Intern Med* 1995; 123:754–762.
27. Weir MR. Diabetes and hypertension: how low should you go and with which drugs? *Am J Hypertens* 2001; 14:17S–26S.
28. UK Prospective Diabetes Study Group. Tight blood pressure control and risk of macrovascular and microvascular complications in type 2 diabetes: UKPDS 38. *Br Med J* 1998; 317:703–713.
29. Strippoli GF, Craig M, Schena FP, Craig JC. Antihypertensive agents for primary prevention of diabetic nephropathy. *J Am Soc Nephrol* 2005; 16:3081–3091.
30. Bakris GL, Weir MR, Sowers JR. Therapeutic challenges in the obese diabetic patient with hypertension. *Am J Med* 1996; 101:33S–46S.
31. Viberti G, Mogensen CE, Groop LC, Pauls JF. European Microalbuminuria Captopril Study Group. Effect of captopril on progression to clinical proteinuria in patients with insulin-dependent diabetes mellitus and microalbuminuria. *JAMA* 1994; 271:275–279.
32. Ravid M, Lang R, Rachmani R, Lishner M. Long-term renoprotective effect of angiotensin-converting enzyme inhibition in non-insulin-dependent diabetes mellitus. A 7-year follow-up study. *Arch Intern Med* 1996; 156:286–289.

33. Heart Outcomes Prevention Evaluation Study Investigators. Effects of ramipril on cardiovascular and microvascular outcomes in people with diabetes mellitus: results of the HOPE study and MICRO-HOPE substudy. *Lancet* 2000; 355:253–259.
34. Parving HH, Lehnert H, Brochner-Mortensen J, Gomis R, Andersen S, Arner P. The effect of irbesartan on the development of diabetic nephropathy in patients with type 2 diabetes. *N Engl J Med* 2001; 345:870–878.
35. Rossing K, Schjoedt KJ, Jensen BR, Boomsma F, Parving HH. Enhanced renoprotective effects of ultrahigh doses of irbesartan in patients with type 2 diabetes and microalbuminuria. *Kidney Int* 2005; 68:1190–1198.
36. Viberti G, Wheeldon NM. Microalbuminuria reduction with valsartan in patients with type 2 diabetes mellitus: a blood pressure-independent effect. *Circulation* 2002; 106:672–678.
37. Lewis EJ, Hunsicker LG, Bain RP, Rohde RD, The Collaborative Study Group. The effect of angiotensin-converting-enzyme inhibition on diabetic nephropathy. *N Engl J Med* 1993; 329:1456–1462.
38. Lewis EJ, Hunsicker LG, Clarke WR *et al.* Renoprotective effect of the angiotensin-receptor antagonist irbesartan in patients with nephropathy due to type 2 diabetes. *N Engl J Med* 2001; 345:851–860.
39. Brenner BM, Cooper ME, de Zeeuw D *et al.* Effects of losartan on renal and cardiovascular outcomes in patients with type 2 diabetes and nephropathy. *N Engl J Med* 2001; 345:861–869.
40. Thurman JM, Schrier RW. Comparative effects of angiotensin-converting enzyme inhibitors and angiotensin receptor blockers on blood pressure and the kidney. *Am J Med* 2003; 114:588–598.
41. Wolf G, Ritz E. Combination therapy with ACE inhibitors and angiotensin II receptor blockers to halt progression of chronic renal disease: pathophysiology and indications. *Kidney Int* 2005; 67:799–812.
42. Mogensen CE, Neldam S, Tikkanen I *et al.* Randomised controlled trial of dual blockade of renin-angiotensin system in patients with hypertension, microalbuminuria, and non-insulin dependent diabetes: the candesartan and lisinopril microalbuminuria (CALM) study. *Br Med J* 2000; 321:1440–1444.
43. Hebert LA, Falkenhain ME, Nahman NS Jr, Cosio FG, O'Dorisio TM. Combination ACE inhibitor and angiotensin II receptor antagonist therapy in diabetic nephropathy. *Am J Nephrol* 1999; 19:1–6.
44. Hamroff G, Katz SD, Mancini D *et al.* Addition of angiotensin II receptor blockade to maximal angiotensin-converting enzyme inhibition improves exercise capacity in patients with severe congestive heart failure. *Circulation* 1999; 99:990–992.
45. Ruilope LM, Aldigier JC, Ponticelli C, Oddou-Stock P, Botteri F, Mann JF. European Group for the Investigation of Valsartan in Chronic Renal Disease. Safety of the combination of valsartan and benazepril in patients with chronic renal disease. *J Hypertens* 2000; 18:89–95.
46. Russo D, Pisani A, Balletta MM *et al.* Additive antiproteinuric effect of converting enzyme inhibitor and losartan in normotensive patients with IgA nephropathy. *Am J Kidney Dis* 1999; 33:851–856.
47. Pohl MA, Blumenthal S, Cordonnier DJ *et al.* Independent and additive impact of blood pressure control and angiotensin II receptor blockade on renal outcomes in the irbesartan diabetic nephropathy trial: clinical implications and limitations. *J Am Soc Nephrol* 2005; 16:3027–3037.
48. Berl T, Hunsicker LG, Lewis JB *et al.* Impact of achieved blood pressure on cardiovascular outcomes in the Irbesartan Diabetic Nephropathy Trial. *J Am Soc Nephrol* 2005; 16:2170–2179.
49. Bakris GL, Weir MR, Shanifar S *et al.* Effects of blood pressure level on progression of diabetic nephropathy: results from the RENAAL study. *Arch Intern Med* 2003; 163:1555–1565.
50. Yusuf S, Sleight P, Pogue J, Bosch J, Davies R, Dagenais G. The Heart Outcomes Prevention Evaluation Study Investigators. Effects of an angiotensin-converting-enzyme inhibitor, ramipril, on cardiovascular events in high-risk patients. *N Engl J Med* 2000; 342:145–153.
51. Estacio RO, Jeffers BW, Hiatt WR, Biggerstaff SL, Gifford N, Schrier RW. The effect of nisoldipine as compared with enalapril on cardiovascular outcomes in patients with non-insulin-dependent diabetes and hypertension. *N Engl J Med* 1998; 338:645–652.
52. Dahlof B, Devereux RB, Kjeldsen SE *et al.* Cardiovascular morbidity and mortality in the Losartan Intervention For Endpoint reduction in hypertension study (LIFE): a randomised trial against atenolol. *Lancet* 2002; 359:995–1003.
53. Pfeffer MA, Braunwald E, Moye LA *et al.* The SAVE Investigators. Effect of captopril on mortality and morbidity in patients with left ventricular dysfunction after myocardial infarction. Results of the survival and ventricular enlargement trial. *N Engl J Med* 1992; 327:669–677.
54. GISSI-3. Effects of lisinopril and transdermal glyceryl trinitrate singly and together on 6-week mortality and ventricular function after acute myocardial infarction. Gruppo Italiano per lo Studio della Sopravvivenza nell'infarto Miocardico. *Lancet* 1994; 343:1115–1122.

55. ISIS-4 (Fourth International Study of Infarct Survival) Collaborative Group. A randomised factorial trial assessing early oral captopril, oral mononitrate, and intravenous magnesium sulphate in 58,050 patients with suspected acute myocardial infarction. *Lancet* 1995; 345:669–685.
56. The CONSENSUS Trial Study Group. Effects of enalapril on mortality in severe congestive heart failure. Results of the Cooperative North Scandinavian Enalapril Survival Study (CONSENSUS). *N Engl J Med* 1987; 316:1429–1435.
57. The SOLVD Investigators. Effect of enalapril on mortality and the development of heart failure in asymptomatic patients with reduced left ventricular ejection fractions. *N Engl J Med* 1992; 327:685–691.
58. Jafar TH, Stark PC, Schmid CH *et al.* Progression of chronic kidney disease: the role of blood pressure control, proteinuria, and angiotensin-converting enzyme inhibition: a patient-level meta-analysis. *Ann Intern Med* 2003; 139:244–252.
59. Jafar TH, Stark PC, Schmid CH *et al.* Proteinuria as a modifiable risk factor for the progression of non-diabetic renal disease. *Kidney Int* 2001; 60:1131–1140.
60. The GISEN Group (Gruppo Italiano di Studi Epidemiologici in Nefrologia). Randomised placebo-controlled trial of effect of ramipril on decline in glomerular filtration rate and risk of terminal renal failure in proteinuric, non-diabetic nephropathy. *Lancet* 1997; 349:1857–1863.
61. Cosio FG, Dillon JJ, Falkenhain ME *et al.* Racial differences in renal allograft survival: the role of systemic hypertension. *Kidney Int* 1995; 47:1136–1141.
62. Cosio FG, Pelletier RP, Sedmak DD, Pesavento TE, Henry ML, Ferguson RM. Renal allograft survival following acute rejection correlates with blood pressure levels and histopathology. *Kidney Int* 1999; 56:1912–1919.
63. Mange KC, Cizman B, Joffe M, Feldman HI. Arterial hypertension and renal allograft survival. *JAMA* 2000; 283:633–638.
64. Opelz G, Wujciak T, Ritz E. Collaborative Transplant Study. Association of chronic kidney graft failure with recipient blood pressure. *Kidney Int* 1998; 53:217–222.
65. Weir MR. Blood pressure management in the kidney transplant recipient. *Adv Chronic Kidney Dis* 2004; 11:172–183.
66. Sica D, Carl D. Pathologic basis and treatment considerations in chronic kidney disease-related hypertension. *Semin Nephrol* 2005; 25:246–251.

12

Are there consequences for attempting to achieve blood pressure goals in the first week after a stroke?

L. L. Pedelty, P. B. Gorelick

INTRODUCTION

Stroke is the most important preventable neurological disease of adult life [1–9]. It has earned this reputation because it has an associated high burden of illness, disability rate and economic cost, together with well-defined modifiable risk factors and proven efficacy of interventions in primary and secondary prevention.

Hypertension stands out as the most important modifiable risk factor for stroke. It is estimated that 25–50% of strokes may be attributed to hypertension. Hypertension is associated with an estimated 3–4-fold increase in risk of stroke – the risk is increased for systolic, diastolic and combined systolic and diastolic hypertension – and a substantial lowering of stroke risk is seen with blood pressure reduction. The increased risk of stroke with hypertension is universal, holding for both sexes and for most geographic regions and ethnic groups that have been studied.

We have begun to shift our conceptualization of risk associated with blood pressure from a *threshold concept* implicating a certain 'hypertensive' blood pressure level above which stroke and other cardiovascular risks increase, to a *continuum concept* recognizing a stepwise increase in risk as blood pressure increases from even normal or pre-hypertensive levels [10]. The continuum concept is further supported by studies demonstrating that the relationship between stroke risk and blood pressure is continuous down to blood pressures as low as 115/75 mmHg (e.g. [11]) and that the majority of strokes occur in individuals with only mild elevation of blood pressure or pre-hypertension [2], and by clinical trials showing benefit of blood pressure-lowering agents on reduction of stroke and other key cardiovascular risk outcomes even among individuals classified as 'non-hypertensive' [12, 13].

Overall, then, as we consider future stroke and cardiovascular disease prevention, we are shifting our risk assessment and treatment focus to *absolute blood pressure* level and associated cardiovascular risk factors (e.g. the components of the metabolic syndrome) [2], and blood pressure lowering is well-established as an important strategy to reduce the long-term risk of first or recurrent stroke [1–3]. Chronic management of blood pressure to

Laura L. Pedelty, PhD, MD, Assistant Professor of Neurology, Department of Neurology and Rehabilitative Medicine, The University of Illinois at Chicago, Chicago, Illinois, USA

Philip B. Gorelick, MD, MPH, John S. Garvin Professor and Head, Director, Centre for Stroke Research, Department of Neurology and Rehabilitative Medicine, The University of Illinois at Chicago, Chicago, Illinois, USA

recommended target goals is accepted as a safe and effective means for reducing stroke and cardiovascular disease burden in the long term.

Management of blood pressure in the acute phase after stroke, however, remains controversial. Hypertension is common in acute stroke, with an estimated 75–80% of stroke patients, including those with no prior history of hypertension, manifesting elevated blood pressures in the days following acute stroke [14–17]. There are, however, no clear evidence-based guidelines for management of blood pressure in acute stroke. Current guidelines are derived predominantly from large-scale clinical trials, and data regarding the consequences of elevated blood pressure in this phase are not consistent.

OBSERVATIONAL DATA

Observational studies of the relationship of acute blood pressure to outcome have revealed conflicting findings. Some investigators have documented better outcome in association with higher acute blood pressure [18, 19], while others have demonstrated improved functional recovery and lower incidence of oedema associated with a 20–30% drop in mean arterial pressure (MAP) [20], even when blood pressure reduction was not the result of active treatment [21]. In a consecutive series of 240 patients presenting with first ischaemic stroke, elevated blood pressure was associated higher odds of cerebral oedema, and failure of blood pressure to decline was seen in the patients with oedema formation but not in those without [22]. A meta-analysis of 32 studies including 10 892 patients concluded that elevated blood pressure in ischaemic stroke and primary intracerebral haemorrhage is associated with higher rate of death, death or dependency, and death or deterioration [23].

Still other studies report a complex pattern, with poor outcomes at extremes of the spectrum [16, 24–26]. Castillo and colleagues [24] report such a pattern in a series of 304 patients, with increased infarct volume, increased risk of neurological deterioration and poorer neurological outcome and increased death rate as systolic blood pressure (SBP) rose above or fell below an inflection point of 180 mmHg. In the International Stroke Trial (IST; n = 17 398), high blood pressure on admission was associated with poor outcome independent of other prognostic factors including age, atrial fibrillation, and stroke severity; low blood pressure was also independently associated with poor outcome, and the best outcomes were seen in patients with moderately elevated or high normal pressures [16]. Vemmos and associates similarly report increased mortality and morbidity for low as well as high acute blood pressure values in a series of 1121 patients, with an inflection point at 130 mmHg.

Non-uniformity of study design and reporting makes it difficult to draw conclusions from observational data. Studies vary in the type of stroke studied (ischaemic vs. haemorrhagic vs. both), in the timing of and procedure for measurement of blood pressure, and in selection criteria. Not all studies control for other comorbid factors such as coronary artery disease and atrial fibrillation, and findings may be different for individuals with diagnosed hypertension who were receiving blood pressure-lowering therapy on presentation than for individuals who had been untreated. Finally, the pathophysiology underlying poor outcome and deterioration at the two ends of the spectrum may not be uniform. In Vemmos and associates' study revealing a U-shaped curve for outcome vs. blood pressure, poor outcome associated with low vs. high blood pressures was associated with different mechanisms: low blood pressures were associated with heart failure and coronary artery disease, while high blood pressures were associated with increased incidence of death due to cerebral oedema [26].

PATHOPHYSIOLOGY

Blood pressure elevations in acute stroke may be mediated by a variety of mechanisms, including pre-existing hypertension, but also stress associated with the acute illness and hospitalization, increased sympathetic drive with catecholamine and cortisol release, activation of the renin–angiotensin–aldosterone system, and the Cushing reflex in cases of markedly increased intracranial pressure (ICP) due to intracerebral haematoma or oedema [27–29]. In addition, transient elevation in blood pressure may in some cases be compensatory: Lindsberg [30] and Mattle and co-workers [31] report findings that blood pressure elevations are seen with vascular occlusion and normalize following recanalization of the occluded vessel.

The natural history of elevated blood pressure in acute stroke is for spontaneous reduction over the course of days or weeks [17, 32]. The question thus arises whether elevated blood pressure in acute stroke needs to be treated at all. Theoretical arguments exist both for and against acute blood pressure reduction.

Current conceptualization of ischaemic stroke recognizes the existence of an ischaemic penumbra, an area surrounding the ischaemic core with impaired blood flow that is marginally maintained by collateral perfusion and potentially viable [33–35]. Under normal conditions, brain tissue requires perfusion of 50 ml/100 mg/min. Below approximately 20 ml/100 mg/min tissue is 'stunned', with impaired or absent electrical activity but preserved cellular integrity and, thus, capable of recovery if perfusion is restored. Below 10–12 ml/100 mg/min, cellular integrity is compromised, ion pumps fail, and irreversible damage occurs [34, 36]. The ischaemic penumbra thus represents tissue that is nonfunctional due to impaired blood flow, but alive and salvageable if adequate blood flow is restored.

Cerebral blood flow (CBF) is dependent on cerebral perfusion pressure (CPP) and cerebrovascular resistance (CVR): CBF = CPP/CVR. CPP represents the difference between MAP and intracerebral pressure (ICP), which under normal conditions is constant and small; CPP is therefore roughly equal to arterial blood pressure. Cerebral blood flow is thus regulated via changes in CVR, mediated by small capacitance arterioles.

In the healthy brain, cerebral blood flow is maintained constant over a wide range of systemic blood pressures; the term 'autoregulation' refers to this independence of CPP from systemic pressure [37]. Autoregulation is largely a function of the small capacitance arterioles, which dilate in response to a decrease in systemic blood pressure, increasing blood flow to the brain, and constrict, limiting blood flow, in the face of increased systemic blood pressure. In non-hypertensive individuals, autoregulation is maintained over a range of systemic blood pressure from 60 to 150 mmHg: below this range, perfusion pressure drops and tissue is susceptible to ischaemia; above it, the blood–brain barrier fails, with resultant oedema and tissue damage. In individuals with chronic hypertension, the autoregulatory curve is shifted to the right (Figure 12.1), so that the lower and upper limits of autoregulatory failure occur at higher systemic blood pressures than in non-hypertensive individuals [38].

In the setting of acute stroke, autoregulation is impaired [36], and cerebral blood flow becomes passively dependent on systemic blood pressure. Thus with high blood pressures, there is, in addition to the risk of ongoing vascular damage due to chronic hypertension, at least a theoretical risk of increased oedema, extension of the infarct, and haemorrhagic transformation [36]. With hypotension there is a risk of hypoperfusion and resultant tissue ischaemia with conversion of the penumbra to a non-viable state [34, 36, 39]. Patients with chronic hypertension may be at risk of hypoperfusion and infarct extension even at 'normal' blood pressure levels due to their shifted autoregulatory curve. In addition, low perfusion pressures could contribute to poor outcome via failure of delivery of antithrombotic medications or via impaired washout of small emboli or increased propogation of thrombus due to stasis, resulting in larger stroke volumes [40].

Systemic blood pressure response to acute stroke and effects of blood pressure reduction may vary depending on the pathophysiology of the stroke. Several studies (e.g. [18, 41]) suggest that lacunar infarcts may be associated with a higher incidence of elevated blood pressure and with a better long-term outcome; blood pressure was observed to normalize more rapidly for larger artery atherothrombotic and lacunar strokes carrying better prognosis,

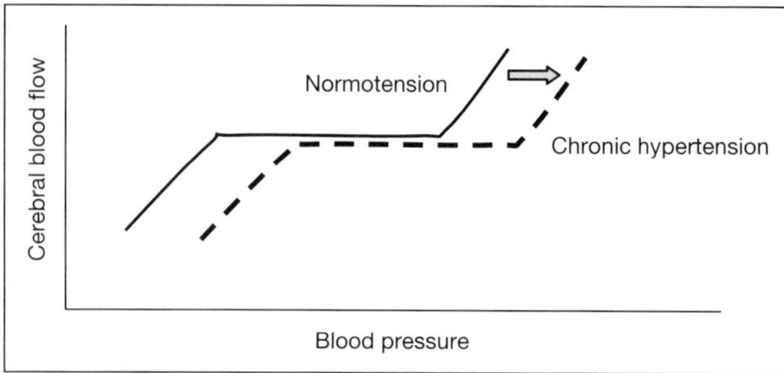

Figure 12.1 Autoregulation: in normotension, cerebral blood flow is maintained at a constant level over a range of MAP ~60–150 mmHg. In hypertension, the upper and lower limits of autoregulation are shifted to a higher MAP.

while blood pressure following embolic strokes (which may be associated with a greater risk of oedema) fell more slowly [41]. Posterior circulation strokes presenting with low blood pressure were associated with a poorer outcome [41].

The pathophysiology of cerebral perfusion in primary intracerebral haemorrhage is complex. In addition to increased ICP due to mass effect from the haematoma, there may be a perihaematomal 'penumbra' due to local tissue pressure in the perihaematoma zone [36]. While the primary concerns in intracerebral haematoma are to minimize clot expansion and rebleeding due to elevated blood pressure among other factors and to treat increased ICP [42], impaired autoregulation may alter the response to blood pressure lowering [43]. Chronic hypertension is a potent risk factor for primary intracerebral haemorrhage, and patients are likely to have shifted autoregulatory curves. Blood pressure management in primary intracerebral haemorrhage is thus potentially another double-edged sword: on the one hand, elevated blood pressures may put the individual at risk for expansion of the haematoma [44] and continued increased ICP; on the other, too rapid or aggressive blood pressure reduction may compromise blood flow, both globally and locally (to the compromized tissue surrounding the haematoma), especially in the setting of increased ICP due to mass effect from the haematoma and associated oedema and in patients with shifted autoregulatory curve due to chronic hypertension. While one set of investigators report impaired autoregulation in intracerebral haemorrhage (ICH) with a drop in MAP of >20% or below 110 mmHg [43], another study [45] demonstrated preservation of autoregulation in patients presenting with small to medium-sized ICH when MAP was lowered up to 15%, suggesting that under these conditions in any case, moderate blood pressure lowering may be safe.

PHARMACOTHERAPY

There is little firm evidence to date regarding the effects of individual classes of blood pressure-lowering agents in acute stroke, but theoretical considerations and limited observational evidence suggest that the agent employed may affect the outcome, independent of blood pressure lowering [14, 46, 47]. The commonly used agents are reviewed below.

BETA-BLOCKERS

While beta-receptor antagonists could theoretically improve outcome by reducing metabolic demands of ischaemic tissue and catecholamine-induced cardiac and neurological damage, administration of labetolol and atenolol was associated with a non-significant increase in mortality and poor functional outcome at 6 months in one randomized clinical trial [48]. The combined alpha- and beta-receptor antagonist labetolol was used in the National Institute for Neurological Disorders and Stroke (NINDS) trial of thrombolysis with intravenous (IV) recombinant tissue plasminogen activator (r-tPA), and was associated with a reduction in death in the placebo group not undergoing thrombolysis [49].

CALCIUM CHANNEL BLOCKERS

Calcium channel antagonists have been extensively tested in randomized clinical trials, both as blood pressure-lowering agents and as potentially neuroprotective agents, given their potential capacity to limit neuronal damage due to post-ischaemic intracellular calcium influx. Some agents also have preferential vasodilatory effect on central nervous system (CNS) vessels, which could potentially exacerbate increased ICP in intracerebral haemorrhage. A meta-analysis of 29 randomized clinical trials of calcium channel antagonists in acute stroke, however, showed no benefit and in fact revealed a non-significant trend towards increased death and disability [50]. The Blood Pressure in Acute Stroke Collaboration similarly found a non-significant trend toward increased death and disability associated with calcium channel antagonists administered orally in 11 trials [51], and the Intravenous Nimodipine West European Trial (INWEST) demonstrated neurological deterioration associated with lowering of diastolic blood pressure (DBP) with administration of IV nimodipine [52, 53].

NITRATES

Nitric oxide donors are cerebral vasodilators that maintain cerebral perfusion while lowering blood pressure in experimental stroke, and may be neuroprotective through other mechanisms as well, including antiplatelet activity and N-methyl-D-aspartate (NMDA) receptor blockade. Triglyceryl nitrate has shown promise in small trials [54], and is currently being investigated in a large randomized clinical trial [55].

ANGIOTENSIN CONVERTING ENZYME INHIBITORS AND ANGIOTENSIN RECEPTOR BLOCKADE

Angiotensin-converting enzyme inhibitor (ACE-I) and angiotensin receptor blockade (ARBs) modify the activity of the renin–angiotensin system and shift the autoregulatory curve to the left, potentially allowing sustained cerebral perfusion with lowering of systemic blood pressure. Captopril and perindopril, both ACE-I agents, have been studied in acute stroke and have been demonstrated to reduce blood pressure with no associated increase in death or disability in small series [56, 57], and perindopril has been shown to be safe and effective in secondary stroke prevention [3, 12]. The Acute Candesartan Cilexetil Evaluation in Stroke Survivors (ACCESS) trial has investigated the use of the ARB candesartan in hypertensive acute stroke patients and demonstrated a significant reduction in death and cerebrovascular and cardiovascular events in the treatment arm, but was halted early with no significant findings for the primary outcome of death or disability at 3 months [58]. Losartan, another ARB, has been shown to lower blood pressure without adverse effects on regional cerebral blood flow in the first week after stroke [59].

DIURETICS

While thiazide diuretics, particularly in combination with ACE-I agents, have proven efficacy in secondary stroke prevention [3], limited studies to date with the thiazide diuretic bendrofludrazine showed no significant blood pressure-lowering effect in the first week after stroke [60].

Observations of improved outcome with higher systemic blood pressure levels, along with the theoretical arguments discussed above, have raised speculation about whether intervention in the opposite direction, i.e. pharmacological elevation of blood pressure, might be beneficial in acute stroke. The IST suggested that systolic hypertension was not associated with cerebral haemorrhage [16, 30]. Although drug-induced hypertension may improve CBF and lessen neurological consequences of stroke [61, 62], further testing is needed before it can be recommended as a routine therapy. Complications may include cardiac arrhythmias or ischaemia, increased risk of cerebral oedema, hypertensive encephalopathy, and haemorrhagic transformation of cerebral infarction.

CLINICAL TRIALS

Debate thus continues about whether blood pressure should be lowered or elevated in acute ischaemic stroke and how this should be accomplished [39, 63]. To guide optimal evidence-based practice, clinical trials are needed to address questions regarding: (1) whether and when to attempt blood pressure reduction in acute stroke; (2) if blood pressure lowering is undertaken, how much reduction should be attempted and at what rate; (3) which agents should be employed; and (4) how acute blood pressure management should be transitioned into chronic management. In addition, many patients presenting with acute stroke do so in the context of diagnosed and treated hypertension. It is unclear whether these patients should be maintained on antihypertensive therapy, or whether antihypertensive medications should be held in the setting of acute stroke, both to allow increase in blood pressure and thus, potentially, perfusion pressure, and to avoid potentially deleterious outcomes associated with certain classes of drugs.

Bath and co-workers [63] captured the key elements of this discussion in a communication from an *ad hoc* workshop at the World Stroke Conference, Melbourne, November 2000: (1) hypertension is commonly associated with ischaemic and haemorrhagic stroke and may be associated with poor outcome which may be related to development of reinfarction, cerebral oedema, or haemorrhagic transformation; (2) differences in the pharmacologic mechanisms of different classes of blood pressure-lowering agents may be important, as there may be multimodal actions; and (3) agents which cause extreme changes in blood pressure or which have limiting features of their delivery system (e.g. IV delivery which may delay or limit early mobilization) might not be optimal for acute stroke treatment.

Clearly, additional carefully done, large-scale clinical trials are needed to determine the best practice for blood pressure management in acute ischaemic stroke or acute ICH. Boysen has nicely summarized the existent data including a Cochrane Review of five small trials suggesting that a limited amount of data makes it difficult to assess the relationship between blood pressure and clinical outcome [64, 65]. Select ongoing or completed recent clinical trials of blood pressure lowering or blood pressure elevation in acute ischaemic stroke are reviewed in Table 12.1. These include three small studies of the CCB nicardipine in haemorrhagic as well as ischaemic stroke (CARING, ATACH, and HASTE), and a large-scale study of outcomes related to maintaining vs. discontinuing antihypertensive medications in treated hypertensives presenting with acute stroke (COSSACS).

In the meantime, best practice in the treatment of blood pressure after acute stroke must be guided by existing data, theoretical motivation, and clinical judgment [66]. There are certain cardiovascular emergencies in which rapid reduction of blood pressure is indicated (Table 12.2). When these conditions are absent, most current guidelines recommend against treating elevated blood pressure in the acute phase, though the upper limits for observation vary. The American Heart Association (AHA) [66] and European Stroke Initiative recommend observation without intervention for SBP ≤220 mmHg and DBP ≤120 mmHg. Following NINDS guidelines, it is recommended that patients undergoing antithrombolytic therapy with r-tPA maintain SBP ≤185 mmHg and DBP ≤110 mmHg.

Bath and the International Society of Hypertension Writing Group [14] point out that the pathophysiology of stroke is complex, and suggest that, rather than recommending strict cutoff points and target goals for treating elevated blood pressure in all stroke patients, characteristics of the stroke and the patient be taken into account, and targets be couched in

Table 12.1 Select ongoing or recently completed randomized clinical trials of blood pressure lowering or elevation in acute stroke

The Control of Hypertension and Hypotension Immediately Post-Stroke Trial (CHHIPS Trial) [70]
A multicentre, prospective, randomized, double-blind, placebo-controlled, dose titration clinical trial to assess whether hypertension or hypotension should be used after acute stroke. The main study sites are in the United Kingdom in acute stroke units. About 2000 adults will be enrolled within 24 h of onset of suspected stroke who have either mean SBP >160 mm Hg or mean SBP <140 mmHg. The study has two main treatment arms: (1) Depressor Arm-Hypertensive (oral lisinopril 5 mg or oral labetolol 50 mg or matching placebo, or sublingual lisinopril or IV labetolol for dysphagic patients): if SBP is not <150 mmHg in 4 h, further lisinopril and labetolol will be administered and repeated in 4 h if SBP remains elevated. Treatment will continue for 2 weeks; and (2) Pressor Arm-Hypotension: those without ICH will be recruited within 12 h and treated with IV phenylephrine or matching placebo for up to 24 h after stroke onset to reach a SBP goal of 150 mmHg or a 15 mmHg increase over baseline. The primary objective of the study is to determine how acute pressor (0–12 h) and depressor (0–24 h) therapy will influence neurological deterioration (<72 h) and death and dependency (at 2 weeks).
Status: Ongoing*

Continue or Stop Post-Stroke Antihypertensives Collaborative Study (COSSACS) [71]
A multicentre, prospective, randomized, open, blinded endpoint study to determine whether existing antihypertensive therapy should be continued or not within 24 h of stroke onset and for the next 2 weeks. The main study sites are in the United Kingdom in acute stroke units. About 2900 adults will be enrolled within 24 h of onset of suspected stroke and within 36 h of the last dose of antihypertensive medication (thiazides, diuretics, beta-blockers, calcium antagonists, ACE-I, angiotensin II antagonists, alpha blockers, and centrally acting agents). Study subjects will be randomized to continue or discontinue their current antihypertensive medications. The primary objective of the study is to assess the short-term (2 weeks) and long-term (6 months) rates of death and disability including stroke recurrence.
Status: Ongoing*

Efficacy of Nitric Oxide in Stroke (ENOS) Trial [55]
The primary objective of the study is to determine if nitric oxide, a multimodal molecule given as glyceryl trinitrate (GTN), is safe and effective in improving outcome after acute stroke. The study is a prospective, international, multicentre, randomized, parallel-group, blinded, controlled, factorial trial of an anticipated 5000 ischaemic or haemorrhagic stroke patients with SBP 140–220 mmHg and studied within 48-h of onset. Patients will be randomized to receive 7 days of transdermal GTN or control, and those taking prior antihypertensives will be randomized to continue or stop for 1 week. The primary outcome is death and disability at 3 months as judged by the modified Rankin Scale.
Status: Ongoing*

Open-Label Prospective Study to Evaluate the Efficacy and Safety of Double or Triple Concentrated Intravenous Nicardipine for Treatment of Hypertension in Patients with Ischemic Stroke, Intracerebral Hemorrhage, or Subarachnoid Hemorrhage – The CARING Trial [72]
The trial is a phase IV, prospective, open-labelled study of patients with ischaemic stroke, ICH, or subarachnoid hemorrhage (SAH) who require blood pressure control. Twenty-five patients will receive a double concentrate dose of nicardipine and 25 patients will receive a triple concentrate dose of nicardipine. The study will evaluate the rate of peripheral IV phlebitis or irritation in double or triple concentrated nicardipine infusion and the time and dosage needed to reach the target blood pressure range.
Status: Ongoing*

Antihypertensive Treatment in Acute Cerebral Hemorrhage (ATACH) [73]
The purpose of the study is to evaluate the treatment feasibility and safety of antihypertensive treatment with nicardipine in patients with acute hypertension associated with ICH. Three levels of antihypertensive therapy will be assessed based on pre-specified SBP range. The primary outcome will be the treatment feasibility of antihypertensive therapy's ability to reach and maintain the pre-specified blood pressure goals. The primary safety outcome will be neurological deterioration defined by a decline in the Glasgow Coma Scale by 2 points or greater or an increase in the NIH Stroke Scale by ≥4 points. Three-months functional outcome will also be assessed.
Status: Completed*

Table 12.1 (continued)

Hypertension in Acute Stroke Treatment (HASTE) [74] The primary objective of this feasibility study is to evaluate the safety and tolerability of treatment to achieve and maintain SBP goals with IV nicardipine infusion in patients with ischaemic stroke who present within 3-h of symptomatic onset. Up to 25 patients will be enrolled and follow-up will occur at 90 days post treatment. The primary safety outcome is a decline in the Glasgow Coma Scale of ≥2 points or an increase in the NIH Stroke Scale of ≥2 points. The secondary outcome is the rate of serious adverse events related to nicardipine infusion (e.g. death, life-threatening adverse event, prolongation of hospitalization, or persistent or significant disability). The tertiary outcome is functional outcome (modified Rankin Scale and Barthel Index) at 3 months post event. *Status*: Ongoing*
*According to The Internet Stroke Center at www.strokecenter.org as of March, 2006

Table 12.2 Indications for aggressive treatment of elevated blood pressure

Aortic dissection
Pulmonary oedema
Acute renal failure
Hypertensive encephalopathy
Acute myocardial infarction
Left ventricular failure

proportional terms (e.g. a goal of 20% reduction in blood pressure in primary intracerebral haemorrhage [67]) rather than as strict target values. Blood pressure lowering should be guided by the clinical scenario, should proceed cautiously, avoiding precipitous drops in MAP, and should employ agents that have good CNS availability, are readily titrated, and have minimal potential for worsening outcome.

The AHA/American Stroke Association (ASA) guidelines for blood pressure management of arterial hypertension in acute ischaemic stroke [66], summarized in Table 12.3, stratify patients according to eligibility for thrombolytic therapy and offer specific algorithms for treatment of arterial hypertension.

Thus for patients otherwise eligible for thrombolytic therapy, with *pre-treatment* SBP >185 mmHg or DBP >110 mmHg, IV labetalol is recommended to bring the SBP or DBP within the range acceptable for administration of thrombolytic therapy. For elevated blood pressure *during* or *after* thrombolytic treatment, the following is recommended: if DBP is >140 mmHg, IV nitroprusside; if SBP is >230 mmHg or DBP is 121–140 mmHg, IV labetalol or IV nicardipine; and if SBP is 180–230 mmHg or DBP is 105–120 mmHg, IV labetalol.

Patients *not* eligible for thrombolytic therapy are monitored up to SBP ≤ 220 mmHg or DBP of 120 mmHg unless there is a compelling indication for treatment (Table 12.2). If SBP ≥220 mmHg or DBP ≥121–140 mmHg, IV labetalol or IV nicardipine are recommended, aiming for an initial blood pressure reduction of 10–15% of the MAP. For DBP ≥140 mmHg, IV nitroprusside is recommended, aiming for a blood pressure reduction of 10–15% of the MAP.

Table 12.3 Summary of AHA/ASA guidelines for treatment of elevated blood pressure in acute ischaemic stroke. With permission [66].

	Comment
Not eligible for thrombolytic therapy	
SBP ≤220 mmHg or DBP ≤120 mmHg	Observe unless compelling indication for treatment*
SBP ≥220 mmHg or DBP 121–140 mmHg	IV labetalol or IV nicardipine
DBP >140 mmHg	IV nitroprusside
Eligible for thrombolytic therapy	
Pretreatment:	
SBP >185 mmHg or DBP >110 mmHg	IV labetalol
During or after treatment:	
DBP >140 mmHg	IV nitroprusside
SBP >230 mmHg or DBP 121–140 mmHg	IV labetalol or IV nicardipine
SBP 180–230 mmHg or DBP 105–120 mmHg	IV labetalol

*Compelling indications may include aortic dissection, acute myocardial infarction, pulmonary edema, or hypertensive encephalopathy.

AHA guidelines for management of blood pressure in spontaneous intracerebral haemorrhage [42] recommend that blood pressure be titrated to a CPP (calculated as MAP − ICP, where MAP is mean arterial pressure and ICP is intracranial pressure as measured by ICP monitor) of ≥70 mmHg in patients with ICP monitor, and that MAP otherwise be maintained below 130 mmHg in individuals with prior history of hypertension. MAP should be maintained below 110 mmHg in the post-operative period, and pressors are recommended if systolic arterial pressure falls below 90 mmHg [29, 42].

Following blood pressure management in acute stroke, chronic blood pressure management will eventually need to be initiated for secondary prevention. For this, we recommend following the guidelines of the Seventh Report of the Joint National Committee on Prevention, Detection, Evaluation, and Treatment of High Blood Pressure (JNC 7 Report) [68] and the National Stroke Association (NSA) Work Group on Recurrent Stroke Prevention [69]. There is controversy about the timing of institution of chronic blood pressure-lowering therapy [1], with some experts recommending initiation of chronic blood pressure-lowering therapy for secondary prevention as early as the first several days after stroke and others recommending waiting up to a month. Ideally, initiation of blood pressure-lowering therapy would be deferred until stable collateral circulation has been established, but this is a determination that is difficult to make clinically. Some experts may recommend initiating chronic blood pressure-lowering therapy after acute ischaemic stroke, if there are no postural symptoms (e.g. worsening of neurological impairment or development of new neurological impairment or symptoms on sitting or standing) to suggest pressure-dependent deterioration.

In summary, elevated blood pressure is common in the setting of acute stroke. Current data regarding optimal management of blood pressure in the first week after stroke are inconclusive. Several clinical trials currently underway should help establish guidelines for raising or lowering blood pressure in the acute setting. Until such evidence-based guidelines are available, it is recommended that blood pressure be treated judiciously and that management of blood pressure takes into account individual characteristics such as a prior history of hypertension and stroke mechanism and location, and follow the AHA guidelines for management of blood pressure in acute stroke [66].

REFERENCES

1. Pedelty L, Gorelick PB. Chronic management of blood pressure after stroke. *Hypertension* 2004; 44:1–5.
2. Gorelick PB. The future of stroke prevention by risk factor management. In: Bogousslavsky J, Fisher M (eds). *Handbook of Clinical Neurology: Stroke* (in press).
3. Gorelick PB. New horizons for stroke prevention: progress and hope. *Lancet Neurol* 2002; 1:149–156.
4. Gorelick PB. Stroke prevention beyond antithrombotics: unifying mechanisms in ischemic stroke pathogenesis and implications for therapy. An invited review. *Stroke* 2002; 33:862–875.
5. Gorelick PB. An integrated approach to stroke prevention. In: Chalmers J (ed.). *Clinican's Manual on Blood Pressure and Stroke Prevention*, 3rd edition. Scientific Press, London, 2002, pp 55–65.
6. Gorelick PB, Sacco RL, Smith DB *et al*. Prevention of a first stroke. A review of guidelines and multidisciplinary consensus statement from the National Stroke Association. *JAMA* 1999; 281:1112–1120.
7. Gorelick PB. Stroke prevention: windows of opportunity and failed expectations? A discussion of modifiable cardiovascular risk factors and a prevention proposal. *Neuroepidemiology* 1997; 16:163–173.
8. Gorelick PB. Stroke prevention. *Arch Neurol* 1995; 52:347–355.
9. Gorelick PB. Stroke prevention: an opportunity for efficient use of health care resources in the coming decade. *Stroke* 1994; 25:220–224.
10. MacMahon S, Neal B, Rodgers A. Hypertension: time to move on. *Lancet* 2005; 365:1108–1109.
11. Lawes CMM, Bennett DA, Feigin VL, Rodgers A. Blood pressure and stroke. An overview of published reviews. *Stroke* 2004; 35:1024–1033.
12. PROGRESS Collaborative Group. Randomized trial of a perindopril-based blood pressure-lowering regimen among 6105 individuals with previous stroke or transient ischemic attack. *Lancet* 2001; 358:1033–1041.
13. The Heart Outcome Prevention Evaluation Study Investigators. Effects of angiotensin-converting enzyme inhibitor, ramipril, on cardiovascular events in high-risk patients. *N Engl J Med* 2000; 342:145–153.
14. International Society of Hypertension Writing Group. Statement on the management of blood pressure in acute stroke. *J Hypertens* 2003; 21:665–672.
15. CAST (Chinese Acute Stroke Trial) Collaborative Group. CAST: randomized placebo-controlled trial of early aspirin use in 20,000 patients with acute ischemic stroke. *Lancet* 1997; 349:1641–1649.
16. Leonardi-Bee J, Bath PMW, Philips SJ *et al*. Blood pressure and clinical outcomes in the International Stroke Trial. *Stroke* 2002; 33:1315–1320.
17. Britton M, Carlsson A, de Faire U. Blood pressure course in patients with acute stroke and matched controls. *Stroke* 1986; 17:861–841.
18. Semplicini A, Maresca A, Boscola G *et al*. Hypertension in acute ischemic stroke: a compensatory mechanism or an additional damaging factor? *Arch Intern Med* 2003; 163:211–216.
19. Yong M, Diener HC, Kaste M, Mau J. Characteristics of blood pressure profiles as predictors of long-term outcome after acute ischemic stroke. *Stroke* 2005; 36:2619–2625.
20. Chamorro A, Vila N, Ascaso C, Elices E, Schonewille W, Blane R. Blood pressure and functional recovery in acute ischemic stroke. *Stroke* 1998; 29:1850–1853.
21. Oliveira-Filho J, Silva SC, Trabuco CC, Pedreira BB, Sousa EU, Bacellar A. Detrimental effect of blood pressure reduction in the first 24 hours of acute stroke onset. *Neurology* 2003; 61:1047–1051.
22. Vemmos KN, Tsivgoulis G, Spengos K *et al*. Association between 24-h blood pressure monitoring variables and brain oedema in patients with hyperacute stroke. *J Hypertens* 2003; 21:2167–2173.
23. Willmot M, Leonardi-Bee J, Bath P. High blood pressure in acute stroke and subsequent outcome: a systematic review. *Hypertension* 2004; 43:18–24.
24. Castillo J, Laira R, Garcia MM, Serena J, Blanco M, Davalos A. Blood pressure decrease during the acute phase of ischemic stroke is associated with brain injury and poor stroke outcome. *Stroke* 2004; 35:520–527.
25. Okumura K, Ohya Y, Maehara A, Wakugami K, Iseki K, Takishita S. Effects of blood pressure levels on case fatality after stroke. *J Hypertens* 2005; 23:1217–1223.
26. Vemmos KN, Tsivgoulis G, Spengos K *et al*. U-shaped relationship between mortality and admission blood pressure in patients with acute stroke. *J Intern Med* 2004; 255:257–265.
27. Myers MG, Norris JW, Hachinski VC, Weingert ME, Sole MJ. Cardiac sequelae of acute stroke. *Stroke* 1982; 13:838–842.
28. Bath P. High blood pressure as a risk factor and prognostic predictor in acute ischemic stroke: when and how to treat it? *Cerebrovasc Dis* 2004; 17(suppl 1):51–57.

29. Aiyagari V, Ruland S, Gorelick PB. Neurogenic hypertension including following stroke and with spinal cord injury. In Feehally J, Floege J, Johnson RJ. *Comprehensive Clincial Neurology*, 3rd edition. Philadelphia: Elsevier (in press).
30. Lindsberg PJ. High blood pressure after acute cerebrovascular occusion: risk or risk marker? *Stroke* 2005; 36:268–269.
31. Mattle HP, Kappeler L, Arnold M *et al*. Blood pressure and vessel recanalization in the first hours after ischemic stroke. *Stroke* 2005; 36:267–272.
32. Wallace JD, Levy LL. Blood pressure after stroke. *JAMA* 1981; 246:2177–2180.
33. Fisher M. The ischemic penumbra: identification, evolution and treatment concepts. *Cerebrovasc Dis* 2004; 17(suppl 1):1–6.
34. Goldstein L. Blood pressure management in patients with acute ischemic stroke. *Hypertension* 2004; 43:137–141.
35. Astrup J, Siesjo BK, Symon L. Thresholds in cerebral ischemia – the ischemic penumbra. *Stroke* 1981; 12:723–725.
36. Powers WJ. Acute hypertension after stroke: the scientific basis for treatment decisions. *Neurology* 1993; 43:461–467.
37. Strandgaard S, Paulson OB. Cerebral autoregulation. *Stroke* 1983; 15:413–416.
38. Baumbach GL, Heistad DD. Cerebral circulation in chronic arterial hypertension. *Hypertension* 1988; 12:89–95.
39. Johnston KC, Mayer SA. Blood pressure reduction in acute stroke: a two-edged sword? *Neurology* 2003; 61:1030–1031.
40. Sedlazek O, Caplan L, Henrici M. Impaired washout – embolism and ischemic stroke: further examples and proof of concept. *Cerebrovasc Dis* 2005; 19:369–401.
41. Vemmos KN, Tsivgoulis G, Spengos K *et al*. Blood pressure course in acute ischemic stroke in relation to stroke subtype. *Clin Methods Pathophysiol* 2004; 9:107–114.
42. Broderick JP, Adams HP, Barsan W *et al*. Guidelines for the management of spontaneous intracerebral hemorrhage: a statement for healthcare professionals from a special writing group of the Stroke Council, American Heart Association. *Stroke* 1999; 30:905–915.
43. Kuwatawa N, Kuroda K, Funoyama M, Sato N, Kubo N, Ogawa A. Dysautoregulation in patients with hypertensive intracerebral hemorrhage. A SPECT study. *Neurosurg Rev* 1995; 18:237–245.
44. Ohwaki K, Yano E, Nagashima H, Hirata M, Nakagomi T, Tamura A. Blood pressure management in acute intracerebral hemorrhage: relationship between elevated blood pressure and hematoma enlargement. *Stroke* 2004; 35:1364–1367.
45. Powers WJ, Zazulia AR, Videen TO *et al*. Autoregulation of cerebral blood flow surrounding acute (6 to 22 hours) intracerebral hemorrhage. *Neurology* 2001; 57:18–24.
46. Robinson TG, Potter JF. Blood pressure in acute stroke. *Age Aging* 2004; 33:6–12.
47. Straandgard S, Paulson OB. Antihypertensive drugs and cerebral circulation. *Eur J Clin Invest* 1996; 26:625–630.
48. Barer DH, Cruickshank JM, Ebrahim SB, Mitchell JR. Low-dose beta-blockade in acute stroke ('BEST' trial): an evaluation. *Br Med J* 1988; 296:737–741.
49. Brott T, Lu M, Kothari R *et al*. Hypertension and its treatment in the NINDS r-tPA stroke trial. *Stroke* 1998; 29:1504–1509.
50. Horn J, Limburg M. Calcium antagonists for ischemic stroke. A systematic review. *Stroke* 1991; 32:570–576.
51. Blood Pressure in Acute Stroke Collaboration (BASC). Vasoactive drugs for acute stroke. *Cochrane Database Syst Rev* 2005; 4.
52. Wahlgren NG, MacMohan DG, De Keyser J *et al*. Intravenous Nimodipine West European Stroke Trial (INWEST) of nimodipine in the treatment of acute ischemic stroke. *Cerebrovasc Dis* 1994; 4:204–210.
53. Ahmed N, Nasman P, Wahlgren NG. Effect of intravenous nimodipine on blood pressure and outcome after acute stroke. *Stroke* 2000; 31:1250–1255.
54. Bath PM, Pathansali R, Iddenden R, Bath FJ. The effect of transdermal glyceryl nitrate, a nitric oxide donor, on blood pressure and platelet function in acute stroke. *Cerebrovasc Dis* 2001; 11:265–272.
55. ENOS Trial. enos@nottingham.ac.uk or http://www.enos.ac.uk. 2006.
56. Waldemar G, Vorstrup S, Andersen AR, Pedersen H, Paulson OB. Angiotensin-converting enzyme inhibition and regional cerebral blood flow in acute stroke. *J Cardiovasc Pharmacol* 1989; 14:722–729.

57. Dyker AG, Grosset DG, Lees KR. Perindopril reduces blood pressure but not cerebral blood flow in patients with recent cerebral ischemic stroke. *Stroke* 1997; 28:580–583.
58. Schrader J, Cuders S, Kulschewski A *et al*. The ACCESS Study. Evaluation of acute candesartan cilexetil therapy in stroke survivors. *Stroke* 2003; 34:1699–1703.
59. Nazir FS, Overell JR, Bolster A, Hilditch JE, Reid JL, Lees KR. The effect of losartan on global and focal cerebral perfusion and on renal function in hypertensives in mild early ischemic stroke. *J Hypertens* 2004; 22:989–995.
60. Eames PJ, Robinson TG, Panerai RB, Potter JF. The systemic hemodynamic and cerebral autoregulatory effects of bendrofluaride in the subacute post-stroke period. *J Hypertens* 2004; 22:2017–2024.
61. Marzan AS, Hungerbuhler HJ, Studer A, Baumgartner RW, Georgiadis D. Feasibility and safety of norepinephrine-induced arterial hypertension in acute ischemic stroke. *Neurology* 2004; 62:1193–1195.
62. Hillis AE, Barker PB, Beauchamp NJ, Winters BD, Mirski M, Wityk RJ. Restoring blood pressure reperfused Wernicke's area and improved language. *Neurology* 2001; 56:670–672.
63. Bath P, Boysen G, Donnan G *et al*. Hypertension in acute stroke: what to do (letter). *Stroke* 2001; 32:1697–1698.
64. Boysen G. Persisting dilemma: to treat or not to treat blood pressure in acute ischemic stroke. *Stroke* 2004; 35:526–527.
65. Blood Pressure in Acute Stroke Collaboration (BASC). Interventions for deliberately altering blood pressure in acute stroke (Cochrane Review). The Cochrane Library. Update Software, Oxford, 2005.
66. Adams H, Adams R, Del Zoppo G *et al*. Guidelines for the early management of patients with ischemic stroke. 2005 guidelines update. A scientific statement from the Stroke Council of the American Heart Association/American Stroke Association. *Stroke* 2005; 36:916–921 (with correction *Stroke* 2005; 36:1352).
67. Morgenstern LB. Lowering blood pressure in acute cerebral hemorrhage. Safe, but will it help? *Neurology* 2001; 57:5–6.
68. Chobanian AV, Bakris GL, Black HR *et al*. The Seventh Report of the Joint National Committee on Prevention, Detection, Evaluation, and Treatment of High Blood Pressure. The JNC 7 Report. *JAMA* 2003; 289:2560–2572.
69. Hanley D *et al*. Determining the appropriateness of selected surgical and medical management options in recurrent stroke prevention: a guideline for primary care physicians from the National Stroke Association Work Group on Recurrent Stroke Prevention. *J Stroke Cerebrovasc Dis* 2004; 13:196–207.
70. CHHIPS Trial. www.le.ac.uk/cv/research/CHHIPS/HomePage.html. 2006.
71. COSSACS Trial. www.le.ac.uk/cv/research/COSSACS/COSSACShome.html. 2006.
72. Wang DZ *et al*. Open-Label Prospective Study to Evaluate the Efficacy and Safety of Double or Triple Concentrated Intravenous Nicardipine for Treatment of Hypertension in Patients with Ischemic Stroke, Intracerebral Hemorrhage, or Subarachnoid Hemorrhage – The CARING Trial. The American Stroke Association International Stroke Conference, Ongoing Clinical Trials Session (poster). New Orleans, LA, 2005.
73. Qureshi AI. Antihypertensive treatment in acute cerebral hemorrhage. In: The American Stroke Association International Stroke Conference, Ongoing Clinical Trials Session (poster). New Orleans, LA, 2005.
74. Kirmani JR. Acute stroke treatment (HASTE). In: The American Stroke Association International Stroke Conference, Ongoing Clinical Trials Session (poster). New Orleans, LA, 2005.

13

Diagnostic and therapeutic strategies in renal artery stenosis

S. I. McFarlane, M. O. Salifu, G. L. Bakris

INTRODUCTION

Renal artery stenosis (RAS) was first described by Harry Goldblatt in 1934 and is defined as narrowing of the renal artery lumen. Atherosclerosis and fibromuscular dysplasia (FMD) are the most common causes for RAS [1]. Based on angiographic feature of the stenosis, RAS is generally classified as ostial, non-ostial, or branch stenoses. Ostial lesions are defined as those in which the leading edge of the stenosis is within 5 mm of the opacified aortic lumen [2]. Non-ostial stenoses are contained entirely within the main renal artery with the leading edge of the lesion beginning >5 mm from the aorta. Branch stenoses on the other hand are lesions in which any component of the stenosis extends into the divisional or segmental arterial branches [2].

RAS may occur as an isolated anatomical abnormality, without functional significance (reduction of renal blood flow) or may present as one of the clearly defined syndromes such as ischaemic renal disease, hypertension (renovascular hypertension [RVHI]), recurrent ('flash') pulmonary oedema, end-stage renal disease and a situation of high cardiovascular risk [2, 3]. All of these syndromes, however, may co-exist, and the presence of hypertension does not necessarily result from RAS. Furthermore, in bilateral RAS renal function or blood pressure may actually be normal, posing diagnostic and therapeutic challenges for the treating physicians [3].

With the rising cardiovascular disease prevalence rate over the last several decades, RAS prevalence is bound to increase [4]. Also, given the alarming rate of chronic kidney disease [5], which precludes the use of nephrotoxic contrast material, physicians are going to be faced with the dilemma of diagnoses and management of this disease [3].

PREVALENCE OF RAS

The prevalence of this disease in the population is undefined because there is no simple and reliable test that can be applied on a large scale. Among all causes of secondary hypertension, RAS is considered the most common, representing 5–10% of all cases [6]. Autopsy data in mixed populations including 1,788 cases during the 12-year period between 1981 and 1992 at the National Cardiovascular Centre Hospital, showed that the frequency of RAS can

Samy I. McFarlane, MD, MPH, Associate Professor, Chief, Division of Endocrinology, Diabetes and Hypertension, SUNY-Downstate and Kings County Hospital, Brooklyn, New York, USA

Moro O. Salifu, MD, MPH, FACP, Associate Professor, Program Director, Division of Nephrology, SUNY-Downstate Medical Center, Brooklyn, New York, USA

George L. Bakris, MD, Professor and Vice-Chairman, Department of Preventive Medicine, Director, Hypertension/ Clinical Research Center, Rush University Medical Center, Chicago, Ilinois, USA

vary from 4–53% [7]. However, the prevalence of RAS may be as low as 1% in cases of mild hypertension but may also be as high as 40–60% in patients with severe or refractory hypertension unresponsive to medical management and in patients over 70 years of age [3]. Furthermore, during routine diagnostic cardiac catheterisation, RAS has also been documented incidentally. For example, in a study involving 1,302 patients undergoing cardiac catheterisation [8], RAS was identified in 30% of the patients. Insignificant RAS was found in 15% and significant (≥50% diameter narrowing) stenosis was found in another 15% of the study population [8]. Significant unilateral disease was present in 11%, and bilateral disease was present in 4% of the cohort. These data demonstrate the high prevalence of undiagnosed RAS, particularly in high-risk populations.

CLINICAL SIGNIFICANCE OF RAS

Inter-observer variability in the angiographic assessment of RAS has been demonstrated in the DRASTIC (Dutch Renal Artery Stenosis Intervention Cooperative) study [9]. In this study, in which 312 angiograms using the intra-arterial digital subtraction technique were obtained from 289 consecutive patients, agreement among radiologists about the presence and the number of arteries stenosed was reasonable; however, agreement about the location and aspect of stenosis was rather poor, highlighting the difficulties, in diagnosing RAS even with the use of angiography, long considered the gold standard [9]. What is certain, however, is that the more severe the stenosis, the more likely it is to be clinically significant [10]. Haemodynamically significant stenosis, however, is generally present when there is a demonstrable pressure gradient of about 40% in renal perfusion pressure. Though a pressure gradient has been documented in stenosis of up to 50% [10], the currently accepted cut-off for haemodynamically significant stenosis is >75%, which results in an ~40% reduction in renal perfusion pressure, leading to loss of renal autoregulation [11]. This level of stenosis is considered 'critical' as glomerular filtration rate (GFR) is solely dependent on perfusion pressure, which induces progressive pathologic changes that will be further detailed in the following sections.

PATHOPHYSIOLOGICAL CLASSIFICATION RAS

ATHEROSCLEROTIC RAS

This entity is by far the commonest type of lesion found in RAS, accounting for about 90% of cases [3]. Figure 13.1 illustrates bilateral atherosclerotic RAS with renal atrophy, most notably in the right kidney [3]. Although diffuse intrarenal atherosclerotic lesions have been well-documented, atherosclerotic RAS usually involves the ostium, either focally or as an extension from an aortic plaque and proximal third of the main renal artery and perirenal aorta [3]. The prevalence of atherosclerotic RAS generally increases with age, affecting men over the age of 45 years with high predilection among those with diffuse atherosclerotic disease as well as those with diabetes [3, 4, 6].

Atherosclerotic renovascular disease usually occurs in parallel with systemic atherosclerosis and generally progresses with the progression of atherosclerosis [12], although partial remission has been observed with control of cardiovascular risk factors [13].

FIBROMUSCULAR DYSPLASIA

Although uncommon, fibromuscular dysplasia (FMD) is the second most common cause of RAS and typically involves white women in their third and fourth decades of life [14]. Although the aetiology of FMD is largely unknown, genetic predisposition, abnormalities of the vasa vasorum, hormonal factors and smoking [15] have been postulated as the most important.

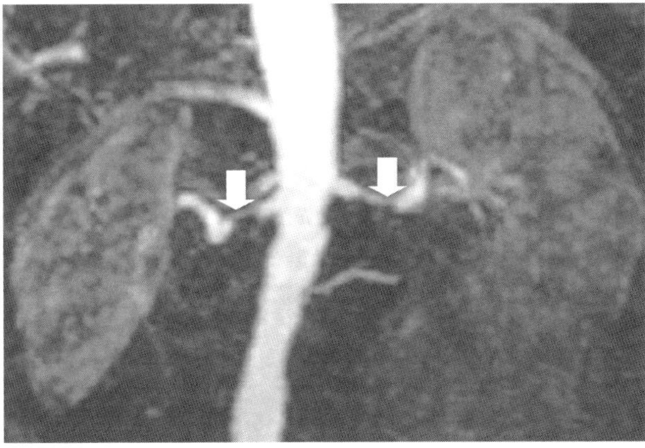

Figure 13.1 Bilateral atherosclerotic renal artery stenosis (arrows), demonstrated by gadolinium-enhanced MRA. Courtesy of Jonathan S. Deitch.

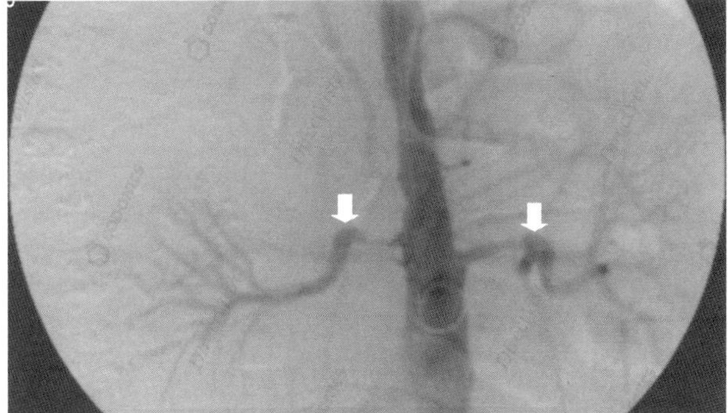

Figure 13.2 Angiographic representation of bilateral FMD of the renal arteries with 'beaded appearance', arrows and post-stenotic aneurysmal dilatation.

FMD is usually bilateral in about two-thirds of cases and involves the distal two-thirds of the main renal artery or its intra-renal branches. It is classified into three subtypes; intimal, medial and peri-adventitial, with the medial subtype being the most common, accounting for nearly 70–90% of cases [16]. FMD typically appears as a 'string of beads' on angiography, as a result of alternating areas of stenoses and aneurysmal dilatation. It usually involves the intrarenal branches as well, as demonstrated in Figure 13.2 [3]. The intimal subtype of FMD is a highly localised stenotic lesion associated with post-stenotic dilatation, whereas the periadventitial variety is characterised by small 'string of beads' appearance [3].

FMD may progress to unilateral renal infarction, particularly that of the periadventitial or intimal subtypes, though bilateral renal infarction due to medial FMD has also been reported [17]. Thrombosis associated with aneurysmal dilatation with subsequent embolisation or vascular occlusion is generally the underlying cause of renal infarction associated with FMD [3].

TRANSPLANT RENAL ARTERY STENOSIS

Transplant renal artery stenosis (TRAS) is a potentially curable cause of post-transplant arterial hypertension, allograft dysfunction, and graft loss and usually occurs in the first

2 years post-transplantation [18]. TRAS results from *de novo* atherosclerosis in the recipient or progressive atherosclerotic disease of donor origin. Immunological vascular injury as well as ischaemia reperfusion injury is also among cited pathophysiological mechanisms. TRAS is usually associated with frequent rejection episodes and its incidence ranges from 1–23%, depending on the diagnostic modality used. Transplant iliac artery or suprarenal stenosis are more common forms that compromise transplant renal blood flow, leading to similar clinical manifestations as those observed with TRAS [19].

TRAS generally presents clinically as severe hypertension with or without allograft dysfunction. Hyperkalaemia and oedema are usually apparent between 3 months and 2 years after renal transplantation, in contrast to suprarenal stenosis, which generally presents 2–6 years post-transplantation. Due to the frequent presence of turbulent flow in the iliac or femoral arteries, bruits are not characteristic features of TRAS.

UNCOMMON FORMS OF RAS

Vasculitis such as Takayasu arteritis, neurofibromatosis, congenital bands, extrinsic compression, emboli, aortic dissection, and arteriovenous malformations are uncommon causes of RAS. Diagnostic modalities employed for RAS are generally useful in diagnosing these uncommon forms of the disease and treatment is generally tailored towards the primary cause of the disease [3].

CLINICAL SYNDROMES ASSOCIATED WITH RAS

RENOVASCULAR HYPERTENSION

Activation of the renin–angiotensin–aldosterone system (RAAS) is the pathophysiologic hallmark of RAS (Figure 13.2). Impaired renal perfusion in haemodynamically significant RAS stimulates juxtaglomerular cells to release renin, which in turn catalyses the breakdown of angiotensin I to angiotensin II (Ang II) and the subsequent release of aldosterone, which is produced by the zona glomerulosa of the adrenal cortex. Ang II and aldosterone mediate vasoconstriction as well as salt and water retention, together with sympathetic stimulation leading to elevated blood pressure (Figure 13.3). These pathophysiological changes are particularly pronounced in people with diabetes [20]. Unilateral RAS is associated with volume expansion, which suppresses renin in the normal kidney leading to 'pressure diuresis' with sodium and water loss. Therefore, in unilateral RAS, hypertension is 'renin-mediated' and/or due to vasoconstriction. In the bilateral form of the disease, or in RAS associated with a solitary kidney, excretion of salt and water is impaired, thus hypertension is generally due to both volume and vasoconstriction [3].

Angiotensin II induces vasoconstriction of the glomerular mesangium as well as of both afferent and efferent arterioles, but more so of the efferent arterioles due to their smaller diameter. This results in restoration of the GFR in the ischaemic kidney *via* efferent arteriolar and mesangial constriction, leading to increased glomerular capillary hydrostatic pressure. Thus, removal of the efferent arteriolar vasoconstrictive effect by Ang II blockade by the use of angiotensin-converting enzyme inhibitors (ACE-I) or Ang II receptor blockers (ARB) may result in a reduction of the GFR and deterioration of renal function, especially in patients with critical and bilateral stenosis of the renal arteries [21, 22].

ISCHAEMIC NEPHROPATHY

Activation of the RAS system and Ang II stimulation leads to a strong inflammatory response induced by factors such as vascular smooth muscle cell growth factor, platelet aggregation, generation of superoxide radicals, activation of adhesion molecules, stimulation of macrophages, induction of gene transcription for proto-oncogenes, oxidation of low-density

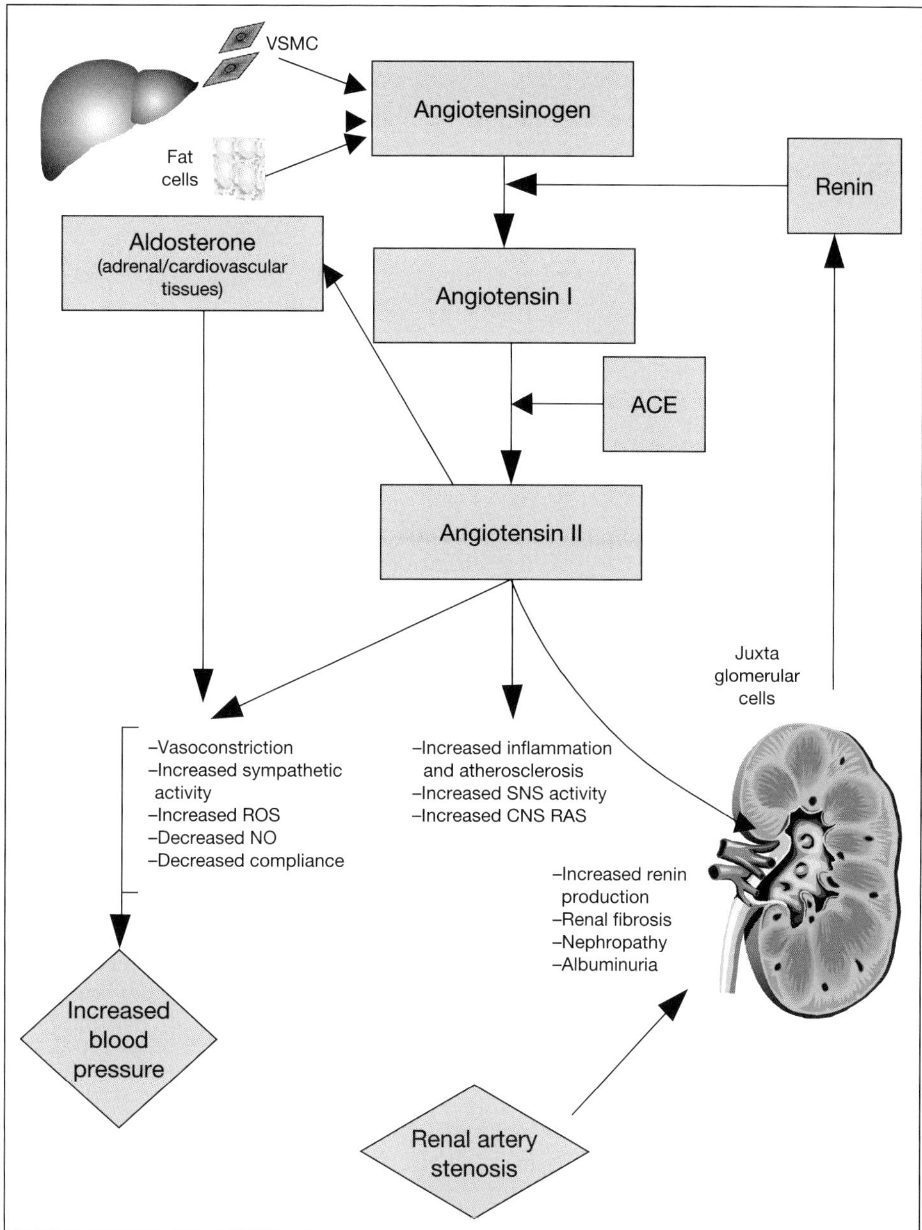

Figure 13.3 Activation of the renin-angiotensin system (RAS) by renal artery stenosis: Effects of Angiotensin II on various organ systems. ROS = reactive oxygen species, NO = nitric oxide, SNS = sympathetic nervous system, CNS = central nervous system.

lipoproteins and other mediators [11]. This inflammatory response results in loss of renal mass, which may be reversible in the early stages but may progress to irreversible nephron loss and renal atrophy with continued RAS [23]. Compensatory glomerular hypertrophy with hyperfiltration of the remaining nephrons occurs as a result of loss of renal mass [24].

The tubules are the hardest hit from ischaemic injury, producing patchy or diffuse interstitial fibrosis and tubular atrophy. However, other histological lesions such as atrophy of the glomerular capillary tuft, thickening and duplication of the Bowman capsule, arteriolosclerosis, cortical infarcts emanating from severely damaged medium-sized upstream vessels, cholesterol atheroembolism from plaques and segmental glomerulosclerosis can be seen [3]. The stenosis can progress over 5 years in up to 30% of patients [25] leading to intractable hypertension (8–10%) or progressive renal insufficiency (<10%) [26].

NEPHROTIC SYNDROME

Atherosclerotic RAS can lead to biopsy-proven focal and segmental glomerulosclerosis [27]. The pathogenesis of this entity is not clearly understood, however, it might involve embolisation of cholesterol crystals, platelet thrombi and other debris into the glomerular microcirculation. Nephrotic syndrome seen in these patients has a tendency to remit after correction of the stenosis [28]. Presumably, these patients have a severe form of Ang II-dependent glomerulopathy [3].

FLASH PULMONARY OEDEMA

Acute hypertensive episodes, attributed to sodium retention and increased permeability of pulmonary microcirculation promoted by Ang II, are associated with flash pulmonary oedema. While an acute coronary event is usually absent, most patients have atherosclerotic heart disease [29]. The high prevalence (34%) of RAS in patients with congestive heart failure and the resolution of flash pulmonary oedema after revascularisation in patients with bilateral RAS [30] provide evidence of the association of RAS and flash pulmonary oedema. Furthermore, patients with CHF and bilateral RAS are at risk of acute renal failure due to ACE-I, ARB or diuretic use, thus underscoring the importance or pursuing the diagnosis of RAS in patients with CHF [3].

CLINICAL FEATURES OF RAS

Combining clinical data with diagnostic studies helps to improve the diagnostic accuracy of RAS. In non-black elderly men, atherosclerotic RAS is more common than in young Caucasian women, who are more likely to have an FMD subtype. RAS of any aetiology often manifests with hypertension and hypokalaemia due to aldosterone excess. While oedema is uncommon in unilateral RAS, due to pressure diuresis of the normal kidney, oedema is evident in bilateral RAS [3].

The diagnosis of RAS should be highly suspected when hypertension occurs with progressive azotaemia, i.e. >40% rise in serum creatinine within 3 weeks that does not plateau over the ensuing weeks. In addition, hypertension associated with an asymmetric kidney documented on ultrasound (>1.5 cm variance), paradoxical worsening of hypertension with diuretic therapy, worsening of azotaemia and hyperkalaemia with the use of ACE-I and ARBs [31] and recurrent pulmonary oedema, especially in patients with atherosclerosis elsewhere or an absence of family history of hypertension further increases the suspicion of RAS.

On physical examination, hypertensive or atherosclerotic retinal disease might be evident of fundoscopic examination. A clinical feature suggestive of congestive heart failure such as pulmonary rales as well as abdominal bruit, which is characteristically persistent in both systole and diastole, is heard in up to 46% of patients with RAS. Renal infarction in patients with RAS may present with abdominal pain [31].

Urine examination in patients with ischaemic nephropathy can be either normal or similar to that of acute tubular necrosis with tubular epithelial cells, red blood cells and broad waxy casts. Ischaemic nephropathy can also manifest as nephrotic syndrome with varying

Table 13.1 Clinical clues suggesting the presence of renal artery disease as the cause of hypertension and CKD

Age at onset of hypertension < 30 years or > 55 years
Abrupt onset of hypertension
Acceleration of previously well-controlled hypertension
Hypertension refractory to an appropriate three-drug regimen
Accelerated hypertensive retinopathy
Malignant hypertension
History of tobacco use
Systolic–diastolic abdominal bruit
Flash pulmonary oedema
Evidence of generalized atherosclerosis obliterans
Asymmetry in kidney size on imaging studies
Acute kidney failure with treatment by an angiotensin-converting enzyme inhibitor or angiotensin receptor blocker
Adapted with permission [55].

degrees of proteinuria. Chemical analysis reveals azotaemia, hypokalaemia, metabolic alkalosis and hyperreninaemic hyperaldosteronism. Lactate dehydrogenase enzyme is usually elevated in renal infarction [31].

CLINICAL PREDICTION RULES FOR RAS

Table 13.1 summarises the clinical clues associated with a high probability of RAS. Derived from well-designed clinical trials, prediction rules have been created to aid in the diagnosis of RAS given a set of known cardiovascular risk factors. These prediction rules help increase the pretest probability of the various screening tests [3]. In a time-honoured Cooperative Study on Renovascular Hypertension [32] involving 339 patients with essential hypertension who were compared with 175 surgically treated RAS cases, age, short duration of hypertension, accelerated nature of hypertension, presence of retinopathy, presence of coronary, peripheral and cerebrovascular disease were predictive of RAS. In the DRASTIC study, using angiographic data in 477 patients [33] age, gender, atherosclerosis elsewhere, body mass index, presence of abdominal bruit, serum cholesterol and creatinine level were predictors of RAS. These clinical predictions are helpful, particularly in atherosclerotic RAS, for identifying patients at high risk for the disease. However, it is important to emphasise that these predictors have not been validated in prospective trials. Table 13.2 summarises the predictive score for renal arterial disease.

NON-INVASIVE EVALUATION OF RAS

Non-invasive imaging of the renal arteries requires confirmation with angiography to determine gradient, location of lesion and location for possible angioplasty or stenting [3].

CAPTOPRIL RENOGRAPHY

The decline in GFR classically noted with Ang II blockade is used as a basis for captopril renography. At least 48 hours before the test, volume depletion and drugs that block the RAAS should be avoided. A baseline study without captopril, using radionuclide technetium mertiatide, technetium-labelled diethylenetriaminepentaacetate (DTPA), Tc-(99 m) mercaptoacetyl triglycine (MAG3) or hippuran is performed, after which captopril (25–50 mg)

Table 13.2 Scoring algorithm for clinical prediction rule for diagnosis of RAD

Predictor	*Score*[1]	
	Non-smoker	*Former or current smoker*
Age (years)		
20	0	3
30	1	4
40	2	4
50	3	5
60	4	5
70	5	6
Female gender	2	2
Signs and symptoms of atherosclerotic vascular disease[2]	1	2
Onset of hypertension within 2 years	1	1
Body mass index <25 kg/m^2	2	2
Presence of abdominal bruit	3	3
Serum creatinine concentration (mg/dl)[3]		
0.45	0	0
0.68	1	1
0.90	2	2
1.13	3	3
1.70	6	6
2.26	9	9
Serum cholesterol level[4] >252 mg/dl (6.5 mmol/l) or cholesterol-lowering therapy	1	1

[1]The sum score is obtained by adding all relevant scores. The sum score can be used to obtain the predicted probability of renal artery stenosis.
[2]Femoral or carotid bruit, angina pectoris, claudication, myocardial infarction, cerebrovascular accident, or vascular surgery.
[3]For intermediate values, the score can be linearly interpolated; to convert serum creatinine from mg/dl to μmol/l, multiply by 88.4.
[4]To convert serum cholesterol from mg/dl to mmol/l, multiply by 0.026

Adapted with permission [55].

is given orally 1 hour before radionuclide injection. A decline of about 10% in the GFR of the stenotic kidney denotes significant stenosis (>50%). The sensitivity of captopril renography is 85–90% and specificity is 93–98% in picking up high-grade stenosis [34]. This is reduced in patients with bilateral disease or renal impairment [35] as well as use of antihypertensive medication (diuretics, β-blockers, ACE-I, calcium channel blockers) 48 hours before the test. Captopril renography is now considered a secondary modality in patients known to have RAS because newer and more sensitive tests are currently available. This test may, however, be helpful in predicting the beneficial impact of captopril treatment in hypertensive patients with diabetic nephropathy [36]. A positive test requires angiographic conformation. A negative test with a high index of suspicion warrants angiography. A negative test in a patient with low index of suspicion warrants no further investigation (Figure 13.4).

DUPLEX ULTRASOUND OF RENAL ARTERIES

This test is the least expensive and provides useful information regarding peak systolic and end diastolic velocities, renal-to-aortic ratios, resistive index, kidney size, degree of stenosis aneurysms and obstruction. In a study of 102 consecutive patients (44 men and 58 women) who had both duplex ultrasound scanning of the renal arteries and renal arteriography and showed a high pretest probability of having RAS, the overall sensitivity of duplex ultrasound was 98%, specificity 98%, positive predictive value 99%, and negative predictive value 97% [37] compared with arteriography. A renal-to-aortic ratio >3.5 and peak systolic velocity >200 cm/s and resistive index <0.5 defines stenosis of 60–99%. Duplex ultrasonography may also help predict which patients will demonstrate an improvement in blood pressure control or renal function after renal artery angioplasty and stenting [3]. The entire renal artery can be imaged despite the presence of a metallic endoprosthesis. Patients who have undergone percutaneous renal revascularisation [38] should be placed in a surveillance program at 6 months, 1 year, and each year thereafter (Figure 13.4).

Duplex ultrasound of the renal arteries is highly operative-dependent and requires expertise. In obese persons, it is often difficult to perform and sensitivity and specificity

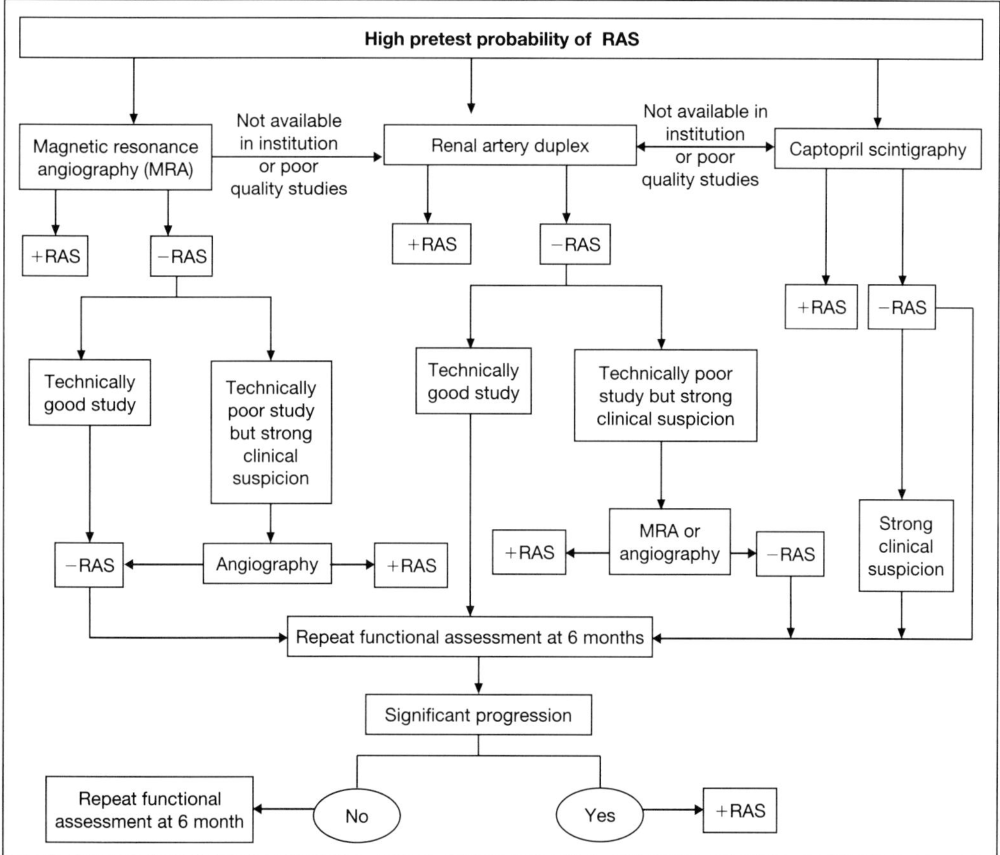

Figure 13.4 Diagnostic strategies in renal artery stenosis.

of identifying accessory renal arteries is decreased to about 60%. A positive test requires angiographic conformation. A negative test which is technically poor in a patient with a high index of suspicion also warrants magnetic resonance angiography (MRA) or radiocontrast angiography. With a technically good study, no further testing is usually necessary [3].

MAGNETIC RESONANCE ANGIOGRAPHY

Gadolinium enhanced MRA has a sensitivity of 97% and specificity of 93% and identifies accessory renal arteries 82% of the time [3, 39]. However, MRA does not yield adequate quantitative analysis of the stenosis and is not useful for monitoring patients after renal artery angioplasty and stenting because of artefacts produced by the stent. History of metallic implants such as pacemaker or aneurysm clip and a history of claustrophobia are among the limiting factors of MRA angiography. A positive test requires angiographic conformation. A negative test which is technically poor in a patient with a high index of suspicion also warrants angiography (Figure 13.4). No further testing is necessary in a technically good study [39].

SPIRAL CT ANGIOGRAPHY

Spiral CT angiography has a sensitivity of 98% and specificity of 94% in diagnosing RAS >50% [40]. In this test, contrast material is injected into a peripheral vein and X-ray pictures are assembled into three-dimensional images. In patients with a plasma creatinine concentration over 1.7 mg/dl the test carries a sensitivity of 93% and a specificity of only 81%. Various newer modalities of angiography such as multidetector computed tomography (MDCT) and 3D electron beam computed tomography (EBCT) have been evaluated in some studies yielding mixed results, though they appear to be comparable with CT angiography.

INVASIVE EVALUATION OF RAS

RADIOCONTRAST ANGIOGRAPHY

Renal angiography is considered the 'gold standard' for evaluation of RAS [41]. It is performed by percutaneous intra-luminal renal artery catherisation via femoral access with radiocontrast injection. Subsequently, digital subtraction angiography (DSA) uses a computer to 'subtract' the bones and tissues in the region being viewed, leading to visualisation only of the contrast-filled vessels.

Contrast nephropathy in patients with azotaemia is a limiting factor in the use of radiocontrast angiography. Therefore, with modern non-invasive imaging techniques being increasingly available, the need for renal radiocontrast arteriography has been much reduced and it is mainly reserved for use in lesions that can potentially be treated by interventional techniques or to analyse renal vasculature pre-operatively [41].

CARBON DIOXIDE DSA

This technique is safe and uses carbon dioxide as an alternative to iodinated contrast medium in DSA. The CO_2 gas acts as a negative contrast agent, i.e. more radiation hits the receptor behind the vessels filled with gas. Following brief displacement of blood, the CO_2 is completely dissolved in the blood and is expired by the lungs. Possible candidates for CO_2 DSA are patients with known reactions to iodinated contrast media and patients with renal insufficiency [42]. Results from animal studies indicate that there is a possibility for neurotoxicity with the use of CO_2 DSA in the cerebral vasculature [43].

GADOLINIUM DSA

This modality is often used as an alternative to iodinated radiocontrast angiography. It is non-allergenic and safer than radiocontrast material, however, gadolinium administration may be associated with acute renal failure in up to 3.5% of patients [44].

CHOICE OF IMAGING MODALITY

The choice of imaging modality depends on the pretest probability (see clinical prediction rules above) and the presence or absence of renal insufficiency. In patients with normal renal function and high pretest probability, the screening method of choice (Figure 13.4) includes MRA or Renal Artery Duplex though captopril renography can be used if MRA or duplex is not available [45]. A positive test requires confirmation with angiography and possible intervention. In patients with progressive renal insufficiency, renal transplant, recurrent episodes of flash pulmonary oedema or uncontrolled hypertension, the preferred modality of screening is duplex ultrasound, MRA or CO_2 angiography [3].

THERAPEUTIC OPTIONS FOR RAS

Renal size is one of the major determinants of the management strategies of RAS (Figure 13.5) [46]. If the kidneys are already atrophic (<8 cm), interventional or surgical procedures are generally not indicated. If kidney size is relatively preserved (>8 cm) and stenosis is not haemodynamically significant, i.e. no significant post-stenotic gradient is present, medical management is the mainstay of therapy for the treatment of hypertension. However, if renal size is relatively preserved and stenosis is haemodynamically significant, invasive intervention is indicated. Moreover, if renal size is >8 cm, irrespective of hypertension, stenting should be considered for revascularisation and preservation of kidney function.

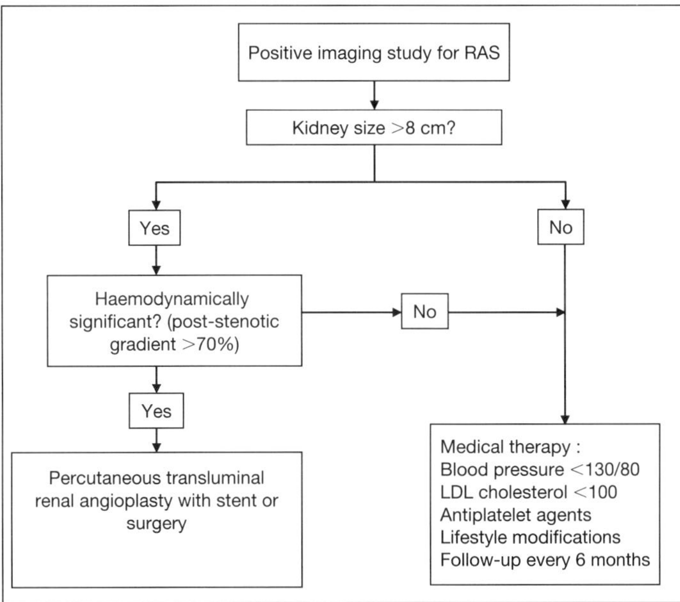

Figure 13.5 Therapeutic strategies in patients with positive imaging study for RAS for reduce blood pressure. With permission from [46].

FIBROMUSCULAR DYSPLASIA

Treatment of choice in FMD is percutaneous transluminal renal angioplasty (PTRA) with or without stenting, because of the high cure rate associated with this intervention. However, it is important to note that up to 25% of patients will have restenosis after 1 year and some patients may still require some anti-hypertensive therapy. Nevertheless, profound pressure response and recurrent hypertension in patients with FMD treated with angioplasty supports the notion that hypertension in these patients has a renovascular aetiology [47]. Surgical intervention is reserved for more complex lesions though this may not be successful. In one patient with complex lesions not amenable to surgery under our observation, anti-thrombotic and anti-hypertensive therapy has stabilised renal function at 5 years of follow-up [17]. Patients with RAS due to FMD are generally younger than those with atherosclerotic RAS; therefore, optimum medical management of their hypertension is essential in order to minimise their lifetime cardiovascular risk.

ATHEROSCLEROTIC RENOVASCULAR DISEASE

MEDICAL MANAGEMENT

No invasive intervention is indicated if RAS is not haemodynamically significant or if the kidneys are already atrophic. In these cases, medical management that encompasses aggressive control of hypertension, lipids, blood sugar, use of anti-platelet agents and lifestyle modification is the treatment of choice. Any anti-hypertensive agent can be used. ACE inhibitors are safe and effective in patients with unilateral RAS, however, these drugs should be started at low doses and renal function tested after 3–5 days, and then after subsequent dose increments. Any anti-hypertensive drug can reduce the GFR in critical stenosis and a 30% increase in serum creatinine from baseline with or without hyperkalaemia raises the probability of bilateral RAS [48]. However, diuretic-induced volume contraction or congestive heart failure should be investigated and treated. ACE-I and ARBs are generally contraindicated in bilateral RAS. Hyperkalaemia *per se* (unless >6 mEq/l) is not an indication to stop ACE-I or ARB therapy and can usually be managed with potassium binding resins, reduction in potassium intake and use of loop diuretics [3]. Patients undergoing solely medical management should be carefully followed for progression of disease using duplex ultrasonography every 6 months–1 year (Figure 13.5).

PERCUTANEOUS TRANSLUMINAL RENAL ANGIOPLASTY

PTRA, with or without stenting, provides a non-surgical option for the treatment of RAS. A diagnostic arteriography should be performed along with angioplasty and stenting when BP is uncontrolled, renal function progressively deteriorates, or a non-invasive study suggests the progression of stenosis. Reduction in anti-hypertensive medications is generally observed 48 hours after a successful procedure [49]. Technical success rates vary with the site of the lesion. Total occlusions and ostial lesions generally do not respond well to angioplasty alone and these are associated with a high rate of restenosis. Ostial lesions can be successfully treated in most patients with angioplasty followed by stent placement, which has become the treatment of choice [50]. In azotaemic patients awaiting PTRA, prophylaxis to reduce the risk of contrast-induced nephropathy is mandatory [51].

SURGICAL INTERVENTIONS IN RAS

The use of bypass grafting or endarterectomy is generally reserved for unreachable ostial lesions, critical bilateral stenosis or in cases of stent failure [52]. It involves bypassing the stenotic segment or removing the small atrophic kidney following complete arterial occlusion. Surgery is generally more effective than angioplasty in the treatment of atherosclerotic disease, with cure of or improvement in the hypertension occurring in 80–95%.

Finally, it is important to note that despite many technological advances over the years, randomised trials [53, 54] have failed to demonstrate any difference in blood pressure control and/or renal function preservation when invasive therapy is compared with medical therapy. In the absence of data supporting invasive therapeutic approaches for RAS, the decision to recommend revascularisation remains a difficult balance between the risks and expense of the procedure and the undoubted benefits that accrue if renal function is successfully stabilised [3]. Thus, it is prudent to try medical management and reserve invasive therapy for those with truly critical stenosis, uncontrolled hypertension, flash pulmonary oedema, azotaemia and preserved renal size (Figure 13.5). On the other hand, the benefit of revascularisation in FMD is significant and should be the treatment of choice unless revascularisation is unsuccessful.

SUMMARY

RAS is the most common cause of surgically/interventionally correctable hypertension, which in the case of FMD is potentially curable. The most common pathophysiological entities of RAS are FMD and atherosclerotic types. RAS manifests with varying clinical presentations ranging from asymptomatic disease to intractable hypertension, ischaemic nephropathy, nephritic syndrome and flash pulmonary oedema. Age, sex and race, as well as the presence of atherosclerotic disease in other organs, together with hypertension and hypokalaemia and worsening azotaemia are among the clinical predictors of RAS. Diagnostic modalities in RAS include invasive as well as non-invasive testing. The choice of therapeutic options depends on the size of the kidney and the haemodynamic significance of the stenosis. Invasive intervention is indicated in patients with preserved kidney size and haemodynamically significant RAS. Physicians should be familiar with clinical predictors of the risk of RAS in order to initiate diagnostic work-up with interventions that could potentially cure hypertension and preserve kidney functions.

REFERENCES

1. Rundback JH, Sacks D, Kent KC *et al*. Guidelines for the reporting of renal artery revascularization in clinical trials. American Heart Association. *Circulation* 2002; 106:1572–1585.
2. Baumgartner I, von Aesch K, Do DD, Triller J, Birrer M, Mahler F. Stent placement in ostial and nonostial atherosclerotic renal arterial stenoses: a prospective follow-up study. *Radiology* 2000; 216:498–505.
3. Salifu MO, Haria DM, Badero O, Aytug S, McFarlane SI. Challenges in the diagnosis and management of renal artery stenosis. *Curr Hypertens Rep* 2005; 7:219–227.
4. Kassab E, McFarlane SI, Sower JR: Vascular complications in diabetes and their prevention. *Vasc Med* 2001; 6:249–255.
5. Levey AS, Coresh J, Balk E *et al*. National Kidney Foundation practice guidelines for chronic kidney disease: evaluation, classification, and stratification. *Ann Intern Med* 2003; 139:137–147.
6. Zoccali C, Mallamaci F, Finocchiaro P. Atherosclerotic renal artery stenosis: epidemiology, cardiovascular outcomes, and clinical prediction rules. *J Am Soc Nephrol* 2002; 13(suppl 3):S179–S183.
7. Uzu T, Inoue T, Fujii T *et al*. Prevalence and predictors of renal artery stenosis in patients with myocardial infarction. *Am J Kidney Dis* 1997; 29:733–738.
8. Harding MB, Smith LR, Himmelstein SI *et al*. Renal artery stenosis: prevalence and associated risk factors in patients undergoing routine cardiac catheterization. *J Am Soc Nephrol* 1992; 2:1608–1616.
9. van Jaarsveld BC, Pieterman H, van Dijk LC *et al*. Inter-observer variability in the angiographic assessment of renal artery stenosis. DRASTIC study group. Dutch Renal Artery Stenosis Intervention Cooperative. *J Hypertens* 1999; 17(pt 1):1731–1736.
10. Wasser MN, Westenberg J, van der Hulst VP *et al*. Hemodynamic significance of renal artery stenosis: digital subtraction angiography versus systolically gated three-dimensional phase-contrast MR angiography. *Radiology* 1997; 202:333–338.

11. Textor SC, Wilcox CS: Renal artery stenosis: a common, treatable cause of renal failure? *Annu Rev Med* 2001; 52:421–442.
12. Pillay WR, Kan YM, Crinnion JN, Wolfe JH. Prospective multicentre study of the natural history of atherosclerotic renal artery stenosis in patients with peripheral vascular disease. *Br J Surg* 2002; 89:737–740.
13. Khong TK, Missouris CG, Belli AM, MacGregor GA. Regression of atherosclerotic renal artery stenosis with aggressive lipid lowering therapy. *J Hum Hypertens* 2001; 15:431–433.
14. Anderson CA, Hansen KJ, Benjamin ME, Keith DR, Craven TE, Dean RH. Renal artery fibromuscular dysplasia: results of current surgical therapy. *J Vasc Surg* 1995; 22:207–215; discussion 215–216.
15. Bofinger A, Hawley C, Fisher P, Daunt N, Stowasser M, Gordon R. Increased severity of multifocal renal arterial fibromuscular dysplasia in smokers. *J Hum Hypertens* 1999; 13:517–520.
16. Luscher TF, Lie JT, Stanson AW, Houser OW, Hollier LH, Sheps SG. Arterial fibromuscular dysplasia. *Mayo Clin Proc* 1987; 62:931–952.
17. Salifu MO, Gordon DH, Friedman EA, Delano BG. Bilateral renal infarction in a black man with medial fibromuscular dysplasia. *Am J Kidney Dis* 2000; 36:184–189.
18. Bruno S, Remuzzi G, Ruggenenti P. Transplant renal artery stenosis. *J Am Soc Nephrol* 2004; 15:134–141.
19. Aslam S, Salifu MO, Ghali H, Markell MS, Friedman EA. Common iliac artery stenosis presenting as renal allograft dysfunction in two diabetic recipients. *Transplantation* 2001; 71:814–817.
20. McFarlane SI, Sowers JR. Cardiovascular endocrinology 1:aldosterone function in diabetes mellitus: effects on cardiovascular and renal disease. *J Clin Endocrinol Metab* 2003; 88:516–523.
21. Mangrum AJ, Bakris GL. Angiotensin-converting enzyme inhibitors and angiotensin receptor blockers in chronic renal disease: safety issues. *Semin Nephrol* 2004; 24:168–175.
22. Riley DJ, Weir M, Bakris GL. Renal adaptation to the failing heart. Understanding the cascade of responses. *Postgrad Med* 1994; 95:141–146, 149–150.
23. Nawar T, Lefebvre R, Rojo-Ortega JM, Cartier P, Genest J. Reversal of ischemic tubular atrophy. *Ann Intern Med* 1970; 72:529–532.
24. Remuzzi G, Bertani T. Pathophysiology of progressive nephropathies. *N Engl J Med* 1998; 339:1448–1456.
25. Caps MT, Perissinotto C, Zierler RE *et al.* Prospective study of atherosclerotic disease progression in the renal artery. *Circulation* 1998; 98:2866–2872.
26. Chabova V, Schirger A, Stanson AW, McKusick MA, Textor SC. Outcomes of atherosclerotic renal artery stenosis managed without revascularization. *Mayo Clin Proc* 2000; 75:437–444.
27. Gephardt GN, Tubbs RR, Novick AC, McMahon JT, Pohl MA. Renal artery stenosis, nephrotic-range proteinuria, and focal and segmental glomerulosclerosis. *Cleve Clin Q* 1984; 51:371–376.
28. Zimbler MS, Pickering TG, Sos TA, Laragh JH. Proteinuria in renovascular hypertension and the effects of renal angioplasty. *Am J Cardiol* 1987; 59:406–408.
29. Pickering TG, Herman L, Devereux RB *et al.* Recurrent pulmonary oedema in hypertension due to bilateral renal artery stenosis: treatment by angioplasty or surgical revascularisation. *Lancet* 1988; 2:551–552.
30. MacDowall P, Kalra PA, O'Donoghue DJ, Waldek S, Mamtora H, Brown K. Risk of morbidity from renovascular disease in elderly patients with congestive cardiac failure. *Lancet* 1998; 352:13–16.
31. Hricik DE, Browning PJ, Kopelman R, Goorno WE, Madias NE, Dzau VJ. Captopril-induced functional renal insufficiency in patients with bilateral renal-artery stenoses or renal-artery stenosis in a solitary kidney. *N Engl J Med* 1983; 308:373–376.
32. Maxwell MH, Bleifer KH, Franklin SS, Varady PD. Cooperative study of renovascular hypertension. Demographic analysis of the study. *JAMA* 1972; 220:1195–1204.
33. Krijnen P, van Jaarsveld BC, Steyerberg EW, Man in 't Veld AJ, Schalekamp MA, Habbema JD. A clinical prediction rule for renal artery stenosis. *Ann Intern Med* 1998; 129:705–711.
34. Nally JV Jr, Clarke HS Jr, Grecos GP *et al.* Effect of captopril on 99mTc-diethylenetriaminepentaacetic acid renograms in two-kidney, one clip hypertension. *Hypertension* 1986; 8:685–693.
35. Bongers V, Bakker J, Beutler JJ, Beek FJ, De Klerk JM. Assessment of renal artery stenosis: comparison of captopril renography and gadolinium-enhanced breath-hold MR angiography. *Clin Radiol* 2000; 55:346–353.
36. Lin CC, Shiau YC, Li TC, Kao A, Lee CC. Usefulness of captopril renography to predict the benefits of renal artery revascularization or captopril treatment in hypertensive patients with diabetic nephropathy. *J Diabetes Complications* 2002; 16:344–346.
37. Olin JW, Piedmonte MR, Young JR, DeAnna S, Grubb M, Childs MB. The utility of duplex ultrasound scanning of the renal arteries for diagnosing significant renal artery stenosis. *Ann Intern Med* 1995; 122:833–838.

38. Napoli V, Pinto S, Bargellini I *et al.* Duplex ultrasonographic study of the renal arteries before and after renal artery stenting. *Eur Radiol* 2002; 12:796–803.
39. Tan KT, van Beek EJ, Brown PW, van Delden OM, Tijssen J, Ramsay LE. Magnetic resonance angiography for the diagnosis of renal artery stenosis: a meta-analysis. *Clin Radiol* 2002; 57:617–624.
40. Olbricht CJ, Paul K, Prokop M *et al.* Minimally invasive diagnosis of renal artery stenosis by spiral computed tomography angiography. *Kidney Int* 1995; 48:1332–1337.
41. Olin JW, Kaufman JA, Bluemke DA *et al.* Atherosclerotic Vascular Disease Conference: Writing Group IV: imaging. *Circulation* 2004; 109:2626–2633.
42. Hawkins IF Jr, Wilcox CS, Kerns SR, Sabatelli FW. CO_2 digital angiography: a safer contrast agent for renal vascular imaging? *Am J Kidney Dis* 1994; 24:685–694.
43. Wilson AJ, Boxer MM. Neurotoxicity of angiographic carbon dioxide in the cerebral vasculature. *Invest Radiol* 2002; 37:542–551.
44. Sam AD 2nd, Morasch MD, Collins J, Song G, Chen R, Pereles FS. Safety of gadolinium contrast angiography in patients with chronic renal insufficiency. *J Vasc Surg* 2003; 38:313–318.
45. Carman TL, Olin JW. Diagnosis of renal artery stenosis: what is the optimal diagnostic test? *Curr Interv Cardiol Rep* 2000; 2:111–118.
46. Bloch MJ, Basile J. Clinical insights into the diagnosis and management of renovascular disease. An evidence-based review. *Minerva Med* 2004; 95:357–373.
47. Birrer M, Do DD, Mahler F, Triller J, Baumgartner I. Treatment of renal artery fibromuscular dysplasia with balloon angioplasty: a prospective follow-up study. *Eur J Vasc Endovasc Surg* 2002; 23:146–152.
48. van de Ven PJ, Beutler JJ, Kaatee R, Beek FJ, Mali WP, Koomans HA. Angiotensin converting enzyme inhibitor-induced renal dysfunction in atherosclerotic renovascular disease. *Kidney Int* 1998; 53:986–993.
49. Bonelli FS, McKusick MA, Textor SC *et al.* Renal artery angioplasty: technical results and clinical outcome in 320 patients. *Mayo Clin Proc* 1995; 70:1041–1052.
50. van de Ven PJ, Kaatee R, Beutler JJ *et al.* Arterial stenting and balloon angioplasty in ostial atherosclerotic renovascular disease: a randomised trial. *Lancet* 1999; 353:282–286.
51. Asif A, Epstein M. Prevention of radiocontrast-induced nephropathy. *Am J Kidney Dis* 2004; 44:12–24.
52. Libertino JA, Beckmann CF. Surgery and percutaneous angioplasty in the management of renovascular hypertension. *Urol Clin North Am* 1994; 21:235–243.
53. Plouin PF, Chatellier G, Darne B, Raynaud A. Blood pressure outcome of angioplasty in atherosclerotic renal artery stenosis: a randomized trial. Essai Multicentrique Medicaments vs Angioplastie (EMMA) Study Group. *Hypertension* 1998; 31:823–829.
54. Webster J, Marshall F, Abdalla M *et al.* Randomised comparison of percutaneous angioplasty vs continued medical therapy for hypertensive patients with atheromatous renal artery stenosis. Scottish and Newcastle Renal Artery Stenosis Collaborative Group. *J Hum Hypertens* 1998; 12:329–335.
55. Kidney Disease Outcomes Quality Initiative (K/DOQI). K/DOQI Clinical Practice Guidelines on Hypertension and Antihypertensive Agents in Chronic Kidney Disease. *Am J Kidney Dis* 2004; 43(suppl 1):S1–S290.

Abbreviations

4D	Die Deutsche Diabetes Dialyze
4S	Scandinavian Simvastatin Survival Study
AASK	African American Study of Kidney Disease and Hypertension
ABCD	Appropriate Blood Pressure Control in Diabetes
ACC	associated clinical conditions
ACCESS	Acute Candesartan Cilexetil Evaluation in Stroke Survivors
ACCOMPLISH	Avoiding Cardiovascular events through Combination therapy in Patients Living with Systolic Hypertension
ACCORD	Action to Control Cardiovascular Risk in Diabetes
ACE	angiotensin-converting enzyme
ACE-I	angiotensin-converting enzyme inhibitor
ACTION	A Coronary disease Trial Investigating Outcome with Nifedipine
AHA	American Heart Association
AIPRD	ACE Inhibition in Progressive Renal Disease
AIPRI	ACE-Inhibition for Progressive Renal Insufficiency
ALERT	Assessment of Lescol in Renal Transplantation
ALLHAT	Antihypertensive and Lipid Lowering Treatment to Prevent Heart Attack Trial
ANBP-2	Second Australian National Blood Pressure Study
Ang II	angiotensin II
ARB	angiotensin receptor blocker
ARIC	Atherosclerosis Risk in Communities
ASA	American Stroke Association
ASCOT	Anglo-Scandinavian Cardiac Outcomes Trial
ATACH	Antihypertensive Treatment in Acute Cerebral Hemorrhage
ATP	Adult Treatment Panel
AURORA	A study to evaluate the Use of Rosuvastatin in subjects On Regular hemodialysis: An assessment of survival and cardiovascular events
BENEDICT	Bergamo Nephrologic Diabetes Complications Trial
BMI	body mass index
BP	blood pressure
CAMELOT	Comparison of Amlodipine vs. Enalapril to Limit Occurrences of Thrombosis
CAN	chronic allograft nephropathy
CARDS	Collaborative Atorvastatin Diabetes Study
CARING	Clozapine and Agranulocytosis Relationships Investigated by Genetics study
CBF	cerebral blood flow
CCB	calcium channel blocker
CD	cerebrovascular disease
CHD	coronary heart disease

CHF	congestive heart failure
CHHIPS	Control of Hypertension and Hypotension Immediately Post-Stroke Trial
CI	confidence interval
CKD	chronic kidney disease
CNS	central nervous system
CONVINCE	Controlled-Onset Verapamil Investigation of Cardiovascular Endpoints
COOPERATE	Combination Treatment of Angiotensin-II Receptor Blocker and Angiotensin converting-enzyme inhibitor in Non-diabetic
COSSACS	Continue or Stop Post-Stroke Antihypertensives Collaborative Study
CPP	cerebral perfusion pressure
CV	cardiovascular
CVD	cardiovascular disease
CVR	cerebrovascular resistance
DASH	Dietary Approaches to Stop Hypertension
DBP	diastolic blood pressure
DETAIL	Diabetics Exposed to Telmisartan and Enalapril study
DHP	dihydropyridine
DHP-CCB	dihydropyridine CCB
DIABHYCAR	Diabetes Hypertension Cardiovascular events trial
DM	diabetes mellitus
DRASTIC	Dutch Renal Artery Stenosis Intervention Cooperative
DREAM	Diabetes Reduction with Ramipril and Rosiglitazone Medications
DS	Dahl salt-sensitive
DSA	digital subtraction angiography
DTPA	diethylenetriaminepentaacetate
EBCT	3D electron beam computed tomography
eGFR	estimated glomerular filtration rate
ENaC	epithelial sodium channel
ENOS	Efficacy of Nitric Oxide in Stroke
eNOS	endothelial nitric oxide synthase
EPO	erythropoietin
ESH-ESC	European Society of Hypertension-European Society of Cardiology
ESRD	end-stage renal disease
EUROPA	European Reduction of cardiac events with Perindopril in stable coronary Artery disease study
EWPHE	European Working Party on High Blood Pressure in the Elderly
FACET	Fosinopril Amlodipine Cardiac Events Trial
FDA	Food and Drug Administration
FFA	free fatty acid
FFD	fibromuscular dysplasia
GEMINI	Glycemic Effects in Diabetes mellitus Carvedilol–Metoprolol Comparison in Hypertensives trial
GFR	glomerular filtration rate
GTN	glyceryl trinitrate
HASTE	Hypertension in Acute Stroke Treatment
HbA1c	glycated haemoglobin
HDL	low density lipoprotein
HDL_2	HDL subfraction 2
HDL-c	high density lipoprotein cholesterol
HMG-CoA	3-hydroxy-3-methylglutaryl

HOPE	Heart Outcomes Prevention Evaluation
HOT	Hypertension Optimal Treatment study
ICH	intracranial haemorrhage
ICP	intracranial pressure
IDDM	insulin-dependent diabetes mellitus
IDNT	Irbesartan Diabetic Nephropathy Trial
IFG	impaired fasting glucose
IGT	impaired glucose tolerance
INSIGHT	Intervention as a Goal in Hypertension Treatment study
INVEST	International Verapamil/trandolopril Study
INWEST	Intravenous Nimodipine West European Stroke Trial
IRMA2	Irbesartan in Patients with Type 2 Diabetes and Microalbuminuria
ISA	intrinsic sympathomimetic activity
ISH	International Society of Hypertension
ISHIB	International Society on Hypertension in Blacks
IST	International Stroke Trial
IV	intravenous
JNC	Joint National Committee
JNC7	Seventh Report of the Joint National Committee on Prevention, Detection, Evaluation and Treatment of High Blood Pressure
LCAT	lecithin cholesterol acyltransferase activity
LDL	low density lipoprotein
LDL-c	low density lipoprotein cholesterol
LIFE	Losartan Intervention for Endpoint in hypertension study
LLA	lipid-lowering arm
LPL	lipoprotein lipase
LVH	left ventricular hypertrophy
MA	microalbuminuria (not abbreviated in other chaps and MAU in chapter 11)
MAP	mean arterial blood pressure
MARVAL	MAU Reduction with Valsartan in Patients with Type 2 Diabetes Mellitus
MAU	microalbumina
MBP	mean blood pressure
MDCT	multidetector computed tomography
MDRD	Modification of Diet in Renal Disease
MICRO-HOPE	Microalbuminuria, Cardiovascular, and Renal Outcomes substudy of HOPE
MRA	magnetic resonance angiography
MRC	Medical Research Council
MRFIT	Multiple Risk Factor Intervention Trial
MS	metabolic syndrome
NAVIGATOR	Nateglinide and Valsartan in Impaired Glucose (A) Tolerance Outcomes Research trial
NCEP	National Cholesterol Education Program
NHANES	National Health and Nutrition Examination Study
NHEFS	National Health Examination and Follow-up Study
NIDDM	non-insulin-dependent diabetes mellitus
NINDS	National Institute for Neurological Disorders and Stroke
NMDA	N-methyl-D-aspartate
NNT	number needed to treat
NO	nitric oxide

NORDIL	Nordic Diltiazem study
NSA	National Stroke Association
ON TARGET	Ongoing Telmarsartan alone and in Combination with Ramipril Global Endpoint Trial
PEACE	Prevention of Events with Angiotensin Converting Enzyme inhibition
PHT2	Stage 2 pre-hypertension
PP	pulse pressure
PPARα	peroxisome proliferator activated receptor α
PROGRESS	Perindopril Protection against Recurrent Stroke Study
PTRA	percutaneous transluminal renal angioplasty
PWV	pulse wave velocity
RAAS	renin-angiotensin-aldosterone system
RAS	renin-angiotensin system renal artery stenosis
REIN-2	Second Ramipril Efficacy in Nephropathy
RENAAL	Reduction of Endpoints in Non-Insulin Dependent Diabetes Mellitus with the Angiotensin II Antagonist Losartan
ROC	receiver operating characteristic
RR	relative risk
r-tPA	recombinant tissue plasminogen activator
RVHT	renovascular hypertension
SAH	subarachnoid haemorrhage
SBP	systolic blood pressure
SCOPE	Study on Cognition and Prognosis in the Elderly
SHARP	Study of Heart and Renal Protection
SHEP	Systolic Hypertension in Elderly Program
SHR	spontaneously hypertensive rat
STOP-2	Swedish Trial in Old Patients with hypertension-2
Syst-China	Systolic Hypertension in Elderly Chinese trial
Syst-Eur	Systolic Hypertension in Europe trial
TG	triglyceride
TL	TG-rich lipoprotein
TNFα	tumour necrosis factor α
TOD	target organ damage
TOMHS	Treatment of Mild Hypertension Study
TRANSCEND	Telmisartan Randomised Assessment Study in a CE-intolerant subject with Cardiovascular Disease
TRAS	transplant renal artery stenosis
TROPHY	Trial of Preventing Hypertension study
UACR	urine albumin to creatinine ratio
UAE	urinary albumin excretion?
UKPDS	UK Prospective Diabetes Study
UP/Cr	urinary protein: creatinine ratio
VALUE	Valsartan Antihypertensive Long-term Use Evaluation
VLDL	very low density lipoprotein
VSMC	vascular snooth muscle cell
VVANNTT	Verapramil Versus Amlodipine in Non-diabetic Nephropathies Treated with Trandolapril
WHO	World Health Organization

Index